# Register Now for Online Access to Your Book!

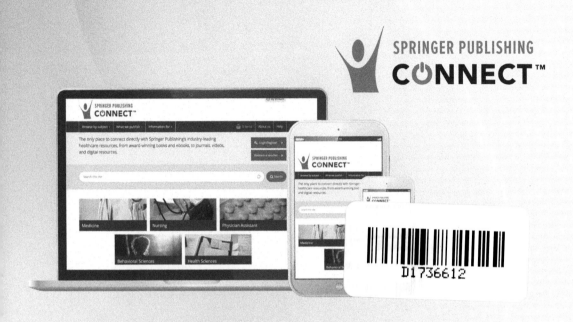

Your print purchase of *Certified Healthcare Simulation Educator (CHSE®) Review, Third Edition,* **includes online access to the contents of your book—** increasing accessibility, portability, and searchability!

## Access today at:
**http://connect.springerpub.com/content/book/978-0-8261-6991-4**
or scan the QR code at the right with your smartphone. Log in or register, then click "Redeem a voucher" and use the code below.

### USHYGULU

**Having trouble redeeming a voucher code?**
Go to https://connect.springerpub.com/redeeming-voucher-code

**If you are experiencing problems accessing the digital component of this product, please contact our customer service department at cs@springerpub.com**

*Scan here for quick access.*

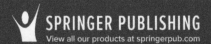

**SPRINGER PUBLISHING**
View all our products at springerpub.com

# Certified Healthcare Simulation Educator (CHSE®) Review

**Linda Wilson, PhD, RN, CPAN, CAPA, NPD-BC, CNE, CNEcl, CHSE-A, FASPAN, ANEF, FAAN, FSSH,** is an assistant dean for continuing education, simulation, and events and a clinical professor in the division of nursing at Drexel University, College of Nursing and Health Professions in Philadelphia, Pennsylvania. Dr. Wilson completed her bachelor of science in nursing (BSN) at Misericordia University in Dallas, Pennsylvania, and her master of science in nursing (MSN) in critical care and trauma at Thomas Jefferson University in Philadelphia. She completed her PhD in nursing research at Rutgers, The State University of New Jersey in Newark. Dr. Wilson has also obtained a postgraduate certificate in epidemiology and biostatistical methods from Drexel University and a postgraduate certificate in pain management from the University of California, San Francisco School of Medicine. She has dual certification in simulation—Certified Healthcare Simulation Educator® (CHSE®; inaugural group) and Certified Healthcare Simulation Educator-Advanced (CHSE-A; inaugural group)—along with several additional certifications. Dr. Wilson was inducted as a fellow in the Society for Simulation in Healthcare Academy in 2023. Dr. Wilson was the project director/primary investigator for SimTeam: The Joint Education of Health Professionals and Assistive Personnel Students in a Simulated Environment, a project funded by the Barra Foundation Inc. She was also the project director/primary investigator for Faculty Development: Integrating Technology Into Nursing Education and Practice, a nearly $1.5 million, 5-year project funded by the Health Resources and Services Administration, Department of Health and Human Services. Dr. Wilson is also the coeditor of *Human Simulation for Nursing and Health Professions, Certified Nurse Educator (CNE/CNEn) Review Manual, Fourth Edition,* and *Certified Academic Clinical Nurse Educator (CNE®cl) Review Manual,* published by Springer Publishing Company.

**Ruth A. Wittmann-Price, PhD, RN, CNS, CNE, CNEcl, CHSE, ANEF, FAAN,** is the dean of the W. Cary Edwards School of Nursing and Health Professions at Thomas Edison State College in Trenton, New Jersey. Dr. Wittmann-Price has been an obstetrical/women's health nurse for 44 years. She received her BSN degree from Felician College in Lodi, New Jersey (1981), and her master's in science as a perinatal clinicial nurse specialist (CNS) from Columbia University, New York, New York (1983). Dr. Wittmann-Price completed her PhD at Widener University, Chester, Pennsylvania (2006), and was awarded the Dean's Award for Excellence. She developed a midrange nursing theory, Emancipated Decision-Making in Women's Health Care. Dr. Wittmann-Price was the coordinator for the nurse educator track in the DrNP program at Drexel University in Philadelphia, Pennsylvania (2007–2010) and the director of nursing research for Hahnemann University Hospital (2007–2010), overseeing all evidence-based practice projects for nursing. The Hahnemann University Hospital was awarded initial Magnet® status (American Nurses Credentialing Center) in December 2009. Dr. Wittmann-Price has taught all levels of nursing students over the past 20+ years (AAS, BSN, MSN, DNP, PhD) and is part of dissertation committees on decisional science. As the founding dean of health sciences at Francis Marion University, Florence, South Carolina, she developed the simulation program, the MSN program, an interprofessional rural health initiative, a physician assistant program, a DNP program, and the speech–language pathology program. She has published over 20 articles, is a coeditor and chapter contributor for 16 books, and is a series editor of Nursing Test Success, a series of unfolding case studies published by Springer Publishing Company. She has presented regionally, nationally, and internationally.

# Certified Healthcare Simulation Educator (CHSE®) Review

## Third Edition

Linda Wilson, PhD, RN, CPAN, CAPA, NPD-BC, CNE, CNEcl, CHSE-A, FASPAN, ANEF, FAAN, FSSH
Ruth A. Wittmann-Price, PhD, RN, CNS, CNE, CNEcl, CHSE, ANEF, FAAN

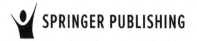 SPRINGER PUBLISHING

Springer Publishing Company, LLC
www.springerpub.com
connect.springerpub.com

*Acquisitions Editor*: Jaclyn Koshofer
*Content Development Editor*: Libby Ornstein
*Compositor*: DiacriTech
*Production Editor*: Ashley Hannen

*ISBN*: 978-0-8261-6990-7
*ebook ISBN*: 978-0-8261-6991-4
*DOI*: 10.1891/9780826169914

23 24 25 26 27 / 5 4 3 2 1

The author and the publisher of this Work have made every effort to use sources believed to be reliable to provide information that is accurate and compatible with the standards generally accepted at the time of publication. Because medical science is continually advancing, our knowledge base continues to expand. Therefore, as new information becomes available, changes in procedures become necessary. We recommend that the reader always consult current research and specific institutional policies before performing any clinical procedure or delivering any medication. The author and publisher shall not be liable for any special, consequential, or exemplary damages resulting, in whole or in part, from the readers' use of, or reliance on, the information contained in this book. The publisher has no responsibility for the persistence or accuracy of URLs for external or third-party Internet websites referred to in this publication and does not guarantee that any content on such websites is, or will remain, accurate or appropriate.

**Library of Congress Cataloging-in-Publication Data**

Contact sales@springerpub.com to receive discount rates on bulk purchases.

*Publisher's Note:* **New and used products purchased from third-party sellers are not guaranteed for quality, authenticity, or access to any included digital components.**

Printed in the United States of America by Hatteras, Inc.

CHSE® is a registered service mark of the Society for Simulation in Healthcare™ (SSH). SSH™ does not sponsor or endorse this resource, nor does it have a proprietary relationship with Springer Publishing.

# Contents

# Contributors

**Denise Antonelle, MS**
Standardized Patient Coordinator/Educator
Clinical Simulation Center Renaissance School of Medicine
Stony Brook University
Stony Brook, New York

**Anthony Battaglia, MS, BSN, RN**
Corporate Counsel
Pocket Nurse
Monaca, Pennsylvania

**Stephanie Blumenfeld, MSN, RN, CHSE**
Director of Interprofessional Simulation Center
La Salle University
Philadelphia, Pennsylvania

**Sevilla Bronson, PhD, MSN, APRN**
Clinical Associate Professor
College of Nursing
University of South Carolina
Columbia, South Carolina

**Brittny D. Chabalowski, RN, MSN, CEN, CNE, CHSE**
Instructor, Program Director
Upper Division/Second Degree Nursing Sequence Coordinator
Undergraduate Simulation
University of South Florida
Tampa, Florida

**Matthew Charnetski, MSMS, NRP, CHSOS, CHSE, FSSH**
Director of Simulation Based Education and Research
Dartmouth Hitchcock Medical Center
Lebanon, New Hampshire

**John T. Cornele, MSN, RN, CEN, EMT-P, CNE**
Adjunct Faculty
Drexel University College of Nursing and Health Professions
Philadelphia, Pennsylvania

**Anthony Errichetti, PhD, CHSE**
Chief of Virtual Medicine, Director, MS in Medical/Health Care Simulation
New York Institute of Technology College of Osteopathic Medicine
Old Westbury, New York

**Karen K. Gittings, DNP, RN, CNE, CNEcl, Alumnus CCRN**
Dean of Health Sciences and Professor of Nursing
Francis Marion University
Florence, South Carolina

**Mary Ellen Smith Glasgow, PhD, RN, ANEF, FAAN**
Dean and Professor
School of Nursing
Vice Provost for Research
Office of Research and Innovation
Duquesne University
Pittsburgh, Pennsylvania

**Maryanne Halligan, DNP, RN, CCRN-K, CNML**
Coordinator Simulation and Clinical Skills, Assistant Professor
Jefferson College of Nursing
Thomas Jefferson University
Philadelphia, Pennsylvania

**Mary Hanson-Zalot, EdD, MSN, RN, CNE**
Associate Dean for Academic Affairs
Jefferson College of Nursing
Thomas Jefferson University
Philadelphia, Pennsylvania

**Bonnie A. Haupt, DNP, RN, CNL, CHSE**
Associate Director for Clinical Training and Engagement
U.S. Department of Veterans Affairs
Simulation Learning, Evaluation, Assessment, and Research Network (SimLEARN), VA
    Healthcare System
San Antonio, Texas

**H. Lynn Kane, MSN, MBA, RN, CCRN**
Clinical Nurse Specialist
Methodist Division
Thomas Jefferson University Hospital
Philadelphia, Pennsylvania

**Beth A. Kuzminsky, MSN, RN SimEMR**
Customer Service and Education Manager
Pocket Nurse
Monaca, Pennsylvania

**Colleen H. Meakim, MSN, RN, CHSE-A, ANEF**
Assistant Professor of the Practice Director, Second Degree BSN Track
M. Louise Fitzpatrick College of Nursing
Villanova University
Villanova, Pennsylvania

**Kymberlee Montgomery, DrNP, WHNP-BC, CNE, FAANP, FAAN**
Vice Dean of Nursing and Student Affairs, Chief Academic Nursing Officer
Drexel University College of Nursing and Health Professions
Philadelphia, Pennsylvania

**Kate Morse, PhD, MSN, RN, AGACNP-Ret**
Assistant Dean for Experiential Learning and Innovation and Associate Clinical Professor
Drexel University College of Nursing and Health Professions
Philadelphia, Pennsylvania

**Nina Multak, PhD, PA-C, DFAAPA**
Professor and Associate Dean, Randolph B. Mahoney Director
School of Physician Assistant Studies
University of Florida College of Medicine
Gainesville, Florida

**Crystal L. Murillo, PhD, RN, CHSE-A, ANEF, FAAN**
Assistant Professor, Director of the Center for Simulation and Experiential Learning (SAEL)
College of Nursing
University of South Carolina
Columbia, South Carolina

**Marilynn Poe Murphy, DNP, RN, CHSE, CNE**
Coordinator of the Simulation and Skills Lab, Assistant Professor
Thomas Jefferson University
Philadelphia, Pennsylvania

**Carol Okupniak, DNP, RN, BC-NI, CHSE**
Associate Professor and Director, Center for Advanced Education, Simulation and Innovation
Jefferson College of Nursing
Thomas Jefferson University
Philadelphia, Pennsylvania

**Fabien Pampaloni, MSN, RN**
Corporate Nurse Educator
Pocket Nurse
Monaca, Pennsylvania

**Arun Ramakrishnan, PhD**
Director of Research Labs
College of Nursing and Health Professions
Drexel University
Philadelphia, Pennsylvania

**Carolyn H. Scheese, DNP, RN, CHSE, CPPS, NE-BC, CAPM**
Assistant Professor, Director, RN to BS in Nursing Program
College of Nursing
University of Utah
Salt Lake City, Utah

**Colette Townsend-Chambers, DNP, MSN, CHSE**
Clinical Associate Professor
College of Nursing
University of South Carolina
Columbia, South Carolina

**Julia Ward, PhD, RN**
Professor and Chair-Undergraduate Programs
Jefferson College of Nursing
Jefferson University
Philadelphia, Pennsylvania

**Dorie L. Weaver, DNP, RN, CNE, FNP-BC**
Assistant Professor and Coordinator of the Nurse Educator Program
Francis Marion University
Florence, South Carolina

**Linda Wilson, PhD, RN, CPAN, CAPA, NPD-BC, CNE, CNEcl, CHSE-A, FASPAN, ANEF, FAAN, FSSH**
Assistant Dean for Continuing Education Simulation and Events
Clinical Professor, Division of Nursing
Drexel University College of Nursing and Health Professions
Philadelphia, Pennsylvania

**Ruth A. Wittmann-Price, PhD, RN, CNS, CNE, CNEcl, CHSE, ANEF, FAAN**
Dean, W. Cary Edwards School of Nursing and Health Professions
Thomas Edison University
Trenton, New Jersey

**Karen Worthy, PhD, MPH, RN, CNE**
Assistant Dean for Undergraduate Studies
Associate Professor
College of Nursing
University of South Carolina
Columbia, South Carolina

# Foreword

*"There are no great men [or women]. Just great challenges which ordinary men [and women], out of necessity, are forced by circumstance to meet."*
—*Admiral William Frederic Halsey, Jr. (WWII)*

Medical knowledge and technology have expanded sufficiently to require interprofessional teams and even whole organizations to deliver quality healthcare. Healthcare simulation is the perfect platform to teach collaboration and provide the ultimate "dress rehearsal" for these predictable interactions and events in healthcare delivery and operations. Over 20 years ago, I was the Chair of Undergraduate Nursing at MCP Hahnemann University, now Drexel University. Our medical students at the time participated in objective standardized clinical exams (OSCEs) under the leadership of Dennis Novack, MD. Dr. Novack emphasized physician/patient communication in addition to clinical skills development and assessment. As I observed the OSCEs, I was struck by how this novel learning experience could improve nursing students' interviewing and assessment skills. So in 2001, Drexel University introduced simulation into the undergraduate nursing curriculum. Working closely with Dr. Novack, we revised the case scenarios to be "nursing focused" rather than medically oriented. We observed increased comfort and proficiency in students' interviewing and assessment skills as a result of the nursing OSCEs.

As a Robert Wood Johnson Executive Nurse Fellow in 2009, I pushed simulation further by creating transdisciplinary simulations for my project, *Educating Professional Nurses and Advanced Practice Nurses for Tomorrow's Complex Clinical Environment and Emerging Demographics: Enhancing Safety and Inter-Professional Communication*. Working with Kym Montgomery, DNP, APRN, and my medical school colleague, Owen Montgomery, MD, we created five scenarios focused on emergent women's health issues in the outpatient area, giving bad news, and critical health situations in the inpatient area, and invited other health professionals to participate. The goal of these simulation educational experiences among multidisciplinary healthcare students was to enhance mutual support and communication in an effort to promote better patient outcomes.

Fast forward, 20+ years in the simulation space, healthcare simulation has evolved to the surprise of many to be a staple in nursing and medical education. We have now honed healthcare simulation education experiences to include multiple disciplines, virtual reality, telehealth, and diverse patient populations, and to encompass ethical dilemmas. I am presently a dean at Duquesne University School of Nursing. One of the faculty, Rebecca Kronk, PhD, CRNP, has incorporated persons with disabilities into the healthcare simulations. These "authentic consultants" assist nursing students in learning how to effectively care for patients with disabilities, understanding their unique care considerations. She also holds a summer theater camp to teach adolescents with disabilities to advocate for their own health by "acting as a patient," a creative use of simulation.

In this review manual, the experienced faculty authors adeptly discuss the essential elements of healthcare simulation from case development to evaluation in an effort to prepare you for the Certified Healthcare Simulation Educator® (CHSE®) exam. Healthcare simulation educators teach students to value teamwork while emphasizing safe clinical practice. Simulation facilitates the preparation of graduates capable of caring for patients in an increasingly complex healthcare environment with exemplary interprofessional collaborative skills. The COVID-19 pandemic has demonstrated the tremendous contributions of the healthcare providers. They have embodied teamwork during this crisis and have met the challenge head-on. Simulation, most likely, played a small part in their comfort of engaging in interprofessional teamwork and responding rapidly in a critical care environment. There is no doubt that there will be new simulation educational experiences as a result of these brave people's clinical knowledge and experiences. They have exhibited extraordinary courage and resilience as they cared for the sick. COVID-19 has shown the world the incredible work of all healthcare providers.

*Mary Ellen Smith Glasgow, PhD, RN, ANEF, FAAN*
Dean and Professor, School of Nursing, Vice Provost for Research, Office of Research and Innovation, Duquesne University, Pittsburgh, Pennsylvania

# Preface

This book was created as part of an interprofessional, international project to assist healthcare simulation educators in becoming certified for the very important work that is being accomplished during every simulation learning and evaluative experience around the world. Simulation is a teaching and assessment modality needed to improve patient safety. Simulation effectively teaches healthcare providers interprofessional collaboration, communication, and cooperation like never before in the history of healthcare. Becoming certified in simulation education is a wonderful step to promoting excellence in healthcare education, and we applaud your efforts.

This book is an invaluable resource in the certification process. The contributing authors have analyzed the certification test plan (Society for Simulation in Healthcare [SSH], 2018) to bring you all the important information that may be presented on the examination. The book is organized in a user-friendly format and the information is divided into short chapters. The authors are simulation and education experts who have added features to this text that will assist in critically analyzing the content.

The feature labeled *Teaching Tips* are provided for educators who would like further explanation and exploration of topics, many of which provide practical hints to incorporate into simulation experiences. *Evidence-Based Simulation Practice* boxes assist you in focusing on the current simulation research and bring you state-of-the art evidence. *Case Studies* and *Practice Questions* at the end of each chapter promote critical thinking and situational decision-making.

Section I of this book includes Chapter 1, which covers the specifics of the examination and the activities needed to reach advanced certification and recertification; and Chapter 2, which concentrates on the current 2018 certification test blueprint. Chapter 3 provides you with test-taking strategies, which are always beneficial for "the student in all of us."

Section II discusses Domain I of the certification examination blueprint (SSH, 2018): Professional Values and Capabilities in relation to teaching with simulation. Chapter 4 covers leadership in educational simulation. Chapter 5 includes special considerations about simulation experiences with learners and describes learning styles. Chapter 6 discusses the wonderful world of interprofessional simulation, while Chapter 7 provides insight into simulation ethics.

Section III addresses Domain II: Healthcare and Simulation Knowledge/Principles. This section reviews foundational knowledge about simulation and includes chapters on specific modalities and integrating simulation education into a professional healthcare curriculum.

Chapters 8 to 13 describe all the current modalities used in a simulation laboratory by experts who use them effectively on a consistent basis. Each modality is given a short chapter explanation that contains the knowledge and principles behind its use. This section addresses human patient simulation, moulage, standardized patients, hybrid simulation, part-task trainers, and the exponentially growing field of virtual reality.

Section IV focuses on Domain III of the certification examination blueprint: Educational Principles Applied to Simulation. In this section of the book, the authors concentrate on the learner and delivering effective simulation by reviewing content on educational theory, curriculum development, debriefing and feedback techniques, planning simulation events, and evaluating learning outcomes.

Section V describes the information in Domain IV: Simulation Resources and Environments. Chapters 22 and 23 discuss simulation laboratory management including personnel and the standards of an accredited simulation environment. Chapter 24 is a simulated practice test, and the answers and rationales appear in Chapter 25. Good luck!

Our hope in developing and revising this review manual is that it will be another valuable tool to assist you in reaching your career goal of recognized excellence. We applaud your efforts as colleagues in the quest to educate the next generation of healthcare workers. We thank you for your efforts to recognize excellence in the simulation field and the very important role simulation plays in patient safety.

*Linda Wilson*
*Ruth A. Wittmann-Price*

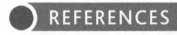

# REFERENCES

Society for Simulation in Healthcare. (2018). *Certified healthcare simulation educator examination blueprint, 2018 version.* Retrieved from http://www.ssih.org/Portals/48/Certification/CHSE_Docs/CHSE_Examination_Blueprint.pdf

# Acknowledgments

To H. Lynn Kane, Helen "Momma" Kane, Linda Webb, and Elizabeth Diaz, thank you for your amazing friendship and for being my family. To Lou Smith, Evan Babcock, Steve Johnson, Trish Costa-DePena, and Fabien Pampaloni, thank you for your friendship and support. To the Philadelphia Eagles, thank you for your inspiration.

—*Linda Wilson*

Thank you to Dr. Julia Ward for her mentorship and friendship.

—*Ruth A. Wittmann-Price*

# Pass Guarantee

If you use this resource to prepare for your exam and do not pass, you may return it for a refund of your full purchase price, excluding tax, shipping, and handling. To receive a refund, return your product along with a copy of your exam score report and original receipt showing purchase of new product (not used). Product must be returned and received within 180 days of the original purchase date. Refunds will be issued within 8 weeks from acceptance and approval. One offer per person and address. This offer is valid for U.S. residents only. Void where prohibited. To initiate a refund, please contact Customer Service at csexamprep@ springerpub.com.

# PART I
## Introduction

# Overview of the Certification Examination, Advanced Certification, and Recertification

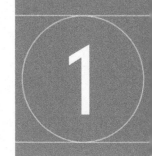

**Ruth A. Wittmann-Price and Brittny D. Chabalowski**

*Do not go where the path may lead, go instead where there is no path and leave a trail.*
*—Ralph Waldo Emerson*

> ▶ LEARNING OUTCOMES
>
> ■ Describe the benefits of certification.
> ■ Review the requirements for initial certification.
> ■ Review the recertification process.
> ■ Describe the requirements for advanced certification.

## ▶ INTRODUCTION

Obtaining specialty certification is a well-recognized method to demonstrate expertise, both in clinical and academic settings. Healthcare educators have used simulation for many years for effective academic and clinical learning and evaluation. Simulation can range from simple part-task trainers (PTTs) to high-fidelity simulated patient care experiences. The goal of complex patient-simulated experiences is to provide learners the opportunity to deliver care in high-risk, low-volume scenarios. These are situations that are seen infrequently in the clinical setting, but require swift and accurate intervention.

Unlike direct patient care encounters, simulation education requires a specialized skill set. Skilled healthcare simulation educators (sometimes referred to as *simulationists*) must be able to develop scenarios that are appropriate for the learners, administer the scenarios in a supportive atmosphere, and debrief the learners appropriately to complete an effective learning experience. It becomes clear that certification assists educators in understanding the need for uniform simulation education and evaluation (Charles & Koehn, 2016).

Recognizing this need, the Society for Simulation in Healthcare (SSH) developed the basic certification examination and the advanced certification standards (SSH, 2019, 2021). The benefits of these certifications go beyond the individual or the individual's organization. One of the goals is to identify, recognize, and pool the knowledge of best practices. This will serve to standardize the unique body of knowledge that belongs to healthcare simulation educators.

## ▶ INITIAL CERTIFICATION (CERTIFIED HEALTHCARE SIMULATION EDUCATOR™)

■ eligibility for initial certification
  ● bachelor's degree or equivalent (any candidate who does not have a bachelor's degree may petition the committee for consideration of equivalency based on experience)
  ● minimum of 2 years' experience in healthcare simulation setting

- able to demonstrate that simulation experience is focused on any level of healthcare learners
- continued use of simulation in healthcare education, research, or administration in the past 2 years (SSH, 2021)
- application for initial certification
  - can be completed online at www.ssih.org/certification/CHSE
  - includes information about simulation experience, education, and employment
  - narrative descriptions required include the following:
    - relevant simulation-based educational activity that demonstrates evidence of the person's capabilities as a simulation-based educator
    - relevant activities that demonstrate the person's advocacy for simulation-based education (this would include activities at the person's place of employment, activities at the local level, as well as activities in professional societies)
    - scholarly activities relevant to simulation-based education (such as participation in research, abstract preparation, publications, posters, workshops, curriculum development, and course construction)
  - contact information for at least three references to complete the Confidential Structured Report of Performance (CSRP) online
  - application processing takes approximately 3 weeks (SSH, 2021).
- fees for initial certification as of 2021
  - $395 for members of the SSH, the Association of Standardized Patient Educators (ASPE), and the International Nursing Association for Clinical Simulation and Learning (INACSL)
  - $495 for all others (SSH, 2021)
- taking the initial certification examination
  - Computer-based testing sites can be located on the ISO Quality Testing, Inc. website at www.isoqualitytesting.com.
  - Examination is scheduled on a space-available basis.
  - Examination must be taken within 90 days of application approval.
  - Candidates are notified of the results at the time of exam completion (SSH, 2021).
- initial certification
  - Certification is valid for 3 years from the successful completion of the exam.
  - The initials of certification "CHSE" (Certified Healthcare Simulation Educator) may be used as a credential after the candidate's name (SSH, 2021).

## ▶ RECERTIFICATION/RENEWAL OF INITIAL CERTIFICATION (SOCIETY FOR SIMULATION IN HEALTHCARE, 2019)

- retake the examination at or near the expiration date *or*
- demonstrate ongoing professional development
  - over the 3-year period, not just activity performed in a narrow time frame
  - in education or simulation-focused activities, including, but not limited to, the following:
    - participation in continuing education (CE) activity such as attending conferences, webinars, or other education events
    - publication of research, such as journal articles, chapters, books, or similar items
    - presenting at educational events, such as conferences
- If the certification expires, candidates must reapply to take the exam and must meet the eligibility requirements in place at that time (SSH, 2019).

# ▶ ADVANCED CERTIFICATION

- eligibility for advanced certification
- possession of basic certification
- participation in healthcare simulation in an educational role
- focused simulation expertise with learners in undergraduate, graduate, allied health, or healthcare courses
- master's degree or equivalent experience (any candidate who does not have a master's degree may petition the committee for consideration of equivalency based on experience)
- 5 years of continued use of simulation in healthcare education, research, or administration
- advanced certification valid for 3 years
- application for advanced certification
- submission of an extensive portfolio, including media submissions and reflective statements
- portfolio to be peer-reviewed and evaluated against the Advanced Standards and Elements (SSH, 2020)

## RECERTIFICATION/RENEWAL OF ADVANCED CERTIFICATION (SOCIETY FOR SIMULATION IN HEALTHCARE, 2015)

- demonstrate ongoing professional development
- over the 3-year period, demonstrate 45 professional development units
- payment of the recertification fee

Professional development units can be awarded for a variety of simulation activities, including the following:

- attending seminars or webinars
- participating in professional development
- presenting
- publishing

Advanced activities submitted to the SSH must span all  five domains of simulation education:

- displaying professional values and capabilities
- knowledge of simulation principles, practice, and methodologies
- education and assessment of learners using simulation
- managing simulation resources and environments
- engaging in scholarly activities (SSH, 2022)

# ▶ SUMMARY

Deciding to take an initial certification examination or apply for an advanced certification will enhance your knowledge and ability as you achieve personal and professional goals. Both the initial and advanced certifications promote facilitation of learning of future healthcare providers, and becoming certified will ultimately benefit patients receiving care. Congratulations on choosing to study and become a Certified Healthcare Simulation Educator. You will promote quality education that will benefit healthcare students and all their patients.

# REFERENCES

Charles, S., & Koehn, M. (2016). Using peer study to prepare for Certified Healthcare Simulation Educator Certification. *Clinical Simulation in Nursing, 12*(6), 202–208. https://doi.org/10.1016/j.ecns.2016.02.009

Society for Simulation in Healthcare. (2022). *Certified healthcare simulation educator advanced-renewal materials.* https://www.ssih.org/Portals/48/Certification/CHSE-A_Docs/CHSE-A%20Recert%20Packet.pdf

Society for Simulation in Healthcare. (2019). *Certified healthcare simulation educator renewal & recertification materials.* http://ssih.org/Portals/48/Certification/CHSE_Docs/CHSERecertPacket.pdf

Society for Simulation in Healthcare. (2020). *SSH certified healthcare simulation educator-advanced handbook.* http://ssih.org/Portals/48/Certification/CHSE-A_Docs/CHSE-A%20Handbook.pdf

Society for Simulation in Healthcare. (2021). *SSH certified healthcare simulation educatorhandbook.* http://www.ssih.org/Portals/48/Certification/CHSE_Docs/CHSE%20Handbook.pdf

# The Certification Examination Test Plan

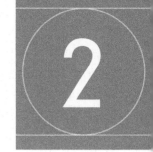

Ruth A. Wittmann-Price

*We learn by example and by direct experience because there are real limits to the adequacy of verbal instruction.*

—*Malcolm Gladwell*

> ▶ **LEARNING OUTCOMES**
>
> ■ Discuss the importance of certification in simulation for healthcare educators.
> ■ Review the specifics of the certification test plan.
> ■ Interpret case studies and practice questions as learning tools to promote success.

## ▶ INTRODUCTION

For many reasons, simulation in healthcare education is needed in today's healthcare educational environment now more than ever. Simulation learning experiences provide a wealth of student benefits that translate into best patient care practices. The Society for Simulation in Healthcare (SSH) has developed the initial and advanced certifications to recognize expert simulation educators in this important and expanding field. Simulation learning can promote student understanding and competence in all aspects of healthcare delivery and ultimately improve patient safety.

The test plan for the certification examination was developed in 2011 and revised in 2018 and can be found on the SSH website (SSH, 2021). There are four broad topic areas included in the initial and advanced certification examinations, which are professional values and capabilities, healthcare and simulation knowledge/principles, educational principles applied to simulation, and simulation resources and environments. The largest number of questions on the test (40%) concentrates on educational principles. Professional values and capabilities comprise 18% of the test items, and simulation resources and environments comprise 14%. Healthcare and simulation knowledge/principles comprise the last 28% of the test (SSH, 2021).

These four major test areas are further broken down into criteria that are more specific and therefore easier to dissect and understand. Each of the specific areas is discussed. It is understood that not all healthcare educators who teach in simulation laboratories are experts in all four areas; however, for the test, each educator needs a working knowledge of the areas. For example, a healthcare educator working in a large simulation laboratory may not be responsible for the stocking, ordering, or maintenance of the laboratory, but will need to have an understanding of the resources needed and used for simulation education.

## ▶ DOMAIN AREA I: PROFESSIONAL VALUES AND CAPABILITIES

The first area of the test is the display of professional values and capabilities (SSH, 2021). This area includes the following:

- demonstrating leadership
- acting as a simulation advocate

- displaying teamwork
- understanding simulation roles
- understanding regulatory compliance
- participating in quality improvement and evidence-based practices

Professional values and capabilities comprise 18% of the test items, so the candidate can expect 20 to 21 questions pertaining to this area. Part II of this book (Chapter 4, "Leadership in Simulation"; Chapter 5, "Special Learning Considerations in Simulation"; Chapter 6, "Interprofessional Simulation"; and Chapter 7, "Ethical, Legal, and Regulatory Implications in Healthcare Simulation") discusses the professional values and capabilities content areas in depth. The following is a quick synopsis of the major content that falls under Domain I.

## LEADERSHIP

Leadership in simulation is thoroughly addressed in Chapter 4, "Leadership in Simulation."

Transformational leadership, first described by Burns (1978), is the current leadership theory discussed in educational organizations. Transformational leaders are described as exhibiting positive attributes including the following:

- vision for future development
- ability to engage others in the vision
- developing values surrounding the vision
- moving people toward the vision
- effecting positive change (Bass, 1985)

Transformational leadership is different from *transactional leadership*. Transactional leadership is equated to more authoritarian management that directs people without motivating them. Some of the attributes associated with transactional leadership are the following:

- hierarchical decisions
- institution of a reward-and-punishment system
- micromanaging from the top of the organization (Khan et al., 2021)

Instituting an effective simulation program benefits from transformational leadership. The simulation team, when passionate about the learning that takes place in the simulation laboratory, demonstrates the ultimate vision of healthcare competency and quality patient care.

## ADVOCATING FOR SIMULATION

It is generally understood that simulation was developed for two major purposes: (a) to improve healthcare safety and (b) to increase the educational experiences of learners. The National Council of State Boards of Nursing (NCSBN, 2013) simulation study (Rutherford-Hemming et al., 2016) demonstrated, using a multisite project with 666 students, that there was no significant difference in program outcomes among three groups of participants. One group used no simulation, the second group used 25% of simulation, and the third group used 50% of simulation for clinical learning experiences.

Another issue that surrounds the use of simulation learning is the resources needed to maintain a simulation laboratory with equipment and a qualified team. Additionally, simulation learning may be difficult to schedule in traditional healthcare programs that require a vast amount of direct patient care hours. Interprofessional simulation experiences are at times especially difficult to schedule due to the involvement of multiple disciplines.

In addition, simulation experiences can be advocated for and expanded to community activities for both the healthcare communities and the laity. Simulation can be an experience used in acute care, outpatient, and community settings. Disaster planning with simulation has made many groups aware of its educational ability. Whenever possible, all simulation educators should explain and demonstrate the positive learning experiences that can be attained through simulation.

## ▶ DOMAIN AREA II: HEALTHCARE AND SIMULATION KNOWLEDGE/ PRINCIPLES

The second content area covered in the examination makes up 28% of the examination or approximately 32 or 33 questions (SSH, 2021). It is divided into 13 subcriteria. Chapter 8, "Human Patient Simulator Simulation"; Chapter 9, "Moulage in Simulation"; Chapter 10, "Simulation Principles, Practice, and Methodologies for Standardized Patient Simulation"; Chapter 11, "Hybrid Simulation"; Chapter 12, "Part-Task Trainers"; and Chapter 13, "Virtual Reality," address all 13 areas, and before the introduction to each chapter the domain being addressed is stated. The second domain includes topics about simulation research, feedback and debriefing, realism, patient safety, and types of simulation activities including virtual simulation.

## ▶ DOMAIN AREA III: EDUCATIONAL PRINCIPLES APPLIED TO SIMULATION

Domain III is the largest part of the test and comprises approximately 46 (40%) questions (SSH, 2021). This section contains nine major criteria and many subcriteria. The content of this section comprises questions regarding the actual use of simulation with learners. Questions contain education scenarios, and candidates will have to choose the correct assessment, plan, intervention, or evaluation of the situation by the correct combination of educator and learner, learner and learner, learner and standardized patient (SP), or educator and SP. Expect application questions in which knowledge from this area is applied to situations. Each of the criteria is also addressed in Chapter 14, "Educational Theories, Learning Theories, and Special Concepts"; Chapter 15, "Implementing Simulation in the Curriculum"; Chapter 16, "Planning Simulation Activities"; Chapter 17, "Debriefing"; Chapter 18, "Standardized Patient Debriefing and Feedback"; Chapter 19, "Evaluation of Simulation Activities"; Chapter 20, "Fostering Professional Development in Healthcare Simulation"; and Chapter 21, "The Role of Research in Simulation."

## ▶ DOMAIN AREA IV: SIMULATION RESOURCES AND ENVIRONMENTS

Domain IV of the examination is made up of six criteria and comprises 14%, or 16 to 17 questions, of the examination (SSH, 2021). This content area is addressed in depth in Chapter 22, "Operations and Management of Environment, Personnel, and Nonpersonnel Resources," and Chapter 23, "Accreditation of Simulation Laboratories and Simulation Standards." The criteria under this content area include improving outcomes, planning and implementing operational changes in a simulation laboratory, using resources, and understanding risk reduction.

### Simulation Teaching Tip 2.1

Introducing simulation experiences in the first semester of healthcare education may increase learners' comfort level with the methodology as it is repeated semester after semester.

### Evidence-Based Simulation Practice 2.1

Pisciottani et al. (2017) studied the use of in situ CPR teaching to nursing students and compared groups using a researcher-made tool. A student t-test in-group comparison was used to demonstrate students' increased proficiency in the following criteria: ventilation with manual resuscitator, insertion of airway, monitoring and aiding defibrillation, and control of timing.

 CASE STUDY 2.1

An expert clinician is hired as one of three educational coordinators in the simulation laboratory for undergraduate healthcare students. The person hired is an expert in the critical care unit of a local acute care hospital. The expert clinician is assisting in setting up a simulation experience for first-semester healthcare learners. During the experience, using a high-fidelity manikin, the education coordinator uses the computer controls to cause the patient to "code," and then, in the debriefing, acknowledges that they thought the learners would know how to handle it better. How would you address this with the education coordinator using Benner's theory?

1. The priority area in a Certified Healthcare Simulation Educator® (CHSE®) examination is:

   A. Professional values and capabilities
   B. Managing simulation resources
   C. Engaging in scholarship activity
   D. Education and assessment of learners

2. The simulation educator understands that caring for equipment and maintaining a budget are expectations of which of the following criteria?

   A. Professional values and capabilities
   B. Managing simulation resources
   C. Engaging in scholarship activity
   D. Education and assessment of learners

3. The simulation educator is facilitating learning in the simulation laboratory for a group of healthcare students. The students are in a simple simulation scenario and have not enacted a plan of care according to the physical, psychological, and social needs of the patient. The simulation educator understands that the students are at which novice-to-expert level?

   A. Novice
   B. Advanced beginner
   C. Competent
   D. Proficient

4. The novice simulation educator understands the impact of simulation when they state:

   A. "Simulation should be used for difficult-to-find clinical learning experiences."
   B. "Students who are exposed to more simulation than direct patient care may not be able to perform as well in clinical practice."
   C. "Simulation cannot assist educators to teach professional values and standards."
   D. "Simulation should not be limited if it meets the students' learning outcomes."

5. The simulation educator is at a general faculty meeting and describes how simulation can be used as a community liaison tool. The simulation educator is demonstrating which simulation certification examination criteria of professional values and capabilities?

   A. Mentorship
   B. Role modeling
   C. Leadership
   D. Advocating

6. The novice simulation educator needs additional understanding when they state simulation can be an effective learning tool for:

   A. Psychomotor skills
   B. Cognitive decision-making
   C. Affective interactions
   D. Social distancing

(See answers next page.)

## 1. A) Professional values and capabilities
Quality simulation experiences assist learners in becoming competent as professionals and in learning the values of the profession that they have chosen through structured learning and assessment. Managing resources in the simulation laboratory is important but only assists with students' learning of professional values and capabilities. Scholarship activity may or may not be part of students' course learning objectives. Education and assessment of learners are also important, but education and assessment need to take place within the framework of professional values and capabilities.

## 2. B) Managing simulation resources
The resources that are needed to effectively run a simulation laboratory include the budget and equipment maintenance, as well as additional supplies, and most importantly qualified professionals. Professional values and capabilities are a different construct and are enhanced by the resources. Engagement in scholarship is also separate from resources. Education and assessment of learners are what the resources are used for theoretically, as well as the development of professional values and capabilities.

## 3. A) Novice
Novice students should be able to enact a simple plan of care before being exposed to a simulation scenario. Advanced beginners can complete procedural steps. Competent practitioners can detect patterns in caring for patients, while proficient healthcare providers can modify plans as needed.

## 4. A) "Simulation should be used for difficult-to-find clinical learning experiences."
Simulation is a good choice when the faculty cannot find the appropriate hands-on learning experiences in the clinical area to meet healthcare students' course objectives. Having more simulation than direct patient care experiences has not been proven beneficial by evidence. Some studies suggest up to 50% yields the same student learning outcomes; therefore, some limits on simulation may occur due to evidence-based practice (EBP). Simulation is a good place to teach professional values and capabilities.

## 5. D) Advocating
The simulation educator is explaining to the faculty one asset of the simulation program. The simulation educator is advocating for simulation as more than a student learning tool. The simulation educator is not mentoring another person or group. The simulation educator may not be in a leadership role and is not role modeling for students' learning purposes.

## 6. D) Social distancing
Although social distancing can be done in a simulation laboratory, this is not one of the learning domains that simulation learning facilitates. Simulation can and is used to enhance cognitive, psychomotor, and affective competencies of healthcare students.

7. A simulation educator rearranges the simulation space to depict a multicar accident in order to teach triage. The simulation educator is guided by which simulation certification examination criteria?

   A. Professional values and capabilities
   B. Managing simulation resources
   C. Engaging in scholarship activity
   D. Education and assessment of learners

8. A simulation education team from an academic setting is presenting at a national conference. The educators are encouraging which simulation certification examination criteria by their work?

   A. Professional values and capabilities
   B. Managing simulation resources
   C. Engaging in scholarship activity
   D. Education and assessment of learners

9. The students in a simulation learning setting understand that a diagnosis in a patient can elicit therapeutic interventions per a protocol. The simulation educator understands that the students are at which novice-to-expert level in performing physical examination?

   A. Novice
   B. Advanced beginner
   C. Competent
   D. Proficient

10. The simulation educator presents a scheduling plan for the simulation laboratory at a general faculty meeting. The simulation educator is demonstrating which simulation certification examination criteria of professional values and capabilities?

   A. Mentorship
   B. Role modeling
   C. Leadership
   D. Advocating

### 7. D) Education and assessment of learners
Triage teaching is a direct method of educating and/or assessing learners' professional decision-making skills. Professional values and capabilities are part of the learning but the focus is on teaching prioritization and case management. This activity is not scholarly activity but can be used as the foundation of a presentation or a manuscript. Resources are used but management of resources is not the focus.

### 8. C) Engaging in scholarship activity
Presenting at conferences is a great way to disseminate information and is considered scholarship in academic institutions. It is not directly teaching professional values and capabilities, managing resources, or educating and assessing students. Presenting is scholarship.

### 9. B) Advanced beginner
The students are advanced beginners because they are ready to follow procedural steps. A novice healthcare student has limited ability in predicting what comes next, a competent healthcare student has advanced planning and organizational skills, and a proficient student has experience and can see situations as a whole.

### 10. C) Leadership
The simulation educator is taking charge of the simulation laboratory and providing the leadership needed to ensure the operations of the laboratory are organized. The simulation educator is not mentoring another person or role modeling for a person or group. The simulation educator is not advocating but is using leadership skills to disseminate information.

# REFERENCES

Bass, B. M. (1985). *Leadership and performance beyond expectation*. Free Press.

Burns, J. M. (1978). *Leadership*. Harper & Row.

Khan, I. U., Khan, M. S., & Idris, M. (2021). Investigating the support of organizational culture for leadership styles (transformational & transactional). *Journal of Human Behavior in the Social Environment, 31*(6), 689–700. https://doi.org/10.1080/10911359.2020.1803174

National Council of State Boards of Nursing. (2013). *National simulation study*. https://www.ncsbn.org/685.htm

Pisciottani, F., França da Rocha, D., da Costa, M. R., Figueiredo, A. E., & Magalhães, C. R. (2017). In situ simulation in cardiopulmonary resuscitation: Implications for permanent nursing education. *Journal of Nursing UFPE on Line, 11*(7), 2810–2815. https://doi.org/10.5205/reuol.9799-86079-1-RV.1106sup201722

Rutherford-Hemming, T., Lioce, L., Kardong-Edgren, S., Jeffries, P. R., & Sittner, B. (2016). After the National Council of State Boards of Nursing Simulation Study—Recommendations and next steps. *Clinical Simulation in Nursing, 12*(1), 2–7. https://doi.org/10.1016/j.ecns.2015.10.010

Society for Simulation in Healthcare. (2021). *Certified healthcare simulation educator examination blueprint, 2018 version*. http://www.ssih.org/Portals/48/Certification/CHSE_Docs/CHSE_Examination_Blueprint.pdf

Wittmann-Price, R. A. (2012). *Fast facts for developing a nursing academic portfolio*. Springer Publishing Company.

# Test-Taking Strategies

Dorie L. Weaver

*Education is the passport to the future. Tomorrow belongs to those who prepare for it today.*
*—Malcolm X*

> ▶ **LEARNING OUTCOMES**
>
> ■ Identify the process to best prepare for the certification examination.
> ■ Discuss evidence-based study tips for success to enhance understanding of key concepts.
> ■ Describe how to integrate standards from practice into information that is outlined in the examination blueprint.
> ■ Discuss general strategies to reduce test-taking anxiety to promote retention.

## ▶ WHY BECOME CERTIFIED IN SIMULATION?

There is an increasing need to improve both patient care quality and patient safety. Today's clinical opportunities for students are limited based on placement and increased restrictions by practice partners. This presents a challenge and has concerning implications for nursing education. The amount of students' direct hands-on experience has been decreasing over time. Studies show that recent graduate nurses do not possess the essential skills and clinical decision-making that are expected upon graduation. However, increasing the amount of simulation exercises can prove to be an effective strategy to bridge the gap between knowledge and application to clinical setting. Simulation exercises are increasingly being used as a teaching method in both undergraduate and graduate nursing education. Four main themes are associated with simulation: (a) facilitates student-centered learning, (b) promotes reflection, (c) boosts student confidence, and (d) creates a safe environment to learn. Feeling secure is reported to be a key aspect of the simulation learning process (Haddeland et al., 2021).

A student told a nurse educator that they were hired to work in an ICU immediately upon successful completion of the National Council Licensure Examination® (NCLEX-RN®). The first day on the job, the graduate nurse's patient coded. Although management of a patient in cardiac arrest was taught within the classroom through lectures as well as through discussions of a written case study, as a student the graduate was not given any opportunity to actually practice these essential skills in any type of setting. Any patient who experienced cardiac arrest while in the hospital while students were in their clinical learning experience was dealt with by the licensed personnel.

Practicing in a simulation laboratory can better prepare students for these types of situations and ultimately improve patient outcomes. Simulation-based learning (SBL) promotes critical thinking and places students in scenarios that mimic situations they most likely will encounter in practice, as well as situations that are rare. The beneficial component of simulation is that it is carried out in a structured, controlled, and safe environment where mistakes can occur with no punitive damage to patients. The hands-on approach refines learning by helping to process knowledge for long-term retention.

It is common knowledge that there are students who can excel on written exams yet struggle in the clinical learning environment. In addition to skills training, simulation can enhance intraprofessional and interprofessional communication and collaboration. Because lack of communication is one major source of error, SBL can indirectly reduce the number of preventable errors.

Simulation is a teaching methodology where situations are created or replicated in a controlled environment to resemble authentic situations that a new graduate may be faced with in real life. As educators and clinicians, it is our responsibility to provide simulations that develop individual and team skills, as well as promote clinical reasoning, to improve the competency of healthcare providers. Furthermore, simulations are an innovative strategy to help students meet learning outcomes (Mulyadi et al., 2021).

Educators and clinicians with years of experience in simulation can now validate their expertise and knowledge by certification. Obtaining a certification is an invaluable resource for future role models, mentors, and visionaries. Attainment demonstrates one's commitment to the nursing profession along with lifelong learning. In addition, it can provide the practitioner with a sense of both personal and professional accomplishment, competence, and credibility. Being certified can help improve education by having a pool of knowledge related to best practices. It can also play a role in obtaining grants and making educational institutions more competitive in attracting students (Society for Simulation in Healthcare [SSH], 2021).

The following list outlines a few of the ways in which those who are certified can affect the healthcare environment:

- Support patient safety guidelines.
- Close the gap between theory and practice.
- Provide standardization of practice within healthcare.
- Impact patient outcomes and quality improvement.
- Develop evidence-based practice and research.

## ▶ QUALIFICATIONS TO BE A CANDIDATE TO TAKE THE EXAMINATION

Answer the following questions:

- Have I participated in simulation within an educational role?
- Was the simulation developed to focus on learners in undergraduate, graduate, allied health programs, or healthcare practitioners?
- Do I have a baccalaureate degree or an equivalent experience?
- Have I used simulation in healthcare education, research, or administration continuously over the past 2 years?

The certification tests can be intimidating and anxiety-provoking for many candidates. The more prepared one is, the better the chance for success.

## ▶ HOW TO PREPARE FOR SUCCESS

- Study in advance. Avoid cramming because much of the information is rarely converted into long-term memory. Set up a formal study schedule as this will help keep learning on track and will ensure adequate time to cover all the necessary topics. If there is procrastination that gets studying off schedule, forgive yourself for any time wasted. This is crucial in order to release the burden and clear your mind so that studying is effective.

Everyone studies differently, but it is best to set up a study calendar that does not overwhelm. Adjust the study calendar when  content that will take more time. The priority is to make sure there is enough time spent studying before securing an examination date. This can help reduce test anxiety. Print the information that is available from the SSH *Certified Healthcare Simulation Educator™ Handbook* (SSH, 2021) at www.ssih. org/chse/handbook. There are four domains found within the exam (Table 3.1).

- With knowledge of the test design and blueprint, the next step is to think about planning an effective study strategy.
- Maximize study time. Prepare an environment that is conducive to studying. Attempt to remove as many distractors as possible. Set aside a fixed place to study. Ensure adequate lighting and a comfortable temperature. Cooler rooms are better to avoid fatigue.
- It is important to know what time you are most efficient. One should study close to the time period when they are most alert. Study the most difficult material at this time.
- It is essential to take periodic study breaks. This helps the mind to recharge.
- Use charts and diagrams to organize information so you can review at a glance. These visual aids also allow the learner to compare and contrast content. Images with key terms can enhance learning and memory. Effective note-taking is multisensory. It helps to more effectively commit concepts to memory. Organizing notes in a logical sense is crucial to help with retention.
- Quiz yourself periodically. This will help establish how successful your preparation has been. Practice answering questions on a routine basis. This will provide you with the ability to recognize gaps in knowledge. Schedule time to research the content that was incorrect on the practice exams. Be certain to read the rationales to have a better understanding of the correct and incorrect answers.
- Look at the list of examination-preparation references, most of which are journal publications. It is to your advantage to read multiple articles related to the categories that carry the highest percentage of questions on the examination.
- Organize related information into groups. Focusing on one topic at a time will help you remember information by comparing and contrasting content. Use the concept of deep learning approach by critically examining new facts and making links between ideas. It is also helpful to relate new knowledge to previous knowledge. Adequate time management will allow a better understanding of content and promote confidence. Being overworked without enough time to study lends itself to use the surface approach to learning, which is good for short-term memory only. This entails storing new facts as isolated information and may result in high anxiety (LeCun et al., 2015).
- Organize a study group with your colleagues. Studying in groups allows each member to take advantage of others' expertise. Reviewing information while in a group may be worthwhile if all members of the group are committed and prepared for the study sessions. It is essential for the group to stay focused. Group members can support and encourage each other. Studying with representatives from various healthcare disciplines can be a valuable learning experience. Discussion and debate are critical for those who are auditory learners.
- Develop mnemonics, acronyms, or checklists. In order to promote patient safety and standardization of care, mnemonics, acronyms, and checklists have been developed as memory aids in specific situations. For example, mnemonics are used in advanced cardiac life support (ACLS) certification to recall algorithms. Healthcare professionals also use the SBAR mnemonic to promote optimal communication during patient handoff.
  - ❏ **S** = Situation
  - ❏ **B** = Background
  - ❏ **A** = Assessment
  - ❏ **R** = Recommendations

There is a tremendous amount of information to remember, so you may want to develop your own mnemonics or acronyms while you study.

■ Healthcare professionals always care for others; now it is time for self-care. Self-care is crucial for optimal performance. It is important to eat consistent meals and avoid concentrated sweets that can surge and then plunge blood glucose levels. It is best to avoid heavy meals prior to a study session or before the examination. Think energy and brain power. Blueberries, strawberries, red beets, broccoli, tomatoes, pomegranate juice, vegetable juice, and nuts can enhance your brain power. Whole-grain foods, nuts, and legumes have low glycemic index and release glucose into the bloodstream slowly, which provides energy for hours. Stay hydrated by drinking at least eight glasses of water daily (Table 3.2).

■ Impaired sleep can hinder the ability to learn, retain, and recall information. It is imperative to get adequate and consistent sleep especially the evening before the examination. Some healthy sleep patterns include avoiding screen time 2 hours before going to bed, going to bed at the same time each night, implementing white noise, and making sure the room is as dark as possible and that there is sufficient air circulation. Engage in daily physical activity to increase stamina and improve energy levels, and increase mental acuity. Finally, do not ignore leisure time with support system people. This can help reduce your stress level.

**Table 3.1** Four Domains of the Certified Healthcare Simulation Educator™ Exam

| Domain | Weight (%) |
|---|---|
| I: Professional Values and Capabilities | 18 |
| II: Healthcare and Simulation Knowledge/Principles | 28 |
| III: Educational Principles Applied to Simulation | 40 |
| IV: Simulation Resources and Environments | 14 |

**Table 3.2** Key Topics for Discussion in Your Review

| Designing stage | Determine a needs assessment by deciding whether cognitive, behavioral, and technical issues will be incorporated into the scenario.<br>Determine the participants: individual, team, and systems.<br>Define the goals of the activity.<br>Develop measurable learning objectives.<br>Write the scenario and integrate complications, distractions, and roles.<br>Select the tool that will be used to evaluate the participants. |
|---|---|
| Planning stage | Organize the simulation team.<br>Schedule the simulation laboratory with time allocated for setup, scenario, and reorganization of the environment.<br>Determine whether the simulation will be videotaped.<br>Reserve the capital equipment needed for the scenario.<br>Schedule SPs if needed.<br>Plan the scene setting.<br>Determine the type of moulage needed.<br>Make a list of supplies and drugs to be used in the scenario.<br>Prepare written information for the simulation team.<br>Determine how to respond to unforeseen issues during simulation, such as equipment failure, drugs or equipment missing, unprofessional behavior, and knowledge gaps. |

(continued)

**Table 3.2** Key Topics for Discussion in Your Review (*continued*)

| Implementation stage | Provide an overview of the goals and objectives.<br>Orient the participants to the environment and the equipment.<br>Brief the participants about the scenario.<br>Assess the participants related to the objectives. |
|---|---|
| Postsimulation stage | Debriefing can include evaluation by self, peers, or faculty.<br>Provide time and schedule the room to view the video (if indicated).<br>Know the debriefing models.<br>Understand the responsibility of the facilitator. |

SPs, standardized patients.

## ▶ KNOW YOUR EQUIPMENT/TECHNOLOGY

- *Task trainers:* used to practice procedures such as wound care and IV insertion
- *Human patient simulators:* manikin-based equipment in human form
- *Virtual reality simulation:* used to provide a computer-based simulation experience sometimes with the use of an avatar
- *Standardized patients (SPs):* use of actors to simulate patients in a standardized manner
- *Hybrid simulation methodology:* simulation that incorporates multiple types of simulation, with one being used to enhance the other; a task trainer can be used with an SP to provide a hybrid simulation experience
- *Mixed simulation:* simulation that incorporates multiple types of simulation, with each being a tool for educational purposes

### Simulation Teaching Tip 3.1

When designing a simulation experience, think about activities to enhance different types of learning styles. Students can access the VARK (Visual, Aural, Read/Write, Kinesthetic) website (http://vark -learn.com/the-vark-questionnaire/) to determine how they learn best (Fleming, 2001).

## ▶ BECOME FAMILIAR WITH COMPUTERIZED TESTING

- Carefully read directions for answering questions. There is usually a tutorial for you to use to familiarize yourself with the process. Make sure you understand the directions that explain how to pause the test if you need to take a break.
- Pay attention to information such as how to change answers.
- Check the clock intermittently to ensure there is adequate time left to complete the exam. If unable to answer the question within 60 to 90 seconds, eliminate those distractors that are incorrect and guess using the remaining ones. Do not waste precious time. Keep in mind that there is no penalty for guessing. Bookmark the question and come back to it later if time allows. Completing timed practice tests can provide insight into how best to manage time during an actual examination.

# ▶ INCORPORATE STRATEGIES TO EASE THE FEAR OF TEST ANXIETY

It is normal to feel some test anxiety about taking a certification examination.

- Anxiety is a natural response to new challenges in our lives.
- Some anxiety will cause heightened awareness and may improve test taking, whereas anxiety that is uncontrolled will impede the ability to concentrate and think critically. Excessive worrying is the root cause of test anxiety.
- Everyone who takes tests experiences some anxiety; however, recognizing and controlling anxiety is an important factor in success.

Some strategies that can be used to ease test anxiety include the following:

- Reduce anxiety related to time constraints.
  - Schedule the examination when your work schedule is less stressful.
  - Start a study group and plan to meet once a week for 2 hours.
    - ❏ Use a detailed test plan to divide assignments.
    - ❏ Each member of the study group can complete an assignment and share notes with the group.
    - ❏ Each member of the group can also share the sources of information.
- Reduce anxiety related to having limited experience in taking tests.
  - Develop a checklist by writing a list of content that concerns you and cross each item off when you have mastered it.
  - Practice the questions in the book and review the rationales, even if you answered the practice question correctly.
  - Self-evaluation will assist you in refocusing on specific content.
  - Practice will increase your proficiency. It will also boost your confidence level.
- Reduce anxiety related to previous unfavorable testing experience.
  - Stop negative thoughts that begin with "what if." Read or repeat a positive message about being successful. Remember the mind is a powerful tool and can either serve as a motivator or an obstacle. Keep in mind that all the necessary information is presented in the exam question. Do not overanalyze. If specific information is not given, this indicates it is irrelevant and will not affect the answer.
  - Should you reach a point when there are several consecutive difficult questions to answer in a row, do not panic! Practice a calming technique, such as deep breathing.
  - Use positive affirmations about goals, such as "I can answer more questions correctly" or "I understand that information now."
  - Try to avoid perfectionism. It is virtually impossible to know everything. This can lead to negative thinking when a difficult question comes up and may result in self-sabotage. Identify reasonable expectations and maintain sufficient study habits.
  - Take time each day to exercise and practice relaxation techniques, such as yoga or meditation. Avoid excessive caffeine intake while studying and before the exam. Caffeine can cause anxiety and can adversely affect one's ability to maintain focus. Avoid refined sugars and high-fat foods, which can drain one's energy, decreasing concentration levels (Sefcik et al., 2013).

Practice these strategies on a regular basis so that reducing anxiety becomes easy to achieve. Engage in activities that you find relaxing on the evening prior to the examination, such as watching a movie or going out to dinner with friends. Do not attempt to open any books. If you do not know the material by this time, you will not learn it the evening prior to the exam. In addition, you will increase your anxiety level. Relaxation can help you switch your focus from any external stressors. It is essential that you get an adequate amount of sleep the night prior to the exam.

# ▶ USE STRATEGIES TO BE A SAVVY TEST-TAKER

## READ OR MISREAD

A common mistake people make when taking a test is misreading the question. Multiple-choice questions often require critical thinking. Read each question carefully and determine the keywords that provide details for answering the question. Misreading the question can dramatically change the objective of the question. Know what the stem of the question is asking. This is extremely critical as it can help you more easily decide the correct option from a plausible distractor. Answers are written to sound plausible to those who do not know the content. This is done to discriminate between individuals who know the information and those who do not. Use the process of elimination to discard those options that you know are not correct.

Formulate an answer before you look at the available choices. Compare the available options with what you think is the correct response. Be sure to read over all options before answering.

---

### Simulation Teaching Tip 3.2

If you begin to feel panicked because you were just given a few consecutive questions that were extremely difficult, say to yourself that these are experimental questions and will not count against you if you answered incorrectly. Always keep in mind that you devoted sufficient time to studying all the key concepts and that you entered the exam well prepared. Refuse to let the exam defeat you. Believe you have great potential to be successful.

---

## VISUALIZATION

If a simulation is described and you are unsure of the answer, close your eyes. Picture the scenario in your mind prior to answering the question. Keep in mind there are times when something in one of the exam questions will help trigger the correct answer to another question.

## CHANGING ANSWERS

The first answer that comes to mind is usually the correct answer. Do not second-guess your "gut" feeling. If you are sure you need to change an answer, do it. However, if you usually change answers from correct to incorrect, do not do it.

## UNDERSTAND THE TYPES OF QUESTIONS DEVELOPED FROM COGNITIVE LEVELS OF LEARNING

Bloom's taxonomy of learning is used to determine whether the candidate has mastered definitive skills or competencies. The easiest or lower level questions would be within the knowledge or comprehension category. These questions include recalling or demonstrating an understanding of concepts. Chances are you will not be responsible for answering many of these types of questions because of their uncomplicated nature.

For studying—think application. Application questions expect the candidate to provide an intervention to the problem. There is usually a large percentage of these questions. In such questions, it would be important to apply ideas, concepts, principles, or theories to solve a problem. Exhibit 3.1 demonstrates an application question.

---

**EXHIBIT 3.1 APPLICATION QUESTION EXAMPLE**

Example: During a simulation, the learners fail to recognize a negative response after a medication is administered. What action by the simulation facilitator would be most appropriate?

A. Decrease the other distractions in the environment
B. Instruct the confederate to provide some information
C. Continue the simulation as originally planned
D. Stop the simulation

The answer is C (continue the simulation as originally planned because this situation occurs in healthcare frequently).
It is important for the scenario to play out because it is a learning experience. The issue would be addressed and discussed during debriefing.

---

Analysis questions will also be evident. These questions expect a logical response to the detailed cause and effect after examining information or reports. This provides an opportunity to break down the relationship between the parts and decide how the whole functions. Ask yourself why a solution worked or did not work. Conclusions should always be supported by facts or results. Keep this in mind while studying for the certification exam. Exhibit 3.2 is an example of an analysis question.

---

**EXHIBIT 3.2 ANALYSIS QUESTION EXAMPLE**

Example: A human simulation experience was designed as a formative assessment for learners who were midway through the nursing program. The learners stated that the experience was too difficult. Which information about the simulation experience should the educator examine first?

A. Course grades of the learners involved in the simulation
B. Training of the standardized patients (SPs)
C. Planning details of the encounter
D. Feedback from the SPs

The answer is D (feedback from the SPs).
Learners are usually very anxious about simulation, which may alter their evaluation of the experience. Verbal feedback from the SPs as well as the information from the checklists will provide accurate information.

---

Another category with high-level questions is synthesis (Exhibit 3.3). These types of questions are not used frequently in testing situations but could be used in simulation because they require creating plans or constructing solutions to problems. All elements are combined into a unified whole to develop a tool or design a plan. Evaluation will also be tested to provide the candidate with the opportunity to make value judgments based on effectiveness of a simulation design, scenario progression, patient outcomes, or equipment. Exhibit 3.4 provides an evaluation question.

## EXHIBIT 3.3 SYNTHESIS QUESTION EXAMPLE

Example: Data have determined that the patient wait time in the ED has increased by 20% within the last quarter. The patient visits and patient acuity have remained the same. Three extra full-time RNs and one clerk have been hired within the past 11 months. Six months ago, a boarding area was constructed to accommodate patients waiting for inpatient beds to open. The manager decides to design a simulation experience for the team to promote best practice. What should be the focus of the simulation?

A. Perfecting skills
B. Team building
C. Effective communication
D. Use of ancillary staff

The answer is B (team building).
The data that were collected do not reflect the fact that the nursing staff has increased and the boarding area is operational. Staff must communicate effectively, perfect their skills, and use ancillary staff appropriately. These issues would all be encompassed in team building.

## EXHIBIT 3.4 EVALUATION QUESTION EXAMPLE

Example: The RN-to-BSN (registered nurse-to-bachelor of science in nursing) nursing program has 375 learners at present. This is an increase of 20% in 1 year. Approximately 60% of the class attends online. After evaluating the program, determine what equipment/technology should be discussed during the upcoming budget meeting.

A. Nasogastric (NG) and tracheostomy care trainer
B. Harvey, the cardiopulmonary patient simulator
C. Wound care trainer
D. Virtual reality simulation

The answer is D (virtual reality simulation).
Learners attending online classes continue to increase. This technology would be accessible to those attending the classes live as well as those attending online. If the learners are already RNs, they should have the skills to care for patients with NG tubes and tracheostomies. Skills as well as heart and lung sounds are available in most virtual simulation programs.

Keep in mind that the simulation certification is available to all healthcare professionals who have met the eligibility requirements. Therefore, the global approach to reviewing information for this examination is critical. Positive patient outcomes rely on the multidisciplinary approach to quality care. Think about concepts in relation to the types of questions (application, analysis, synthesis, and evaluation) that will be tested. Examine your own activities as an educator and in practice and relate them to the content in the questions.

## CASE STUDY 3.1

A course chair requested that the faculty teaching the course use a simulation the last week of the term. The course had five sections. The goal was to provide a safe environment for learners to use assessment techniques and fundamental nursing skills with the use of a high-fidelity manikin. The educators were provided with a choice of four different scenarios, objectives, lists of equipment, and medications needed for each simulation. A self-evaluation tool was also available for learners to complete after the simulation.

After the completion of the term, the course chair received multiple emails from learners stating that their section never had an opportunity to experience a simulation. The two sections involved were taught by the same educator. How should the course chair approach this issue?

1. Which task is multisensory and plays a significant role in committing information to long-term memory?

   A. Reading books and journals
   B. Watching videos and animations
   C. Taking practice examinations and quizzes
   D. Writing notes in an organized and outlined manner

2. The goal of simulation-based learning is to:

   A. Use technology that students enjoy
   B. Make the students feel secure
   C. Teach safe patient care
   D. Fulfill the course outcomes

3. What is the main purpose of debriefing?

   A. Allows for self-reflection and identification of strengths
   B. Reduces the gap between theory and practice
   C. Helps students identify their weaknesses
   D. Enhances intraprofessional communication and collaboration

4. A faculty member recently earned their simulation education certificate. Which of the following statements made by this faculty member is inaccurate?

   A. "Being certified can make our nursing program a bit more competitive and provides an edge for obtaining grant funding."
   B. "I will be able to improve simulation education through identifying best practices."
   C. "I earned my certification because it shows my commitment to the nursing profession and lifelong learning."
   D. "If you are not certified, you may not understand enough theory to carry out effective simulations."

5. Unforeseen issues may happen in simulation and are best addressed during which simulation phase?

   A. Designing
   B. Planning
   C. Implementation
   D. Post simulation

6. The novice student needs to understand better study habits when they:

   A. Take periodic breaks so that their mind can relax
   B. Study difficult concepts when most alert
   C. Read the rationales only to those questions answered incorrect
   D. Use mnemonics, acronyms, and charts to help retain information

## 1. D) Writing notes in an organized and outlined manner
Studies demonstrate that writing notes in a logical and organized manner increases retention. Other types of learning such as reading books and journals as well as watching videos and animations may not address the content as thoroughly and only encompass one sense. Writing is visual and psychomotor. Videos are visual, as is reading. Taking practice examinations may be visual and psychomotor, but the psychomotor involvement is limited to clicking a button or circling an answer.

## 2. C) Teach safe patient care
The goal of developing a simulation program is to increase patient safety. Students generally do enjoy technology and simulation can increase confidence in clinical situations, but patient safety is the ultimate goal, not just fulfilling the course's student learning outcomes. Making students feel secure is also an effect of simulation, but is not the ultimate goal.

## 3. B) Reduces the gap between theory and practice
Simulation is a learning methodology that assists student development for direct patient practice. It does allow for self-reflection and identifying weaknesses and strengths, and can assist in the development of intraprofessional communication; however, the main goal is to promote positive patient care.

## 4. D) "If you are not certified, you may not understand enough theory to carry out effective simulations."
Being certified does assist simulation educators in understanding the theory and practice of simulation-based learning (SBL), but simulation educators can also understand the practice and theory of SBL without certification. Being certified is an asset for the individual and the organization. Being certified can assist in obtaining simulation grant funding and can open up the door to finding access to best practices. Certification is also a commitment to simulation education.

## 5. B) Planning
During the planning phase, the simulation educator should discuss with the simulation team members what should be done should an unforeseen incident occur. This is not part of the original design and is too late to discuss during the implementation phase. The postsimulation phase is debriefing about what has already occurred.

## 6. C) Read the rationales only to those questions answered incorrect
The rationales for all answers should be read to increase overall understanding of the content. It is good to take breaks, study when alert, and use study aids to assist memorization.

7. The goal of studying for an examination is to convert knowledge to:

   A. Improve test scores
   B. Short-term memory
   C. Question recognition
   D. Long-term memory

8. A good test-taking strategy is to:

   A. Skim the question but thoroughly read all the answer options
   B. Look for the keywords or phrases in the question
   C. Add information to get a more complete picture
   D. Randomly choose an option if unsure of the answer

9. The simulation educator asks the following question on a test: "Identify the best type of simulation for developing interpersonal skills." The answer is "standardized patients." This question is at what level of Bloom's taxonomy?

   A. Understanding
   B. Applying
   C. Comprehending
   D. Analyzing

10. An issue that should be discussed and decided on before the simulation implementation phase is:

   A. Scheduling standardized patients (SPs) as needed
   B. Debriefing using a chosen method
   C. Viewing the video with all participants
   D. Briefing the SPs on the scenario

### 7. D) Long-term memory

The goal of learning is retention of important content and information. Improving test scores, short-term memory, and question recognition are not methods that lead to learning that can eventually be applied in clinical practice.

### 8. B) Look for the keywords or phrases in the question

Looking for key or phrase word clues in the question stem can assist a learner in answering correctly. All questions and distractors should be thoroughly read and only the information presented should be used to answer. Randomly choosing a distractor only provides a 25% chance of choosing the correct answer.

### 9. A) Understanding

Identifying is a lower level verb in Bloom's taxonomy, and verbs that are more interactive with the learner are usually higher on the taxonomy. Applying is used when a question includes a decision about practice. Comprehending is more than just recall; it includes making use of the information understood. Analyzing is looking at a variety of information and then making a decision.

### 10. A) Scheduling standardized patients (SPs) as needed

The SPs need to be scheduled in the planning phase and then briefed during the implementation phase. The video is viewed and the debriefing done during the postsimulation phase.

# REFERENCES

Fleming, N. (2001). *VARK: A guide to learning styles*. http://www.vark-learn.com/english/page.asp?p=categories

Haddeland, K., Slettego, A., & Fossum, M. (2021). Enablers of the successful implementation of simulation exercises: A qualitative study among nurse teachers in undergraduate nursing education. *BMC Nursing, 20*(1). https://doi.org/10.1186/s12912-021-00756-3

LeCun, Y., Bengio, Y., & Hinton, G. (2015). Deep learning. *Nature, 521,* 436-444. https://doi.org/10.1038/nature14539

Mulyadi, M., Tonapa, S. I., Rompas, S. S. J., Wange, R., & Lee, B. (2021). Effects of simulation technology-based learning on nursing students' learning outcomes: A systemic review and meta-analysis of experimental studies. *Nurse Education Today, 107,* Article 105127. https://doi.org/10.1016/j.nedt.2021.105127

Sefcik, D., Bice, G., & Prerost, F. (2013). *How to study for standardized tests*. Jones & Bartlett.

Society for Simulation in Healthcare. (2021). *SSH certified healthcare simulation educator handbook*. http://www.ssih.org/Portals/48/Certification/CHSE_Docs/CHSE%20Handbook.pdf

# PART II
## Professional Values and Capabilities

# Leadership in Simulation

Ruth A. Wittmann-Price and Brittny D. Chabalowski

*The task of the leader is to get people from where they are to where they have not been.*

*—Henry A. Kissinger*

This chapter addresses Domain I: Professional Values and Capabilities (Society for Simulation in Healthcare [SSH], 2021).

> ## ▶ LEARNING OUTCOMES
>
> - Discuss the role of certification in simulation leadership.
> - Identify activities that contribute to leadership in simulation.
> - Review resources available for faculty development in simulation instruction.

## ▶ INTRODUCTION

Simulation in healthcare requires experienced, confident, and well-educated professionals. Simulation educators often participate in various simulation education training programs, conferences, and workshops, all of which enhance the learning and evaluation methods in the simulation laboratory. Experienced educators often pass along the bulk of simulation knowledge to novice educators through mentorship. Demonstration of leadership in the field includes development of future simulation educators.

In addition to building the unique body of simulation knowledge, educators are responsible for understanding and disseminating best practices. Leadership in the field of simulation education includes innovation and collaboration. Activities that demonstrate leadership include publication, presentation, and continued professional development (CPD). Sharing experiences in simulation and novel ideas builds the specialty and improves the delivery of simulation education on a large scale.

As a leader in the field of simulation education, being a champion of this pedagogy is a principal responsibility. The use of simulation as a teaching–learning strategy can be intimidating for experienced educators because many did not use high-fidelity simulation in their own educational process. Being an enthusiastic mentor to novice simulation educators will have a monumental impact on the specialty of simulation education.

## ▶ KNOWLEDGE ACQUISITION

Without a formal training program in place, how did we get to specialty certification? Some excellent ways to improve subject knowledge include the following:

- attending workshops
- working with an experienced individual or observing an experienced individual
- reading about simulation

More articles are appearing in reputable journals that instruct educators on how to set up and organize effective simulation scenarios (Sanner-Striehr, 2017; Watts et al., 2020).

## ▶ FACULTY CONTINUOUS PROFESSIONAL DEVELOPMENT

As stated in Chapter 2, "The Certification Examination Test Plan," the use of Patricia Benner's novice-to-expert theory (1982) has been proposed as a framework for faculty development in simulation education. Using Benner's stages, the Bay Area Simulation Collaborative Model describes the steps for instructor training (Waxman & Telles, 2009):

- novice
  - technical training
  - may include training through the simulator manufacturer
- advanced beginner
  - foundations of simulation methodology
  - may include written or online resources
- competent
  - begins observation with experienced simulation educator
  - collaborates on scenario development
  - practices facilitating simulation with feedback from experienced simulation educator
  - leads debriefing sessions with feedback
  - receives advanced technical training
  - receives discipline-specific training
- proficient
  - facilitates simulations independently
  - gains experience in simulation
  - develops scenarios independently
- expert
  - acts as experienced simulation educator and mentor for novice simulation educators
  - demonstrates innovation in simulation

## ▶ FACULTY MENTORSHIP

In a fashion very similar to designing learning outcomes, mentorship for simulation educators begins with an assessment of learning style and current knowledge. There are a number of resources available, both in print and online, that are useful in the *advanced beginner* stage of training. When the educator moves into the *competent stage*, the mentor provides a comfortable learning environment for the educator.

Simulation should be a safe and supportive environment for the learners and the new simulation educator. As with any new experience, novice simulation educators can become frustrated if they feel they do not have the tools or support necessary to be successful. Some things to consider include:

- Begin with observation of one or more experienced simulation educators.
- Start new simulation educators in their content area "comfort zone."
- Provide the new educator with a clear and concise template for the scenario.
- Allow new educators to engage at their own pace (initial interaction may be as minimal as controlling the technical aspect of a high-fidelity simulator).
- Model positive behaviors with learners.
- Promote a supportive environment for educators and learners.
- Demonstrate effective debriefing techniques.

Once new educators have reached the *proficient level* and are functioning independently, continue to serve as a resource for questions and support the development of innovation. As new simulation educators design and implement new scenarios, be sure to provide continuous guidance. As faculty grow into this role, there is a tendency to try to incorporate too much information into an experience. Emphasis on clear and concise learning outcomes and competencies is key. There should be between three and five outcomes and/or competencies for each scenario. Having more than five learning outcomes diminishes the experience for the learners and they may become overwhelmed.

While transitioning to independence as a new simulation educator, it is easy to fall back onto teaching methods that are more familiar. Experienced clinical faculty who transition to the role of simulation educator tend to interact with the learners during the scenario. This is the method that they may find most comfortable, and they may have difficulty allowing the learners to work independently without "real-time" guidance from the educator. As a mentor in simulation, it is important to continue to provide support. This includes the reassurance that the best learning experience develops by allowing the learners to work with minimal intervention from the educator (Terpstra & King, 2021).

That being said, one of the greatest challenges new simulation educators face when they begin to function independently is making modifications on the fly. What if the scenario does not go as planned? Anticipating and planning for the unexpected during simulation will improve the confidence of the new simulation educator (Schmutz et al., 2018).

Consider whether the learners:

- Do not perform the required behaviors to progress to the next phase of the simulation.
- Make an error that would cause great harm to the patient.
- "Kill" the patient.

As a mentor, it is important to discuss the "what ifs" with the new simulation educator. Although the goal is to provide all learners with a similar simulation experience, this is not always the case. Oftentimes, the learners' behaviors will drive the scenario down an unexpected path. After facilitating a scenario multiple times, the educator can begin to identify the most common errors. Those errors can be anticipated, and cues to refocus the learners can be developed to ensure psychological safety for the learners (Park & Kim, 2021).

There is evidence to suggest that unexpected death in simulation can negatively impact the learning experience. Some studies suggest that unless death is one of the learning objectives, the facilitator should not allow the simulator to "die," but simulation can be an effective method for teaching proper bereavement interactions with families (Colwell, 2017).

Simulation can also be a valuable resource to teach learners how to rescue a patient who is deteriorating (Bennion & Mansell, 2021). Mentoring a new simulation educator should include the development of an escape plan for each scenario. These can include transfer to a higher level of care or intervention by a critical care team.

Mentorship for new simulation faculty is a continuous process. As a certified simulation educator, the expectation regarding leadership and mentorship extends to all levels of simulation. This includes continuing to ensure best practices and serving as a resource for educators, staff, and learners.

## Evidence-Based Simulation Practice 4.1

Teber Betegon et al. (2021) used the lean principles as a quality management mode to gain advanced simulation center certification. The model was based on customers' expectations and risk-taking related to process improvements.

## ▶ RESOURCES FOR CONTINUOUS PROFESSIONAL DEVELOPMENT

As a leader in simulation, development of a formal training program may not be a feasible short-term goal. However, there are a number of training resources available for CPD:

- SSH
  - annual conference—International Meeting on Simulation in Healthcare (IMSH)
- CAE Healthcare
  - annual conference—Human Patient Simulation Network (HPSN)
- National League for Nursing (NLN) Simulation Innovation Resource Center (SIRC)
  - online training modules
  - content continuously updated
  - appropriate for novice-to-expert simulation educators
  - www.sirc.nln.org
- Drexel University's Certificate in Simulation
  - one-week-long training program
  - offered throughout the year
  - onsite at Drexel University in Philadelphia, Pennsylvania
  - www.drexel.edu/cne/conferencesCourses/conferences/Certificate_in_Simulation
- *Simulation in Nursing Education: From Conceptualization to Evaluation*
  - edited by Pamela Jefferies, PhD, RN, FAAN, ANEF
  - published by the NLN, Washington, DC
- *Developing Successful Health Care Education Simulation Centers: The Consortium Model*
  - written by Pamela Jeffries, PhD, RN, FAAN, ANEF, and Jim Battin, BS
  - published by Springer Publishing Company, New Jersey
- *Human Simulation for Nursing and Health Professions*
  - edited by Linda Wilson, PhD, RN, CPAN, CAPA, BC, CNE, CHSE, CHSE-A, ANEF, FAAN, and Leland Rockstraw, PhD, RN
  - published by Springer Publishing Company, New Jersey

## ▶ ADVOCATING FOR SIMULATION

Many healthcare training facilities have incorporated simulation into their programs on some level. However, advocating for simulation means increasing the use of simulation in a curriculum and cultivating new simulation educators. Acceptance of increasing simulation activities may initially be met with some resistance. Some anticipated challenges include the following:

- time to prepare for simulation activities
- lack of training
- belief that it is not a useful teaching method
- lack of space or equipment
- complicated scheduling
- lack of funding
- lack of staffing
- concerns about student engagement (Roh & Jang, 2017)

As a champion for simulation integration, acknowledging and addressing these challenges will be imperative. Some strategies include the following:

- Identify educators who are interested in being educated in simulation learning.
- Meet with content or course leaders to explore opportunities for simulation.

- Suggest simulation activities that do not require elaborate equipment or space (e.g., Second Life simulations or use of standardized patients [SPs]).
- Review course competencies and identify ways to incorporate simulation to meet the student learning outcomes.
- Advocate for simulation as a tool to increase learners' experience with diversity and high-risk, low-volume patient experiences.

## ▶ SUMMARY

The responsibilities of being a certified simulation educator include continuous knowledge development and acquisition of the best practices of simulation. Furthermore, the dissemination of this knowledge serves to develop new simulation educators and the growing field of simulation. Serving as a champion for simulation means:

- mentoring new faculty
- promoting innovation in simulation
- participating in building the specialty

## CASE STUDY 4.1

A new simulation educator is being mentored by an experienced simulation educator and feels ready to start designing and implementing their own simulation scenarios. After reviewing the simulation design, the experienced educator finds there are 15 objectives for the 30-minute activity. What is the best approach to use to mentor the new educator?

1. Leadership in simulation includes which of the following attributes?

   A. Simulation knowledge
   B. Laboratory setup skills
   C. Succession planning
   D. National recognition

2. A leader's moral obligation to simulation learning includes:

   A. Developing scenarios
   B. Debriefing learners
   C. Understanding simulation terms
   D. Disseminating novel ideas

3. A new simulation educator has been orientating with a mentor. The new educator requests to add some detail to the scenario being developed for the advanced practice nurse learners. The new simulation educator is demonstrating that they are at which stage of Benner's development?

   A. Novice
   B. Advanced beginner
   C. Competent
   D. Proficient

4. The expert simulation educator needs more understanding of their mentorship role during orientation when they ask the new simulation educators to:

   A. Observe several simulations
   B. Create a scenario
   C. Demonstrate debriefing
   D. Use an existing scenario

5. At which of Brenner's developmental stages should the simulation educator mentor consider the new simulation educator independent?

   A. Novice
   B. Advanced beginner
   C. Competent
   D. Proficient

6. An important concept in simulation learning is to understand that the simulation educator should:

   A. Coach the students as they move along in the scenario
   B. Provide details about treatments during the scenario
   C. Stop the scenario if it is not meeting the learning objectives
   D. Allow the students to critically think and make decisions

## 1. C) Succession planning

Leaders make short- and long-term goals and are passionate about the organization continuing regardless of whether they are the appointed leader. Setting up laboratory skill stations is a managerial task. Simulation knowledge may be an attribute of many healthcare educators and some may not display leadership qualities. National recognition may be for simulation research, scholarship, or service besides leadership.

## 2. D) Disseminating novel ideas

Simulation leaders have the moral obligation to share new and novel ideas so other simulation educators can have learners benefit. Developing scenarios may only affect the people who use them. Debriefing learners does not take leadership per se, but a trained debriefer. Understanding simulation terminology is the responsibility of everyone who works in a simulation laboratory.

## 3. C) Competent

Competence is the stage at which the person can assist by adding information to a situation. Novice educators are limited in their capacity to change things and may be somewhat inflexible. Advanced beginners can recognize parts of situations. Proficient practitioners can see a big picture and are confident to change plans if needed, not just add to them.

## 4. B) Create a scenario

Creating a scenario should not be part of a new simulation educator's role during orientation. Scenario development should come later. Novice simulation educators should observe simulations being completed and demonstrate debriefing before implementing simulations or debriefing themselves. Using an existing scenario may be more of an obtainable learning session than creating a scenario from scratch. Creating a scenario takes experience.

## 5. D) Proficient

At the proficient stage, the new simulation educator should have completed enough orientation and have received enough mentorship to be independent in the simulation laboratory because they are able to modify plans and are flexible in their teaching techniques. At the novice stage, the simulation educator is inflexible and focused on tasks. The advanced beginner is starting to recognize meaningful pieces of a scenario. A competent educator is able to organize and plan but may not have the ability to know how to do the job and does not have enough experience to be independent.

## 6. D) Allow the students to critically think and make decisions

Simulation learning is hands-on learning in which students are encouraged to make decisions and think about possible solutions to patient issues. Coaching during the simulation scenario may be necessary at times. Providing detail should not be necessary during a scenario because it should be completed during prebriefing. Stopping a scenario should only be a last attempt at getting students on track.

7. An effective method for advocating for simulation would be:

   A. Appointing simulation educators
   B. Designating shared space with other learning activities
   C. Recruiting interested faculty
   D. Reusing equipment to decrease cost

8. A novice simulation educator needs a better understanding of the benefits of simulation learning when they say: "I should use simulation for . . . ":

   A. Common assessments that the students do every day in direct patient care experiences
   B. Hard to acquire patient scenarios that meet the student learning outcomes
   C. Assisting students in understanding a team collaborative approach to patient care
   D. Providing experiences in caring for diverse patients that may not be encountered in direct patient care experiences

9. A method a simulation educator can use to promote student engagement is to:

   A. Use high-tech equipment
   B. Review the pathophysiology
   C. Review the student learning outcomes
   D. Provide a complex scenario

10. A simulation educator is observing the development of a scenario. The simulation educator is most likely in which stage of development?

    A. Novice
    B. Advanced beginner
    C. Competent
    D. Proficient

## 7. C) Recruiting interested faculty

Faculty that are interested are more likely to demonstrate enthusiasm for simulation learning. Appointing faculty may not produce advocacy for simulation education if the faculty are not passionate about simulation. Designing shared space with other learning activities may not keep the simulation equipment safe, and reusing equipment may not produce good results if it is outdated or in poor repair.

## 8. A) Common assessments that the students do every day in direct patient care experiences

A better use of simulation is to expose students to team activity, hard to acquire patient care experiences, and diversity not encountered in direct patient care experiences. Common assessments and competencies that the students do often in direct patient care usually do not need additional practice in the simulation laboratory.

## 9. C) Review the student learning outcomes

Meeting the student learning outcomes will assist in providing a learning experience that is at the appropriate level and using the appropriate content. This will provide students with the best method of engagement because they will make the connection between the learning experience and the learned didactic content. Using high technology does not guarantee results and should be used for scenarios that call for the technology. Reviewing pathophysiology is a good idea but may not stimulate student engagement. Providing complex scenarios is a good engagement process if the students are at a higher level in their education process.

## 10. A) Novice

A simulation educator at the novice level should be observing a seasoned simulation educator to learn proper delivery of learning and evaluation methodologies in the simulation laboratory. Advanced beginner simulation educators can add pieces to the scenario. Competent simulation educators can understand the pattern that the scenario will assume. Proficient simulation educators can modify a scenario as needed.

# REFERENCES

Benner, P. (1982). From novice to expert. *American Journal of Nursing*, *82*(3), 402–407. https://doi.org/10.1097/00000446-198282030-00004

Bennion, J., & Mansell, S. K. (2021). Management of the deteriorating adult patient: Does simulation-based education improve patient safety? *British Journal of Hospital Medicine*, *82*(8), 1–8. https://doi.org/10.12968/hmed.2021.0293

Colwell, P. (2017). Building confidence in neonatal bereavement: The use of simulation as an innovative educational approach. *Journal of Neonatal Nursing*, *23*(2), 65–74. https://doi.org/10.1016/j.jnn.2016.07.005

Park, J. E., & Kim, J. (2021). Nursing students' psychological safety in high fidelity simulations: Development of a new scale for psychometric evaluation. *Nurse Education Today*, *105*, Article 105017. https://doi.org/10.1016/j.nedt.2021.105017

Roh, Y. S., & Jang, K. I. (2017). Survey of factors influencing learner engagement with simulation debriefing among nursing students. *Nursing & Health Sciences*, *19*(4), 485–491. https://doi.org/10.1111/nhs.12371

Sanner-Striehr, E. (2017). Using simulation to teach responses to lateral violence: Guidelines for nurse educators. *Nurse Educator*, *42*(3), 133–137. https://doi.org/10.1097/NNE.0000000000000326

Schmutz, J. B., Kolbe, M., & Eppich, W. J. (2018). Twelve tips for integrating team reflexivity into your simulation-based team training. *Medical Teacher*, *40*(7), 721–727. https://doi.org/10.1080/0142159X.2018.1464135

Society for Simulation in Healthcare. (2021). *Certified healthcare simulation educator examination blueprint, 2018 version*. http://www.ssih.org/Portals/48/Certification/CHSE_Docs/CHSE_Examination_Blueprint.pdf

Teber Betegon, M. A., Baladron Gonzalez, V., Bejarano Ramirez, N., Martinez Arce, A., Rodriquez DeGuzman, J., Redondo, C., & Francisco, J. (2021). Quality management system implementation based on lean principles and ISO 9001: 2015 standard in an advanced simulation centre. *Clinical Simulation in Nursing*, *51*, 28–37. https://doi.org/10.1016/j.ecns.2020.11.002

Terpstra, N., & King, S. (2021). The missing link: Cognitive apprenticeship as a mentorship framework for simulation facilitator development. *Clinical Simulation in Nursing*, *59*, 111–118. https://doi.org/10.1016/j.ecns.2021.06.006

Watts, P. I., Hallmark, B. F., & Beroz, S. (2020). Professional development for simulation education. *Annual Review of Nursing Research*, *39*(1), 201–221. https://doi.org/10.1891/0739-6686.39.201

Waxman, K. T., & Telles, C. L. (2009). The use of Benner's framework in high-fidelity simulation faculty development: The bay area simulation collaborative model. *Clinical Simulation in Nursing*, *5*(6), e231–e235. https://doi.org/10.1016/j.ecns.2009.06.001

# Special Learning Considerations in Simulation

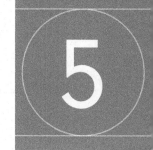

Ruth A. Wittmann-Price

*It is time for parents to teach young people early on that in diversity there is beauty and there is strength.*

—Maya Angelou

This chapter addresses Domain I: Professional Values and Capabilities (Society for Simulation in Healthcare [SSH], 2021).

## ▶ LEARNING OUTCOMES

- Discuss the importance of recognizing diversity in learning styles, teaching styles, and generational differences.
- Develop simulation learning experiences for culturally diverse healthcare students.
- Discuss the enactment of the Americans with Disabilities Act (ADA; 2017) in the simulation laboratory.
- Describe diversity through a case study and practice questions.

## ▶ INTRODUCTION

*Diversity* can be defined as "the condition of having or being composed of different elements" (Merriam-Webster, n.d.). Diversity related to simulation experiences can include any or all of the human attributes, in any combination, listed in Exhibit 5.1. The list is not inclusive of all diversity issues, but demonstrates some of the issues that an individual may have when entering a simulation learning experience.

### EXHIBIT 5.1 DIVERSITY ATTRIBUTES

Diversity attributes can be exhibited by any of the humans or simulated humans, such as the patient (including the family or the community), learner, or educator. The attributes can include any of the following elements:

- demographic
  - age
  - gender
    - ❑ sex
    - ❑ sexual preference
  - ethnicity
  - disabilities
- experiential
  - work–life experiences (e.g., adult learners)

*(continued)*

---

**EXHIBIT 5.1 DIVERSITY ATTRIBUTES (*continued*)**

- ▪ informational
  - ● educational background
  - ● learning–teaching styles
- ▪ fundamental
  - ● different beliefs and values
  - ● relationships with others

---

Simulation experiences used for learning and evaluation must consider the diversity and experiences inherent in all the participants because personal characteristics and past experiences are "brought to the table" within any learning environment. The *realism* created within a simulation environment or scenario can easily trigger personal reactions that are guided by the participants' diversity and/or experiences. Simulation is a *social practice*. Dieckmann (2020) defines it as a contextual event in space and time, conducted for one or more purposes, in which people interact in a goal-oriented fashion with each other, with technical artifacts (the simulator), and with the environment (including relevant devices). This chapter briefly outlines several elements of human diversity and relates them to the simulation environment. The outcome of understanding diversity and experiences and gaining tolerance to human differences can be reached through learning and reflection, which are hallmarks of simulation.

## ▶ DIVERSITY IN LEARNING STYLES

All learners come to the simulation, the skills laboratory, or the virtual environment with their own unique learning styles. A *learning style* refers to the ways and conditions under which learners most prefer to assimilate knowledge.

- ▪ The approach learners take to accomplish different tasks is also important.
- ▪ A learning style is an approach to learning that works for the individual learner.
- ▪ Learners may have more than one learning style (Blevins, 2021).

The four most common learning styles are defined by the acronym VARK, as described by Fleming and Mills (1992).

- ▪ V: visual
- ▪ A: auditory
- ▪ R: read/write
- ▪ K: kinesthetic

### VISUAL OR SPATIAL LEARNERS

- ▪ These learners learn best through what they *see.*
- ▪ Pictures, diagrams, flowcharts, timelines, maps, and demonstrations enhance their ability to learn.
- ▪ A good learning assignment for a visual learner might involve concept mapping using computers and graphics.

- These learners may also be called *graphic* (G) learners.
- It is important to note that visual learners do not usually care to learn by viewing movies, videos, or PowerPoint presentations (Fleming, 2001).

## AURAL OR AUDITORY LEARNERS

- These learners prefer to learn through what is *heard or spoken*.
- They learn best from lectures, tapes, tutorials, group discussions, speaking, web chats, emails, smartphones, and talking things throughout loud.
- By talking about a topic, these learners are able to process the given information (Fleming, 2001).

## READING OR WRITING LEARNERS

- These learners prefer to have the information to be learned displayed as *written words*.
- They prefer text-based input and output in all of its forms.
- Many academics have a preference for this style of learning.
- These learners are often fond of PowerPoint presentations, the internet, lists, dictionaries, thesauri, quotations, or anything else featuring words (Fleming, 2001).

## KINESTHETIC OR ACTIVE LEARNERS

- These learners use their body and sense of touch to enhance learning while engaged in physical activity.
- They like to think about issues while working out or exercising.
- They like to participate, play games, role-play, act, and model experiences.
- They appreciate demonstrations, simulations, videos, and movies of "real things," as well as case studies, practice sessions, and applications (Fleming, 2001).
- Felder and Solomon (1998) refer to these learners as *active learners*.

## MULTIMODAL/MIXTURE (M) LEARNERS

- These learners prefer to learn via two or more styles of learning or using a variety of modes.
- They like information to be context-specific or might choose a single mode to suit a certain occasion or situation.
- They like to gather information from each mode and often have a deeper and broader understanding of topics (Fleming, 2001).

In addition to the previous points, there are labels given to other learning styles by various authors. These include the following:

- verbal (linguistic) learners
- tactile learners
- global learners
- intuitive learners
- sequential learners
- reflective learners
- analytical learners
- accommodative learners

Table 5.1 displays the characteristics of these alternative types of learning styles identified by various learning specialists.

**Table 5.1** Various Diverse Learning Styles

| | |
|---|---|
| **Verbal (linguistic) learners** (similar to auditory learning style) | ■ Learn from spoken words<br>■ Enjoy talking through procedures<br>■ Use recordings of content for repetition<br>■ Frequently use mnemonics to retain information |
| **Tactile learners** | ■ Learn by touching or manipulating objects<br>■ Require movement<br>■ Trace words and use letter tiles to learn to spell words (scrabble) |
| **Global learners** | ■ Make decisions based on their emotions and intuition<br>■ Are spontaneous and focus on creativity<br>■ Do not consider tidiness as important<br>■ Enjoy learning<br>■ Use humor, tell stories, and enjoy group work<br>■ Like to participate in activities<br>■ Tend to absorb materials randomly<br>■ Frequently do not see connections at first, but then suddenly "get it"<br>■ Are able to solve complex problems quickly or put things together in unique ways once they have grasped the big picture, but may have difficulty explaining how they did it<br>■ Lack good sequential thinking abilities (Felder & Solomon, 1998) |
| **Intuitive learners** | ■ Like to discover the possibilities in relationships<br>■ Like solving problems using well-established methods<br>■ Do not like complications or surprises<br>■ Do not like repetition<br>■ Work fast<br>■ Are innovative<br>■ Do not like courses that involve memorization or routine calculations<br>■ Easily become bored<br>■ Are prone to careless mistakes on tests because they are impatient with details, such as checking math calculations (Felder & Solomon, 1998) |
| **Reflective learners** | ■ Prefer to think about new materials by reflecting quietly<br>■ Prefer to work alone, rather than with groups<br>■ Do not like classes that cover large amounts of materials quickly<br>■ Do not like to be asked simply to read and memorize<br>■ Like to stop periodically to review what they have read<br>■ Find it helpful to write short summaries of readings or class notes in their own words to help them retain the material better (Felder & Solomon, 1998) |
| **Analytical learners** | ■ Base all of their decisions on logic<br>■ Plan and organize well<br>■ Focus on details and facts<br>■ Like a tidy, well-organized environment<br>■ Enjoy learning, take sequential steps, and follow "the rules" |
| **Accommodative learners** | ■ Like a combination of concrete experiences and active experimentation<br>■ Complete tasks and are less concerned about the theories<br>■ Are risk-takers<br>■ Solve problems by trial and error<br>■ Are concerned with abstract concepts and assimilate abstract conceptualizations with reflective observations |

## KOLB'S LEARNING STYLES

Kolb describes *experiential learning* (Chapter 6, "Interprofessional Simulation") as a type of learning in which the student is actively engaged in the learning process. Kolb also discusses learning styles in relation to experiential learning. The following are Kolb's four learning styles:

- *Diverging:* This type of learner likes to work in groups and generate ideas. Students are fine with feedback and reflecting on the activities learned. This learning style uses concrete experiences and reflective observation.
- *Assimilating:* This type of learner prefers to read information, be presented with lectures, and then analyze topics. This learning style, according to Kolb, is generated by learners who prefer abstract conceptualization and reflective observation.
- *Converging:* This type of learner likes to put ideas to practical application. This style of learning is generated from those who abstract, conceptualize, and actively experiment.
- *Accommodating:* This type of learner enjoys hands-on work in teams to complete projects. This style of learning is derived from people who use concrete experiences and active experimentation (Kolb, 1984).

### Evidence-Based Simulation Practice 5.1

Cremerius et al. (2021) studied learning styles in relation to three teaching modalities: team-based learning, peer-assisted learning, and conventional didactic learning. Using Kolb's Learning Style Inventory, all three groups were evaluated using objective structured clinical examination (OSCE) performance. The results demonstrated that the team-based learning group significantly acquired more knowledge when compared with the peer-assisted and the conventional learning groups.

### Evidence-Based Simulation Practice 5.2

Carvajal et al. (2021) evaluated Kolb's Learning Style Inventory (LSI) in comparison with a Likert-scale inventory. The LSI uses "forced choice" items, which has been statistically controversial. Studies did not support the four learning styles outlined by Kolb and proposed that the forced choice items rendered artificial results.

## GENERATIONAL LEARNERS

In addition to learning styles, the era or context in which learners were born and reared will affect how they view receiving and retaining information. Just as homogeneous groups of healthcare learners are obsolete, having learners who all fall within one generation in higher education is also not a reality in higher education. Characteristic learning attributes have been noted in different generational learners, but of course, as with any other categorization, individual differences and preferences may override any stereotypical attribute (Hart, 2017). Table 5.2 shows the attributes of generational learners.

**Table 5.2** Generational Learners

| Generational Label | Learner Attributes | What May Facilitate Learning |
|---|---|---|
| **Baby boomers** (born between 1946 and 1964) | ■ Most healthcare educators fall into this category | ■ Respond to competition due to large peer groups (80 million strong)<br>■ Are taught mainly by lecture<br>■ May think technology is nice but not essential |

*(continued)*

**Table 5.2** Generational Learners (*continued*)

| Generational Label | Learner Attributes | What May Facilitate Learning |
|---|---|---|
| **Generation X** (born between 1965 and 1979) | ▪ Challenge authority<br>▪ Are independent problem-solvers<br>▪ Are multitaskers | ▪ Respond to self-learning modules<br>▪ Find demonstration to be useful<br>▪ Are pragmatic and focused on the outcomes of learning<br>▪ Want real-world skills |
| **Generation Y**<br>**Millennials**<br>**Nexters**<br>**MTV generation** (born after 1975 or between 1981 and 1996)<br>This generation is:<br>▪ More culturally diverse<br>▪ One-third raised in single-parent homes<br>▪ 81 million strong | ▪ Need constant stimulation<br>▪ Respond to multimedia and instant information<br>▪ Are critical consumers<br>▪ Expect entertainment<br>▪ Are active, hands-on learners<br>▪ Prefer fast-paced experiences<br>▪ Seek instant gratification<br>▪ Respond to positive reinforcement<br>▪ Are resourceful<br>▪ Like the challenge of problem-solving<br>▪ Prefer group activities<br>▪ May have poor reading and math skills<br>▪ Display poor work habits<br>▪ Are multitaskers<br>▪ Have no time for school<br>▪ Are visual learners due to computers | ▪ Use critical reading<br>▪ Use intertextuality: reading multiple electronic sources to critically appraise the overlap for meaning<br>▪ Display self-preferentiality: are better critiquing topics they are passionate about or can relate to in their own lives<br>▪ Consider different viewpoints or cultural interpretations<br>▪ Journal to foster reflection and critical thinking<br>▪ Like using technology<br>▪ Use concept mapping<br>▪ Respond to simulation of teamwork |
| **Generation Z** (usually born between 1997 and 2012) | ▪ Digital natives<br>▪ Use wearable technology for health and exercise (Kamble et al., 2021)<br>▪ Passionate about equality and social justice (Coplen, 2021)<br>▪ Most racially diverse group | ▪ Virtual learning<br>▪ Use social media as learning tool<br>▪ Focus on critical thinking skills and not information (Edwards-Maddox et al., 2021)<br>▪ Problem-based learning (Siebert, 2021) |

## Evidence-Based Simulation Practice 5.3

Ho et al. (2021) studied the effectiveness of the iLearning application on chest tube care education among nursing students ($N = 107$). Their study used a mobile application for learning with Generation Z students. The quasi-experimental study demonstrated that there was no difference in clinical reasoning and self-directed learning between the intervention group with iLearning and the traditionally taught group of students; however, the intervention group showed significantly higher clinical reasoning and self-directed learning scores than the comparison group ($p < .05$) 1 week and 1 month after the intervention.

# ▶ DIVERSITY IN TEACHING STYLES OF HEALTHCARE EDUCATORS

Jeffries (2007) emphasizes the importance of the teacher's role in simulation as well as the facilitator–learner relationship. Students' perception of teaching effectiveness increases when the faculty use simulation appropriately. The method by which the teacher designs the simulation experience and the educational practices used to organize and deliver the experience will affect the quality of learning (Taha et al., 2021).

The teaching style used during the experience is another variable in the success of a simulation experience. Teaching styles permeate the development and orchestration of the simulation experience and have been classified by many different methods. Simulation healthcare educators rarely ascribe to just one teaching style. Most educators use a variety of styles, even within a single simulation session. Using a mixed style approach can appeal to the variety of learning styles and improve learning outcomes. Reflecting on the type of style used encourages self-understanding the most and may serve to improve effectiveness.

Individual teaching styles involve teaching behaviors and are noteworthy because behaviors have a direct effect on the simulation teaching–learning environment. The next section describes some of the ways teaching styles are categorized and what experts say are good teaching behaviors and personality traits of educators (Table 5.3).

**Table 5.3** Helpful Teaching Strategies and Teacher Characteristics

| Teaching Strategies | Teacher Characteristics |
| --- | --- |
| Uses repeat demonstrations | Knows learners |
| Role-models good communication | Has a welcoming voice and demeanor |
| Is flexible about debriefing method | Dresses the part |
| Repeats instructions | Calm |
| Explains steps | Welcomes learners' questions |
| Does not rush | Experienced and current in practice |
| Discusses worst-case scenarios to alleviate fear | Willing to learn with and from students |
| Provides feedback to learners | Uses teachable moments and errors to learn |
| Maintains civil environment | Communicates well |
| Provides learners with opportunity to think through a situation | Enthusiastic and passionate |
| Role-plays thinking in action | Empathizes with learners' feelings |

## GRASHA'S CLASSIFICATION OF TEACHING STYLES

Grasha's (1996) classification defines teaching styles as expert, formal authority, demonstrator, facilitator, and delegator. The characteristics of each teaching style are unique and are listed in Table 5.4.

**Table 5.4** Grasha's Teaching Styles

| Style | Characteristics |
| --- | --- |
| Expert | ■ Educator uses vast knowledge base to inform learners.<br>■ Educator challenges students to be well-prepared.<br>■ Educator can be intimidating to the learner. |

*(continued)*

**Table 5.4** Grasha's Teaching Styles (*continued*)

| Style | Characteristics |
|---|---|
| **Formal authority** | ▪ Educator is in control of learners' knowledge acquisition.<br>▪ Educator is not concerned with student–teacher relationships.<br>▪ Educator focuses on the content to be delivered. |
| **Demonstrator** | ▪ Educator coaches, demonstrates, and encourages active learning. |
| **Facilitator** | ▪ Learner-centered, active learning strategies are encouraged.<br>▪ Accountability for learning is placed on the learner. |
| **Delegator** | ▪ Educator's role is that of a consultant.<br>▪ Learners are encouraged to direct the entire learning process. |

*Source:* Adapted from Grasha, A. (1996). *Teaching with style.* Alliance.

## QUIRK'S CLASSIFICATION OF TEACHING STYLES

Another useful classification of teaching styles was devised by Quirk in 1994.

- *Assertive:* Communication is usually content-specific and the educator drives the information home.
- *Suggestive:* The educator uses experiences to describe a concept and then requests that the learners seek more information on the subject.
- *Collaborative:* The educator uses skills to promote problem-solving and a higher level of thinking in learners.
- *Facilitative:* The educator challenges the learners to reflect and use affective learning, ask ethical questions, and demonstrate skills in interpersonal relationships and professional behaviors.

## KELLY'S TEACHING EFFECTIVENESS

Kelly (2008) also studied learners' perceptions of teaching effectiveness and found that teaching effectiveness has three main important attributes. The first of these, educator knowledge, was rated the most important and consists of four separate domains, as shown in Figure 5.1.

## HOUSE, CHASSIE, AND SPOHN'S TEACHING BEHAVIORS

House et al. (1999) provide examples of the following behaviors and their effects on learners:

- Making eye contact can encourage learner participation.
- Positive facial expressions that elicit a positive learner response, such as head nodding, can assist learners in feeling comfortable, whereas negative gestures, such as frowning, can discourage learners' participation in class.
- Vocal tone is very important and can easily portray underlying feelings and encourage or discourage learner participation.

## CHOO'S POSITIVE CHARACTERISTICS FOR EDUCATORS

Choo (1996) conducted research on teachers and identified characteristics that students rated positively.

- values learning
- exhibits a caring relationship
- provides learner independence

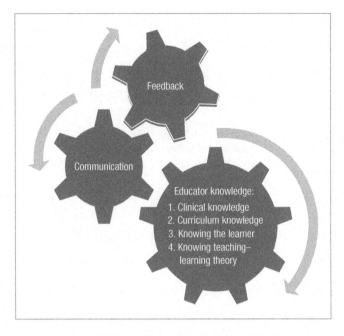

**Figure 5.1** Kelly's attributes for teaching effectiveness.
*Source:* Adapted from Kelly, C. (2008). Students' perceptions of
effective clinical teaching revisited. *Nurse Education Today, 27*(8),
885–892.

- facilitates questioning
- tries different approaches
- accepts differences among learners

## HICKS AND BURKUS

Hicks and Burkus (2011) describe the attributes of "master teachers," which include the following:

- clear communication
- positive role modeling
- professionalism demonstrated in lifelong learning and scholarship
- reflective practice and making adjustments for improvement
- use of philosophical, epistemological, and ontological influences in their practice of education

## STORY AND BUTTS

Story and Butts (2010) discuss teaching delivery in the frame of the four important "Cs" shown in Figure 5.2.

## THE MYERS–BRIGGS TYPE INDICATOR

The Myers–Briggs Type Indicator (MBTI) measures Jung's 16 personality types by classifying them into four bipolar dimensions; the educator's personality also affects instruction.

- extroversion–introversion
- sensing–intuition
- thinking–feeling
- judgment–perception (Schublova, 2017)

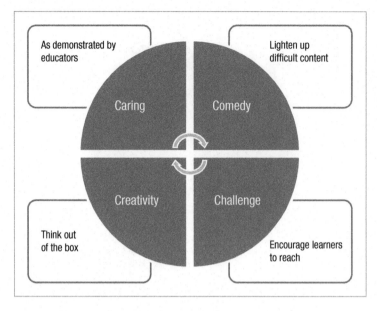

**Figure 5.2** The four "Cs" of teaching methods.
*Source:* Adapted from Story, L., & Butts, J. B. (2010). Compelling teaching with the four Cs: Caring, comedy, creativity, and challenging. *Journal of Nursing Education, 49*(5), 291–294. https://doi.org/10.3928/01484834-20100115-08.

## SILVER, HANSON, AND STRONG

Silver et al. (1996) developed a teaching style inventory (TSI) based on Jung's theory of psychological types or personality types. It tests educators' propensity for one of four types.

- sensing–thinking
- sensing–feeling
- intuitive–thinking
- intuitive–feeling

Looking at all the teaching styles and the preferred attributes of educators is helpful in reflective assessment because there are trends in all the studies listed above. Attributes can be summed up as keeping the student central in the learning environment and communicating clearly during the entire learning experience. The positive attributes identified are congruent with positive simulation learning experiences. Knowing your teaching style and understanding your personality style and how these two personal aspects mix in the simulation or skills environment can be very enlightening. Reflecting on these attributes can assist healthcare educators in providing learners with excellent environments in which to facilitate their knowledge acquisition.

### Simulation Teaching Tip 5.1

Many students learn the content used for simulation learning experiences best through formal delivery and informal practice discussion (Oberai et al., 2021).

## EMOTIONAL NEEDS OF LEARNERS

Developed scenarios may depict situations that learners relate to on an emotional level. This phenomenon may be due to the student experiencing a recent loss of a loved one or because the situation is similar to one that happened to them or to someone they know or a family member. Prebriefing should include a description of what is going to take place, and the simulation educator should request that any student who is uncomfortable with the situation notify them so other arrangements can be made for the student to achieve the learning outcomes (LeBanc & Posner, 2022).

## ▶ CULTURALLY DIVERSE LEARNERS

Each person has an individual culture constructed by unique social determinants. Culture encompasses an individual's values, attitudes, perceptions, interpersonal needs, roles, and cognitive styles. Cultural humility is needed by faculty to fully appreciate the experience of students. It is important for simulation educators to recognize that cultural diversity can influence learning ability and needs and how learning is perceived by individuals. Perceptions of individuals must be considered during any educational session.

Despite the growing diversity of the nation, the healthcare workforce continues to be underrepresented by minorities (Ahmed et al., 2020).

Moreover, culturally diverse learners face certain barriers that may impinge on their ability to achieve success in college. The following are the most common of these barriers:

- lack of ethnically diverse faculty
- finances
- academic preparation
- available role models
- academic support
- family support
- peer support

Many times, the needs of diverse or underrepresented students include the following (Alicea-Planas, 2017):

- personal needs (lack of finances, time issues, family responsibilities and obligations, and difficulties related to language and communication)
- academic needs (large or heavy workload)
- language needs (difficulty reading and understanding assignments, prejudice due to their accents, and verbal communication barriers)
- cultural needs (expectations related to assertiveness and cultural norms, lack of diverse role models, and difficulty with communication)

An important issue among culturally diverse learners is their level of knowledge of the English language, which if inadequate can be problematic. Barriers to progressing in healthcare programs, once accepted, may also exist among English-as-a-second-language (ESL) learners.

Hansen and Beaver (2012) discuss test development for ESL learners and provide the following tips:

- Use short simple sentences.
- Be direct when stating information.
- Use common vocabulary (Lindberg et al., 2021).

## ▶ EFFECT OF DIVERSITY ON SIMULATION SCENARIOS

Culturally and linguistically diverse (CALD) learners often have different learning needs when related to clinical and simulation experiences. There remains a lack of evidence on how best to assist CALD students in order to succeed in healthcare programs. Hari et al. (2021) found that the attributes needed by the faculty were flexibility with assessments, modifying teaching styles according to learning needs, providing appropriate orientation, creating a welcoming environment, providing consistency with resource allocation, and providing appropriate faculty education. Merry et al. (2021) completed a literature review about the challenges of international and migrant healthcare students. The investigators searched 10 databases to examine international and migrant students' mental health, well-being, and academic outcomes, and found that research did not address gender identification. Challenges were identified in the literature related to wearing a hijab and being a "foreign-born male nurse" and viewing nursing as a low-status profession. Additionally, research is needed to identify educational strategies that increase the chance of success of international and migrant students. Simulation has been suggested as a positive intervention. It has been demonstrated to increase cultural confidence and to overcome student and faculty language barriers (Kessler & Kost, 2021).

Dieckmann et al. (2010) discuss simulation *lifesavers* (p. 219), that is, manipulations of a scenario when unexpected situations occur. Unexpected situations are listed in the following, as identified by Dieckmann et al. (2010), and are preempted many times by the diversity of the simulation learners. The following are the causes of unexpected situations:

- differences in cultural understanding
- comprehensiveness of the scenario that is unclear to participants due to poor instructions or ambiguous clues during the scenario
- inability to accept the scenario due to participants' inexperience or distractibility
- unrealistic difficulty level of the scenario which does not match the competency of the participants
- participants in the scenario not following the procedural steps and producing unexpected actions
- participants changing the intended scenario to a familiar scenario that is also plausible

When unexpected occurrences take place during a scenario, debriefing (which will be discussed in depth in Chapter 17) may be affected. The lifesavers are the anticipated actions that may be needed during a scenario. Scenario lifesavers can be used to adapt to the situation or restore the scenario to its original form. Lifesavers can be used to mitigate cultural differences. These scenario-lifesaving actions are identified before the scenario and can come from "within" the scenario or the simulation room itself by altering the patient or providing hints, or it can come from "outside" the scenario by using the director's voice to clarify, stop, or explain the scenario. Some lifesaving techniques are commonly used in many scenarios either to provide the participants with time or to emphasize missed clues, such as the patient asking learners to repeat information. Other lifesavers must be specific to the scenario, such as altering vital signs more drastically to gain learners' attention.

Simulation as a teaching–learning methodology is an excellent platform for students to understand, integrate, and reflect on diversity, equity, and inclusion. Cultural awareness can be used as a simulation framework and healthcare students can and scenario assessments can be easily based on the community's needs assessment. Developing partnerships with diverse patient groups and using diverse standardized patients can enhance student sensitivity (Buchanan et al., 2021).

# ▶ LEARNERS AND LEARNING DISABILITIES

Learning disabilities are the most common type of disability found on college campuses. Although increasing numbers of individuals with physical or affective disabilities are attending higher educational institutions and many disabilities are known and accommodated for before the learner enters college, other learners with learning disabilities begin college without their disability having been detected.

- In healthcare education, these disabilities are often noted when significant differences are noticed between a learner's classroom and simulation or clinical performance. Often, a learner may perform well in the simulation or clinical environment, but may be unable to demonstrate the same ability, skills, and competency in the classroom.
- Healthcare educators should always refer learners they suspect as having a learning disability to the appropriate counselors or office for accommodations for assistance (Joshi & Bouck, 2017). Learners with documented disabilities are entitled to the same access to education as traditional learners. An office of academic services must be available to provide learners with *reasonable accommodations* and support services.
- Accommodations must be made for students with learning disabilities in accordance with the ADA.
- It is important for educators to be aware of learners with physical disabilities, such as those with a documented or apparent physical limitation, substance abuse, chemical or alcohol impairments, and/or mental health problems (Rushton, 2017). Many college students use extended time to complete testing in college, and it is often related to having attention deficit hyperactivity disorder (ADHD) and to taking science, technology, engineering, and mathematics (STEM) courses, which are part of the curricula of healthcare students. When simulation is used as an evaluative tool and not learning, an extended time to complete the assessment may be appropriate (Gelbar & Madaus, 2021).

# ▶ BELONGINGNESS

Learners who are marginalized are less likely to succeed, so simulation and virtual experiences must be inclusive, providing a valued role for each learner. Belongingness is conceptually related to motivation, and students who do not feel they belong may lose motivation to study and prepare for simulation. Additionally, lack of belongingness can have adverse physical consequences on students (Hussain et al., 2021).

# ▶ SIMULATION LEARNING AS A SOCIAL PRACTICE

Goffman (1974) describes social meaning in terms of "frames" that are perceived by the individual about the reality that they are experiencing. Frames help individuals understand what is happening at the moment and make sense of the situation. Goffman breaks experiences down into two types of frames:

- *Primary frames:* Assist the individual to make sense out of the current situation.
- *Modulation frames:* Bring in the individual's perception of the world and therefore will include individual differences (all diversity issues previously discussed). These frames must be addressed to ensure positive learning experiences (Dieckmann et al., 2007).

### Simulation Teaching Tip 5.2

Coretta et al. (2021) successfully used simulation to bring to life the concepts and principles of diversity and inclusion, social determinants of health, and interprofessional team science.

### Evidence-Based Simulation Practice 5.4

Elliot and Sandberg (2021) completed an integrative review of the literature to clarify best practices for teaching social justice. The researchers analyzed coursework, teaching methods, sites for application of learning, and methods to evaluate student learning, and found that junior- and senior-level nursing students applied social justice information in clinical learning experiences where vulnerable populations were served, as well as in simulated environments. The researchers concluded that social justice can be threaded throughout the curriculum with the use of traditional and nontraditional teaching strategies.

## ▶ SOCIALIZATION DURING SIMULATION

Walton et al. (2011) provide results of a classic grounded study with nursing learners that discusses socialization during simulation. Five phases of "negotiating the role of the professional nurses" (p. 301) were identified and are shown in Table 5.5.

**Table 5.5** Five Phases of "Negotiating the Role of the Professional Nurses"

| Phase 1 | Feeling like an imposter (includes anticipation, wanting further instructions, not knowing where to start, and anxiety) |
|---------|---------|
| Phase 2 | Trial and error (includes practice, replaying and reviewing, self-reflection, and mentoring) |
| Phase 3 | Taking the role seriously (includes making the scenario realistic, having dedication to learn, using nursing language, developing team leadership, analyzing, and having a better understanding of the situation) |
| Phase 4 | Transference (includes gaining confidence, socializing into the healthcare role, feeling devastated after failing, then repracticing and rebuilding) |
| Phase 5 | Professionalism (includes growth in role as a nurse and patient advocate, interprofessional collaboration, and career goal building) |

*Source:* Adapted from Walton, J., Chute, E., & Ball, L. (2011). Professional nurse: The pedagogy of simulation: A grounded study. *Journal of Professional Nursing, 27,* 299–310. https://doi.org/10.1016/j.profnurs.2011.04.005.

The socialization aspects of simulation cannot be overlooked. Simulation is a powerful mechanism that provides learning environments in all three domains: cognitive, psychomotor, and affective, or sometimes stated as knowledge, skills, and attitudes.

 CASE STUDY 5.1

A healthcare student tells the simulation educator that they need time and a half to take tests and should have extra time to read and understand the patient history on the simulation scenario that is being used for evaluative purposes in a capstone course. How should the simulation educator respond and what (if any) provisions would be made and under what circumstances?

1. The simulation educator observes a student crying after the death of a cardiac patient portrayed by a manikin in the scenario. The simulation educator understands that this can happen because simulation is:

   A. An unfair social practice
   B. An intense learning experience
   C. An emotionally charged situation
   D. A situation involving students with unpredictable personality types

2. Simulation learning activities can lend themselves to a better understanding of human diversity because:

   A. There are faculty who can adjust scenarios
   B. Many laboratories have diverse manikins
   C. It is a reflective learning environment
   D. Diversity can be discussed during a scenario

3. Student learning styles are important to understand so that educational methodologies can reflect students' preferences. The simulation educator should be aware that preparing the night before the simulation scenario is most likely best suited to learners who prefer which learning style?

   A. Visual
   B. Read/write
   C. Aural
   D. Kinesthetic

4. A simulation educator is facilitating learning about a procedure and one of the learners has difficulty following the steps. The learner may be displaying characteristics of which learning type?

   A. Tactile
   B. Intuitive
   C. Global
   D. Reflective

5. Many simulation educators are baby boomers or Generation Xers, while learners are millennials or Generation Z. One of the learning strategies that millennials and Generation Z respond positively to is:

   A. Modular learning
   B. Lecture before the scenario
   C. Problem-solving
   D. Group activities

### 1. C) An emotionally charged situation

An emotionally charged situation may occur if the learner relates a scenario to a situation that has occurred in their life or that of a friend or family member. The scenario does not depict unfair social practice so this should not be the trigger for the student. Intense learning experiences are usually complex, with many things going on at once, and higher level students should have the resiliency to react in these situations. Unpredictable personality types do not necessarily mean that a student will become emotionally upset.

### 2. C) It is a reflective learning environment

Learning to reflect is a primary simulation experience, and reflection leads to understanding unconscious biases and tolerance and appreciation for diversity, inclusion, and equity. Diverse manikins assist in recognizing diversity as do discussions about diversity. Faculty can adjust a scenario to include diversity, but understanding is really a product of reflection.

### 3. B) Read/write

Learners who primarily use the read/write mode to learn would benefit from having the time to read over the scenario the night before. Visual, aural, and kinesthetic learners are more suited to learn during prebriefing.

### 4. C) Global

Global learners many times will see the big picture before the details and therefore may have a challenge with procedures. Tactile, intuitive, and reflective learners may be more in tune to the procedural steps in a process.

### 5. C) Problem-solving

Both groups learn well by problem-solving. Millennials like teamwork and group activities. Modular learning and lectures are more akin to baby boomers and Generation X students.

6. Grasha's teaching styles describe simulation educators who have different approaches. The BEST approach an educator can have with a group of learners in a simulation scenario is:

   A. Expert
   B. Formal
   C. Demonstrator
   D. Delegator

7. A simulation educator provided students with the topic of the simulation for the following day and asks them to research the patient's care. According to Quirk, which teaching style is this?

   A. Assertive
   B. Suggestive
   C. Collaborative
   D. Facilitative

8. The novice simulation educator is reviewing the characteristics of teaching effectiveness outlined by Kelly (2008) and needs further review when they state that _____ is included as a trait of an effective teacher.

   A. Feedback
   B. Communication
   C. Knowledge
   D. Sensitivity

9. Social determinants that may place a student at risk include:

   A. Lack of friends
   B. Family members
   C. Lack of diverse faculty
   D. Peer support

10. Lifesavers are sometimes needed in a scenario to promote positive learning and to:

    A. Decrease emotions
    B. Understand health and illness concepts
    C. Reach the learning outcomes
    D. Develop a care plan for the patient

### 6. C) Demonstrator

Demonstrators coach, demonstrate, and encourage active learning, which is congruent with simulation learning. Experts, formal, and delegators do not encourage students' active learning directly.

### 7. B) Suggestive

Suggestive educators use experiences to describe a concept and then request that the learners seek more information on the subject. Assertive educators do not use facilitation. Collaborative and facilitative educators use problem-solving and reflective learning as opposed to enhancing students' ownership of learning by suggesting they participate in information finding.

### 8. D) Sensitivity

Sensitivity is not an attribute identified by Kelly (2008). Kelly's research demonstrated that the three main attributes needed for effective teaching are feedback, communication, and knowledge of the content.

### 9. C) Lack of diverse faculty

Lack of diverse faculty is a challenge for diverse at-risk learners. Peer support, friends, and family support may be factors, but lack of diverse faculty has been a well-documented deterrent in at-risk students' success.

### 10. C) Reach the learning outcomes

Changing the scenario to meet students' learning outcomes is needed if learners are offtrack. Decreasing emotions should be handled during prebriefing and debriefing. Content understanding and developing a plan of care can also be addressed during prebriefing or debriefing.

# REFERENCES

Ahmed, S., Birtell, M. D., Pye, M., & Morrison, A. P. (2020). Stigma towards psychosis: Cross-cultural differences in prejudice, stereotypes, and discrimination in White British and South Asians. *Journal of Community & Applied Social Psychology, 30*(2), 199–213. https://doi.org/10.1002/casp.2437

Alicea-Planas, J. (2017). Shifting our focus to support the educational journey of underrepresented students. *Journal of Nursing Education, 56*(3), 159–163. https://doi.org/10.3928/01484834-20170222-07

Americans with Disabilities Act (ADA). (2017). *Information and technical assistance on the American with Disabilities Act.* http://www.ada.gov

Blevins, S. (2021). Learning styles: The impact on education. *MEDSURG Nursing, 30*(4), 285–286.

Buchanan, D. T., & O'Connor, M. R. (2020). Integrating diversity, equity, and inclusion into a simulation program. *Clinical Simulation in Nursing, 49*, 58–65. https://doi.org/10.1016/j.ecns.2020.05.007

Buchanan, H., Newton, J. T., Baker, S. R., & Asimakopoulou, K. (2021). Adopting the COM-B model and TDF framework in oral and dental research: A narrative review. *Community Dentistry & Oral Epidemiology, 49*(5), 385–393. https://doi.org/10.1111/cdoe.12677

Carvajal, C. C., Ximenez Gomex, C., Lay-Lisboa, S., & Briceno, M. (2021). Reviewing the structure of Kolb's learning style inventory from factor analysis and Thurstonian item response theory (IRT) model approaches. *Journal of Psychoeducational Assessment, 39*(5), 593–609. https://doi.org/10.1177/07342829211003739

Choo, L. A. (1996). Reflections: Learning at work. *Professional Nurse (Singapore), 23*(3), 8–11.

Coplen, A. E. (2021). Mentoring the next generation of leaders in dental hygiene. *Journal of Dental Hygiene, 95*(4), 4–5.

Coretta, J., Murillo, C. L., Chew, A. Y., & Barksdale, D. J. (2021). Simulation in PhD programs to prepare nurse scientists as social justice advocates. *Nursing Education Perspectives, 42*(6), E60–E62. https://doi.org/10.1097/01.NEP.0000000000000835

Cremerius, C., Gradl-Dietsch, G., Beeres, F. J. P., Link, B., Hitpa, L., Nebelung, S., Horst, K., Weber, C. D., Neuerburg, C., Eschbach, D., Bliemel, C., & Knobe, M. (2021). Team-based learning for teaching musculoskeletal ultrasound skills: A prospective randomised trial. *European Journal of Trauma & Emergency Surgery, 47*(4), 1189–1199. https://doi.org/10.1007/s00068-019-01298-9

Dieckmann, P. (2020). The unexpected and the non-fitting—considering the edges of simulation as social practice. *Advances in Simulation, 5*(1), 1–4. https://doi.org/10.1186/s41077-020-0120-y

Dieckmann, P., Lippert, A., Glavin, R., & Rall, M. (2010). When things do not go as expected: Scenario life savers. *Simulation in Healthcare, 5*(4), 219–225. https://doi.org/10.1097/sih.0b013e3181e77f74

Dieckmann, P., Manswer, T., Wehner, T., & Rall, M. (2007). Reality and fiction cues in medical patient simulation: An interview study with anesthesiologists. *Journal of Cognitive Engineering Decision Making, 1*(2), 148–168. https://doi.org/10.1518/155534307x232820

Edwards-Maddox, S., Cartwright, A., Quintana, D., & Contreras, J. A. (2021). Applying Newman's theory of health expansion to bridge the gap between nursing faculty and Generation Z. *Journal of Professional Nursing, 37*(3), 541–543. https://doi.org/10.1016/j.profnurs.2021.02.002

Elliot, A., & Sandberg, M. (2021). Teaching social justice in undergraduate nursing education: An integrative review. *Journal of Nursing Education, 60*(10), 545–551. https://doi.org/10.3928/01484834-20210729-04

Felder, R. M., & Solomon, B. A. (1998). *Learning styles and strategies.* http://www4.ncsu.edu/unity/lockers/users/f/felder/public/ILSdir/styles.htm

Fleming, N. (2001). *VARK: A guide to learning styles.* http://www.vark-learn.com/english/page.asp?p=categories

Fleming, N., & Mills, C. (1992). Not another inventory, rather a catalyst for change. In D. Wulff & J. Nygist (Eds.), *To improve the academy: Resources for faculty, instructional, and organizational development* (Vol. 11, pp. 137–155). New Forums.

Gelbar, N., & Madaus, J. (2021). Factors related to extended time use by college students with disabilities. *Remedial & Special Education, 42*(6), 374–383. https://doi.org/10.1177/0741932520972787

Goffman, E. (1974). *Frame analysis: An essay on the organization of experience.* Harper & Row.

Grasha, A. (1996). *Teaching with style*. Alliance.

Hansen, E., & Beaver, S. (2012). Faculty support for ESL nursing students: Action plan for success. *Nursing Education Perspectives, 33*(4), 246–250. https://doi.org/10.5480/1536-5026-33.4.246

Hari, R., Geraghty, S., & Kumar, K. (2021). Clinical supervisors' perspectives of factors influencing clinical learning experience of nursing students from culturally and linguistically diverse backgrounds during placement: A qualitative study. *Nurse Education Today, 102*, 104934. https://doi.org/10.1016/j.nedt.2021.104934

Hart, S. (2017). Today's learners and educators: Bridging the generational gaps. *Teaching & Learning in Nursing, 12*(4), 253–257. https://doi.org/10.1016/j.teln.2017.05.003

Hicks, N. A., & Burkus, E. (2011). Knowledge development for master teachers. *Journal of Theory Construction and Testing, 15*(2), 32–35.

Ho, C., Chiu, W., Li, M., Huang, C., & Cheng, S. (2021). The effectiveness of the iLearning application on chest tube care education in nursing students. *Nurse Education Today, 101*, 104870. https://doi.org/10.1016/j.nedt.2021.104870

House, B. M., Chassie, M. B., & Spohn, B. B. (1999). Questioning: An essential ingredient in effective teaching. *Journal of Continuing Education in Nursing, 21*(5), 196–201.

Hussain, M., Johnson, A. E., Hua, J., Hinojosa, B. M., Zawadzke, M. J., & Howell, J. L. (2021). When belongingness backfires: Experienced discrimination predicts increased cardiomet abolic risk among college students high in social belonging. *Journal of Behavioral Medicine, 44*(4), 571–578. https://doi.org/10.1007/s10865-021-00228-8

Jeffries, P. (Ed.). (2007). *Simulation in nursing: From conceptualization to evaluation*. National League for Nursing.

Joshi, G., & Bouck, E. C. (2017). Examining postsecondary education predictors and participation for students with learning disabilities. *Journal of Learning Disabilities, 50*(1), 3–13. https://doi.org/10.1177/0022219415572894

Kamble, A., Desai, S., & Abhang, N. (2021). Wearable activity trackers: A structural investigation into acceptance and goal achievements of Generation Z. *American Journal of Health Education, 52*(5), 307–320. https://doi.org/10.1080/19325037.2021.1955229

Kelly, C. (2008). Students' perceptions of effective clinical teaching revisited. *Nurse Education Today, 27*(8), 885–892. https://doi.org/10.1016/j.nedt.2006.12.005

Kessler, T. A., & Kost, G. C. (2021). An innovative approach for using cross-cultural, collaborative simulation during undergraduate nursing study abroad exchanges. *Clinical Simulation in Nursing, 61*, 14–22. https://doi.org/10.1016/j.ecns.2021.09.004

Kolb, D. A. (1984). *Experiential learning: Experiences as the source of learning and development*. Prentice Hall.

LeBlanc, V. R., & Posner, G. D. (2022). Emotions in simulation-based education: Friends or foes of learning? *Advances in Simulation, 7*(1), 1–8. https://doi.org/10.1186/s41077-021-00198-6

Lindberg, R., McDonough, K., & Trofimovich, P. (2021). Investigating verbal and nonverbal indicators of physiological response during second language interaction. *Applied Psycholinguistics, 42*(6), 1403–1425. https://doi.org/10.1017/S014271642100028X

Merriam-Webster (n.d.). Diversity. In *Merriam-Webster.com dictionary*. http://www.merriam_webster.com/dictionary/diversity

Merry, L., Vissandjee, B., & Verville-Provencher, K. (2021). Challenges, coping responses and supportive interventions for international and migrant students in academic nursing programs in major host countries: A scoping review with a gender lens. *BMC Nursing, 20*(1), 1–37. https://doi.org/10.1186/s12912-021-00678-0

Oberai, T., Laver, K., Woodman, R., Crotty, M., Kerkhoffs, G., & Jaarsma, R. (2021). The effect of an educational intervention to improve orthopaedic nurses' knowledge of delirium: A quasi-experimental study. *International Journal of Orthopaedic & Trauma Nursing, 42*, 100862. https://doi.org/10.1016/j.ijotn.2021.100862

Olmstead, S. B., Conrad, K. A., & Davis, K. N. (2019, August 29). First-year college students' experiences of a brief sexual health seminar. *Sex Education, 20*(3), 300–315. https://doi.org/10.1080/14681811.2019.1654446

Quirk, M. E. (1994). *How to learn and teach in medical school: A learner-centered approach*. Charles C Thomas.

Rushton, T. (2017). Understanding the experiences of occupational therapy students, with additional support requirements, while studying BSc (hons) in occupational therapy. *British Journal of Occupational Therapy, 80,* 2–3.

Schublova, M. (2017). Learning styles and personality types of freshman level pre-athletic training major students. *Internet Journal of Allied Health Sciences and Practice, 15*(4), 2–7.

Seibert, S. A. (2021). Problem-based learning: A strategy to foster generation Z's critical thinking and perseverance. *Teaching & Learning in Nursing, 16*(1), 85–88. https://doi.org/10.1016/j.teln.2020.09.002

Silver, H., Hanson, J. R., & Strong, R. W. (1996). *Teaching styles and strategies (Unity in Diversity Series, Manual No. 2)*. Silver and Strong.

Society for Simulation in Healthcare. (2021). *Certified healthcare simulation educator examination handbook*. https://www.ssih.org/Portals/48/Certification/CHSE_Docs/CHSE%20Handbook.pdf

Story, L., & Butts, J. B. (2010). Compelling teaching with the four Cs: Caring, comedy, creativity, and challenging. *Journal of Nursing Education, 49*(5), 291–294. https://doi.org/10.3928/01484834-20100115-08

Taha, A. A., Jadalla, A., Bin Ali, W., Firkins, J., Norman, S., & Aza, N. (2021). Structured simulations improves students' knowledge acquisition and perceptions of teaching effectiveness: A quasi-experimental study. *Journal of Clinical Nursing, 30*(21/22), 3163–3170. https://doi.org/10.1111/jocn.15815

Walton, J., Chute, E., & Ball, L. (2011). Professional nurse: The pedagogy of simulation: A grounded study. *Journal of Professional Nursing, 27,* 299–310. https://doi.org/10.1016/j.profnurs.2011.04.005

# Interprofessional Simulation

Kate Morse and Kymberlee Montgomery

*Coming together is a beginning. Keeping together is progress. Working together is success.*
—*Henry Ford*

This chapter addresses Domain II: Healthcare and Simulation Knowledge and Principles (Society for Simulation in Healthcare [SSH], 2021).

## ▶ LEARNING OUTCOMES

- Discuss the history of interprofessional education (IPE) over the past century.
- Define the following IPE principles that foster a climate of patient/population care that is safe, timely, effective, and equitable: values and ethics (VE), roles and responsibilities (RR), interprofessional communication/communication competency (IC/CC), and teams and teamwork (TT).
- Discuss IC techniques in simulation based education (SBE) to translate an improved team approach to daily patient care: application of closed-loop communication techniques in all professional interactions; creation of a climate where providers apply a shared mental model; and support of learner understanding and respect of individual providers' roles and those of other professions to collaboratively address the healthcare needs of patients.
- Discuss barriers and facilitators of effective design and implementation of IPE SBE.

## ▶ HISTORY OF INTERPROFESSIONAL EDUCATION OR IPE

The recognized and often-used acronym *IPE* (interprofessional education) has a variety of meanings and interpretations. The most recognized definition adapted from the Centre for the Advancement of Interprofessional Education (CAIPE) in the United Kingdom and the World Health Organization (WHO) states that IPE occurs when two or more professions learn with, about, and from each other to enable effective collaboration and improve health outcomes (quality of care; CAIPE, 2002; WHO, 2010, p. 7). The National Center for Interprofessional Practice and Education (NEXUS) further enhanced the IPE acronym to include interprofessional *practice* and education that emphasizes support of healthcare professionals, healthcare workers, residents, students, families, patients, and communities to learn together every day to enhance collaboration and improve health outcomes while also reducing costs (NEXUS, 2021).

For many, learning through some type of active participation, experience, and reflection (experiential learning) provides a fresh lens in viewing the educational process (Kolb, 1984). To simulate real-life environments as the backdrop can be even more powerful. Thus, to practice together better, it is imperative that students can collaborate with and learn from one another in a safe educational environment (Montgomery, Griswold-Theodorson, et al., 2012).

## ▶ BACKGROUND

The national recommendations to redesign the health education system to embrace the strengths of multidisciplinary skill sets are certainly not novel, nor were they developed out of a need to comply with the changes derived from healthcare reform. In fact, the origin of this challenge can be traced to the Flexner Report of 1910 (Flexner, 1910), and a call for healthcare educational transformations to include IPE initiatives has been a recurrent theme threaded through the following landmark reports of the Institute of Medicine (IOM) over the past half century (Table 6.1).

- *Educating for the Health Team* (IOM, 1972)
- *To Err Is Human: Building a Safer Health System* (Kohn et al., 2000)
- *Crossing the Quality Chasm: A New Health System for the 21st Century* (IOM, 2001)

**Table 6.1** Historical Landmark Reports That Have Made Recommendations Regarding the Integration of Interprofessional Education to the Healthcare Environment

| Landmark Reports | IPE Recommendations |
|---|---|
| Flexner Report (1910) | Suggests a full redesign of medical school education systems |
| *Educating for the Health Team* (IOM, 1972) | Challenges national healthcare educators and administrators to<br>■ Engage in IPE<br>■ Develop clinical settings to begin interprofessional innovation<br>■ Lobby governmental and professional support of IPE for healthcare delivery teams |
| *To Err Is Human: Building a Safer Health System* (Kohn et al., 2000) | Encourages the reduction of preventable medical errors through<br>■ Provision of support to multidisciplinary teams of researchers, healthcare facilities, and organizations to determine the causes of medical errors<br>■ Development of new knowledge to assist in the creation of demonstration projects |
| *Crossing the Quality Chasm: A New Health System for the 21st Century* (IOM, 2001) | Provisions made to ensure licensing and accreditation organizations begin the evolution of our siloed educational processes through<br>■ Stressing evidence-based practice instruction<br>■ Providing opportunities for interprofessional training |
| *Health Professions Education: A Bridge to Quality* (Greiner & Knebel, 2003) | Reiterates the need for *all* healthcare professionals to be<br>■ Educated to deliver patient-centered care as members of an interprofessional team<br>■ Prepared to use evidence-based practice, quality improvement approaches, and informatics |

*(continued)*

**Table 6.1** Historical Landmark Reports That Have Made Recommendations Regarding the Integration of Interprofessional Education to the Healthcare Environment (*continued*)

| Landmark Reports | IPE Recommendations |
| --- | --- |
| *The Future of Nursing: Leading Change, Advancing Health* (IOM, 2011) | Recommends that nurses need to be an integral part of the healthcare team by<br>▪ Practicing to the full extent of their education and training<br>▪ Intertwining advanced competencies within higher levels of training and education<br>▪ Becoming equal partners in redesigning and improving healthcare<br>▪ Participating in workforce planning and policymaking initiatives |
| *Framework for Action on Interprofessional Education and Collaborative Practice* (WHO, 2010) | Provides strategies to support global health workforce and<br>▪ Identifies the necessity of IPE education and collaboration strategies to increase health profession workforce<br>▪ Defines IPE as the future of health education and essential in the delivery of quality patient care |
| *Health Professionals for a New Century: Transforming Education to Strengthen Health Systems in an Interdependent World* (Frenk et al., 2010) | Suggests that health education reform should<br>▪ Promote interprofessional and transdisciplinary education that breaks down professional siloes<br>▪ Encourage collaborative and nonhierarchical relationships in effective teams<br>▪ Promote a new century of transformative professional education |
| *Measuring the Impact of Interprofessional Education on Collaborative Practice and Patient Outcomes* (IOM, 2015) | Examines the methods necessary to measure IPE impact on collaborative practice and health and system outcomes<br>Develops a model template for the evaluation of an IPE that is adaptable to a particular setting in which it is applied |
| *Assessing Progress on the IOM Report "The Future of Nursing"* (IOM, 2015) | Evaluation of the work completed 5 years after the release of *The Future of Nursing* report<br>▪ Continued work needed to complete the recommendations in *The Future of Nursing* report through the following steps: removal of scope-of-practice barriers and strengthening pathways to higher education with specific emphasis on increasing diversity and continuing competence<br>▪ Data collection on a wide range of outcomes needed, from the education and makeup of the workforce to the services nurses provide and the ways in which they lead<br>▪ Further promotion of nurses' interprofessional and lifelong learning; creation of opportunities for collaboration and education |

IOM, Institute of Medicine; IPE, interprofessional education; WHO, World Health Organization.

Unfortunately, although these reports provided the premise that IPE-based programs would decrease preventable medical errors through increased multidisciplinary team collaboration and communication and improved quality care delivery and patient safety outcomes, these challenges yielded slim results.

Years of escalating governmental spending, rising healthcare costs, numbers of uninsured and underinsured Americans, and fear of an individual's inability to afford basic healthcare spawned a unified consensus among governmental and private foundations to transform both the healthcare and health education system, strongly emphasizing the need for IPE in the United States (Montgomery, Griswold-Theodorson, et al., 2012). Rethinking the IPE's call-to-action initiatives was postulated in three well-respected and nationally recognized sentinel reports:

■ *The Future of Nursing: Leading Change, Advancing Health* (IOM, 2011)
■ "Framework for Action on Interprofessional Education and Collaborative Practice" (WHO, 2010)
■ "Health Professionals for a New Century: Transforming Education to Strengthen Health Systems in an Interdependent World" (Frenk et al., 2010)

Many years after the initial IOM's call to action for collaboration among healthcare professionals, six of the major national healthcare organizations convened an expert panel to produce documents containing the foundation of IPE (Montgomery, Morse, et al., 2012). *Team-Based Competencies: Building a Shared Foundation for Education and Clinical Practice* (Josiah Macy Jr. Foundation, 2011) and *Core Competencies for Interprofessional Collaborative Practice* (American Association of Colleges of Nursing, 2011) define 4 measurable core competency domains and 38 subcompetencies for curriculum foundation for IPE and practice in all healthcare realms:

■ Values and Ethics (VE)
■ Roles and Responsibilities (RR)
■ Interprofessional Communication/Communication Competency (IC/CC)
■ Teams and Teamwork (TT)

See Exhibit 6.1 for further definitions.

Since the development of these competencies, IPE has been gaining popularity and recognition across the country. Increasing accreditation body endorsement, new IPE-specific faculty development and training program offerings, increased dissemination and promotion of IPE competencies, and the opening of the first National Center for Interprofessional Education and Practice (NEXUS) are only a few of the many indications that IPE is the future of healthcare education (Interprofessional Education Collaborative [IPEC], 2016).

In 2016, the IPEC Board, with an additional representation from nine new professions, reconvened to "reaffirm the original competencies, ground the competency model firmly under the singular domain of interprofessional collaboration, and broaden the competencies to better integrate population health approaches across the health and partner professions. This action will enhance collaboration for improving both individual care and population health outcomes" (IPEC, 2016, p. 3). This has resulted in the development of a Josiah Macy Jr. Foundation-funded IPEC Portal, a collection of peer-reviewed educational resources and materials supporting IPE instruction and the redesign of competencies that reflect the inclusion of population health competencies.

---

### EXHIBIT 6.1 IPEC 2016 UPDATE

■ Reaffirm the dissemination and impact of the 2011 core competencies.
■ Reorganize the competencies within the single domain of interprofessional collaboration instead of domains within IPE.
■ Attempt to achieve the Triple Aim (improve the patient experience of care, improve the health of populations, and reduce the per capita cost of healthcare) by expanding the interprofessional competencies with a population health focus.

# ▶ GENERAL INTERPROFESSIONAL EDUCATION COMPETENCIES

The competencies for IPE in health professions were developed by the IPEC, an expert panel that included the American Association of Colleges of Nursing, the American Association of Colleges of Osteopathic Medicine, the American Association of Colleges of Pharmacy, the American Dental Education Association, the Association of American Medical Colleges, and the Association of Schools of Public Health. The overarching goal of this collaboration was to develop individual-level core interprofessional competencies. Originally developed with an authentic patient-practice focus, these definitions are also foundational to IPE in simulated environments. The IPEC defined *interprofessional competencies* in healthcare as the "integrated enactment of knowledge, skills and values/attitudes that define working together across the professions, with other healthcare workers, and with patients, along with families and communities as appropriate to improve health outcomes in specific care contexts" (Josiah Macy Jr. Foundation, 2011, p. 1).

The collaborative identified that core IPE competencies were needed in order to coordinate and direct the curricular revisions needed in health professions, including pedagogy and assessment strategies to promote success, to lay the foundation for a teaching curriculum in IPE that was connected to the development of students' lifelong learning, to foster discussion regarding the divide between authentic patient care demands and IPE core competencies, to identify opportunities to integrate IPE content with current accreditation expectations, to provide a framework of common IPE competencies that would eventually link to a common set of accreditation standards, to provide licensing and credentialing bodies with potential testing content, and to promote the conduct of evaluation and research in this area to support outcomes (IPEC Expert Panel, 2011).

The competencies are based on a single, unifying concept, interprofessionality, which was originally defined as part of the work by Health Canada (D'Amour & Oandasan, 2005). It refers not merely to practicing in the same room or on the same team, but to a deliberate practice of professionals to reflect and develop an integrated practice model focused on addressing needs at the level of patient/family or population. The key elements include constant knowledge sharing between professionals and an emphasis on active patient participation. This is a paradigm shift from traditional care teams and educational models in most health professions. Thus, the development of core IPE competencies to describe the unique attributes of IPE practice was needed. The intent of the publication and competencies was to remain general in nature to provide for individual profession and institutional flexibility. In 2016, as part of the competency's revisions, the four domains listed earlier (VE, RR, IC, TT) now reside under the single domain of interprofessional collaboration (Figure 6.1).

Exhibit 6.2 demonstrates the IPE core competencies from the IPEC (Dieckmann et al., 2009). Of note, in June 2021, the IPEC has begun work to revise the 2016 competencies once again. The core competencies have been crucial to moving the IPE forward. The revisions, to be completed in 2023, will include a "cyclical review on common definitions for competence, competency and competency framework; and ensure that this framework accurately reflects any changes in research, policy, and practice" (IPEC, 2022).

---

**EXHIBIT 6.2 CORE COMPETENCIES FOR INTERPROFESSIONAL COLLABORATIVE PRACTICE FROM THE INTERPROFESSIONAL EDUCATION COLLABORATIVE**

- VE. Work with individuals of other professions to maintain a climate of mutual respect and shared values.
- RR. Use the knowledge of one's own role and those of other professions to appropriately assess and address the healthcare needs of the patients and to promote and advance the health of populations.

*(continued)*

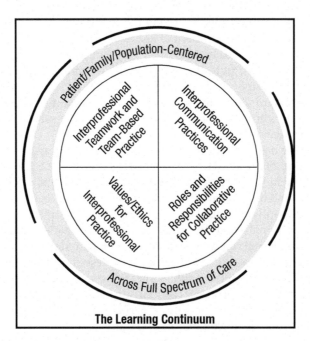

**Figure 6.1** Interprofessional collaborative practice core competency domains.

*Source:* Reprinted under Creative Commons permission from 2016 IPEC©.

Each of the four core competencies or domains is further delineated into specific IPE competencies that are outlined in the following sections.

## DETAILED VALUES AND ETHICS COMPETENCIES

This domain moves beyond the individual's professional ethics and focuses on the development of interprofessional ethics.

■ VE 1. Place the interests of patients and populations at the center of the IPE healthcare delivery and population health programs and policies, with the goal of promoting health and health equity across the life span.

■ VE 2. Respect the dignity and privacy of patients while maintaining confidentiality in the delivery of team-based care.

■ VE 3. Embrace the cultural diversity and individual differences that characterize patients, populations, and the health team.

■ VE 4. Respect the unique cultures, values, roles/responsibilities, and expertise of other health professions and the impact these factors can have on health outcomes.

■ VE 5. Work in cooperation with those who receive care, those who provide care, and those who contribute to or support the delivery of prevention and health service programs.

■ VE 6. Develop a trusting relationship with patients, families, and other team members.

■ VE 7. Demonstrate high standards of ethical conduct and quality of care in one's contribution to team-based care.

■ VE 8. Manage ethical dilemmas specific to interprofessional patient/population-centered care situations.

■ VE 9. Act with honesty and integrity in relationships with patients, families, communities, and other team members.

■ VE 10. Maintain competence in one's own profession appropriate to the scope of practice.

## DETAILED ROLES AND RESPONSIBILITIES COMPETENCIES

The interaction between understanding your own and others' RR within an interprofessional team while providing patient-centered or population-focused care is delineated in the RR-specific competencies. Each profession's RR is delineated within a legal scope of practice that may be significantly influenced by the practice environment, region, or location. However, within the appropriate scope of practice, RR may vary depending on the situation. The following are specific RR subcompetencies:

■ RR 1. Communicate one's RR clearly to patients, families, community members, and other professions.

■ RR 2. Recognize one's limitations in skills, knowledge, and abilities.

■ RR 3. Engage diverse professionals who complement one's own professional expertise, as well as associated resources, to develop strategies to meet specific healthcare needs of patients and populations.

■ RR 4. Explain the RR of other care providers and how the team works together to provide care, promote health, and prevent disease.

■ RR 5. Use the full scope of knowledge, skills, and abilities of professionals from health and other fields to provide care that is timely, safe, effective, and equitable.

■ RR 6. Communicate with team members to clarify each member's responsibility in executing the components of a treatment plan or public health intervention.

■ RR 7. Forge interdependent relationships with other professions within and outside the health system to improve care and advance learning.

■ RR 8. Engage in continuous professional and interprofessional development to enhance team performance and collaboration.

■ RR 9. Use unique and complementary abilities of all members of the team to optimize health and patient care.

■ RR 10. Describe how professionals in health and other fields can collaborate and integrate clinical care and public health interventions to optimize population health.

## DETAILED INTERPROFESSIONAL COMMUNICATION COMPETENCIES

These subcompetencies expound on the critical nature of effective verbal, written, and health literacy communication to promote interprofessional collaboration. This includes using a shared language that is known to all team members. The following is a list of positive communication techniques (Cochrane et al., 1998):

- CC 1. Choose effective communication tools and techniques, including information systems and communication technologies, to facilitate discussions and interactions that enhance team function.
- CC 2. Communicate information with patients, families, community members, and health team members in a form that is understandable, avoiding discipline-specific terminology when possible.
- CC 3. Express one's knowledge and opinions to team members involved in patient care and population health improvement with confidence, clarity, and respect, working to ensure mutual understanding of information and treatment and care decisions, and population health programs and policies.
- CC 4. Listen actively and encourage ideas and opinions of other team members.
- CC 5. Give timely, sensitive, instructive feedback to others about their performance on the team, responding respectfully as a team member to feedback from others.
- CC 6. Use respectful language appropriate for a given demanding situation, crucial conversation, or interprofessional conflict.
- CC 7. Recognize how one's own uniqueness (experience level, expertise, culture, power, and hierarchy within the health team) contributes to effective communication, conflict resolution, and positive interprofessional relationships.
- CC 8. Communicate the importance of teamwork in patient-centered care and population health programs and policies.

Simulation is a well-matched modality to bring together teams in a predictable, reproduceable, learning environment with well-designed cases that promotes learning from, with, and about one another. However, the challenges of creating successful IPE experiences can be daunting. An integrative review of outcomes of IPE simulation in nursing education revealed that, while interest and progress are sustained, more rigorous design, implementation, and analysis of IPE interventions are needed (Horsley et al., 2018). West et al. (2016) described similar barriers in their survey of 16 U.S. medical schools participating in IPE. Foronda et al. (2016) examined IC in healthcare in an integrative review and concluded that the next steps should include adding courses on patient safety, employing interprofessional patient hand-off tools, practicing in simulation, and using virtual technologies to bring together the professions. In a narrative synthesis of barriers and facilitators of IPE simulation, three primary themes were identified: characteristics of learning process, learning outcomes, and interprofessional dynamics (Connolly et al., 2021). These reviews highlight the need for ongoing work in SBE to facilitate a successful IPE.

Simulation Teaching Tip 6.1 outlines the pearls and pitfalls for the simulationist.

## Simulation Teaching Tip 6.1

### Pearls and Pitfalls Implementing Interprofessional Simulation-Based Education

### Pearls

Facilitators of interprofessional education (IPE) simulations include the following:

- creating interprofessional design work teams that reflect the learning teams
- striving to balance interprofessional learning outcomes with individual professional responsibilities and domains of learning (one simulation may not meet all those goals)
- transparent collaboration among the faculty designers focused on interest and outcomes

(continued)

- focusing on psychological safety of all participants throughout the learning process
- using multiple modalities and considering virtual collaboration
- accepting incremental improvement in the IPE program which can lead to critical learning for the design team; perfection should not get in the way of progress

## Pitfalls

The enormity of bringing healthcare providers together to practice without risk to patients and to improve patient care is systematically challenging. The practical issues of scheduling and time commitment may be some of the most significant barriers to successful implementation.
    Other barriers include the following:

- schedule and resource coordination
- lack of resource and financial support from leadership
- interprofessional simulation design and debriefing teams not adequately trained
- multiple interests of different professions not initially negotiated
- realism of the scenarios not effective for all disciplines for optimal engagement
- failure to evaluate outcomes
- different definitions/perceptions of IPE among team members
- fear of relinquishing discipline hierarchical status

## Suggested Enabling Frames for IPE Educator Engagement

- striving for "good," not perfection; messy is okay
- planning for multiple contingencies for scheduling
- staying focused on the interests of the learners
- understanding that multiple perspectives make us better clinicians and educators

## DETAILED TEAMS AND TEAMWORK COMPETENCIES

The last subcompetencies address the concepts of effective team members and team behaviors that may influence, positively or negatively, the team's overall effectiveness.

- TT 1. Describe the process of team development and the roles and practices of effective teams.
- TT 2. Develop consensus on the ethical principles to guide all aspects of teamwork.
- TT 3. Engage health and other professionals in shared patient-centered and population-focused problem-solving.
- TT 4. Integrate the knowledge and experience of health and other professions to inform health and care decisions, while respecting patient and community values and priorities/ preferences for care.
- TT 5. Apply leadership practices that support collaborative practice and team effectiveness.
- TT 6. Engage self and others to constructively manage disagreements about values, roles, goals, and actions that arise among health and other professionals and with patients, families, and community members.
- TT 7. Share accountability with other professions, patients, and communities for outcomes relevant to prevention and healthcare.
- TT 8. Reflect on individual and team performance for individual as well as team performance improvement.

■ TT 9. Use process improvement strategies to increase the effectiveness of interprofessional teamwork and team-based services, programs, and policies.

■ TT 10. Use available evidence to inform effective teamwork and team-based practices.

■ TT 11. Perform effectively on teams and in different team roles in a variety of settings.

## Evidence-Based Simulation Practice 6.1

The impact of teamwork training, including interprofessional education (IPE) principles conducted using simulation and debriefing, has been associated with improved patient care process outcomes (Marr et al., 2012; Riley et al., 2011; Starmer et al., 2014). Although it is extremely difficult to understand the specific methodology used in each of these studies to definitively understand what, when, and how IPE principles practiced outside of the patient care environment led to patient care improvements, the following studies are promising. In 2010, Capella et al. (2010) studied trauma team performance after a simulation-based TeamSTEPPS™ training. In their study, time to CT, time to tracheal intubation, and appropriateness of time to the operating room were all significantly improved after training. Additional studies (Marr et al., 2012; Steinemann et al., 2011) have been able to demonstrate similar patient care process outcomes after multidisciplinary providers practiced high-stress clinical situations in a simulated environment.

Riley et al. (2011) demonstrated that a simulation-based intervention, in addition to interprofessional team training, resulted in a statistically significant improvement of 37% in perinatal morbidity scores. The authors used the Weighted Adverse Outcome Score measure of perinatal morbidity and a culture-of-safety survey (Safety Attitudes Questionnaire) before and after intervention to compare three hospital groups. The first group served as the control, and the second hospital received the U.S. Agency for Healthcare Research and Quality-supported curriculum, the TeamSTEPPS™ didactic training program. The third hospital received both the TeamSTEPPS™ program and a series of in situ simulation training exercises. The authors found that a comprehensive interprofessional team training program using in situ simulation in addition to IPE team training in nontechnical skills improved perinatal safety in the hospital setting. They also reinforced the idea that didactic instruction alone without simulation was not effective in improving perinatal outcomes.

In 2013, Theilen et al. (2013) published a prospective cohort study of all deteriorating inpatients of a tertiary pediatric hospital requiring admission to pediatric ICU the year before and after the introduction of pediatric rapid-response medical emergency team (pMET) and concurrent team training. The article suggests improvements in patient outcomes were specifically related to the in situ simulation training. Lessons learned by ward staff during regular training that brought physicians and nurses together for weekly, in situ team training led to significantly improved recognition and management of deteriorating inpatients with evolving critical illness. A follow-up study published in 2017 (Theilen et al., 2017) demonstrated a sustained improvement in the hospital response to critically deteriorating inpatients, significantly improved patient outcomes, and substantial cost savings after exposure to an IPE simulation education curriculum.

A systematic review and meta-analysis of the effects of IPE on healthcare students concluded that IPE has a positive impact on attitudes, and the development of knowledge, competencies, and collaboration (Marion-Martins & Pinho, 2020). Foronda et al.'s (2016) review of IC in healthcare supports the use of simulation and standardized interprofessional tools to improve communication.

### Pearls to Utilize the Evidence

■ Conduct a review of the literature before designing new outcome tools to assess the impact of simulation-based education (SBE) on IPE behaviors.

● Move beyond measuring learner satisfaction and look for more impactful outcomes.

# CASE STUDY 6.1

A Certified Healthcare Simulation Educator® (CHSE®) is arranging an interprofessional simulation experience with multiple disciplines in a teaching hospital laboratory. All the healthcare professionals are licensed and are needed for the simulation experience of a prolapsed cord in a patient in labor. It is imperative that nursing, medicine, obstetrical operating room team, respiratory, and neonatology disciplines respond. The simulation experience is scheduled at three separate times, and at all three times one of the participants cancels due to "being busy in the labor-and-delivery suites." What pitfall is the CHSE falling into and how can this be overcome?

1. The simulation educator is charged with designing an interprofessional education (IPE) course with medical students, nurses, and pharmacists. Despite reaching out to colleagues, they have been unable to develop a team. The next BEST step is to:

   A. Move forward alone and design scenarios that have a team caring for a patient
   B. Abandon the project and stick to domain-specific learning
   C. Locate an IPE case already designed and implement the program without support from the other disciplines
   D. Reach out to the leadership of each discipline to discuss the needed resources and team members, and understand their interests

2. The simulation educator overhears a participant of the interprofessional education (IPE) experience raising their voice loudly and stating an order to someone in a different discipline without addressing this person by name. The simulation educator would best handle this situation initially by:

   A. Exploring the action observed in the debriefing following the case
   B. Ignoring the behavior and focusing on the medical management of the case in the debrief
   C. Reporting the participant to their supervisor for remediation
   D. Stopping the scenario, removing the participant, and restarting the scenario

3. The simulation educator working in a hospital-based simulation center is leading an interprofessional (IP) team designing a simulation-based education course to improve patient outcomes. To leverage the impact of the educational program, the team wishes to address the most common cause of error in authentic patient care. Which of the following will BEST serve that objective?

   A. Lack of knowledge
   B. Inadequate resources
   C. Lack of communication
   D. Lack of leadership

4. The simulation educator is collaborating with an interprofessional (IP) team to design an interprofessional education (IPE) course. Which of the following modalities will engage learners from all professions?

   A. In a virtual learning environment, learners asynchronously reading case studies and answering questions
   B. In an IP team, seeing standardized patients and codeveloping a plan of care, followed by feedback and debriefing
   C. Seeing a standardized patient by a group of professionals from one discipline and then writing domain-specific care notes
   D. In a virtual reality learning environment where they take turns being the team leader in an advanced cardiac life support (ACLS) case

## 1. D) Reach out to the leadership of each discipline to discuss the needed resources and team members, and understand their interests

Tackling the barrier of needed resources needs leadership support to increase the chance of success. Not partnering with leadership and other professions will not result in optimal IPE simulation. Moving forward alone will not ensure IPE or using an existing scenario if there is no buy-in. Abandoning the project is not an option because communication in the practice area needs to be interprofessional to decrease patient care mistakes.

## 2. A) Exploring the action observed in the debriefing following the case

This is an opportunity to explore their thinking and the impact of their actions on other team members and offer a new way of approaching closed-loop communication. To ignore and not talk about the behavior during the debriefing results in a missed opportunity to discuss interprofessional (IP) team communication. Reporting the participant potentially violates confidentiality and a psychologically safe learning environment, and stopping the scenario potentially breaks psychological safety for all learners.

## 3. C) Lack of communication

Lack of communication in IP teams is the most common cause of patient care errors. Lack of knowledge, inadequate resources, and lack of leadership, while contributing factors, are not the most common cause of patient care errors.

## 4. B) In an IP team, seeing standardized patients and codeveloping a plan of care, followed by feedback and debriefing

Learners are interacting as an IP team and are learning with, from, and about one another with a live patient. Asynchronous learning does not engage the IP team. Seeing a patient with only one profession present does not engage an IP team. Virtual reality can use an IP team, but in person increases interactions in real time.

5. The simulation educator is preparing to be in the role of a debriefer in an interprofessional team simulation. In preparing for their role and reviewing the Institute of Medicine (IOM) report, which of the following should they anticipate including in prebriefing to describe the primary reason the team is practicing:

   A. To decrease attrition from their respective professions
   B. To increase efficiency of patient care
   C. To increase communication across professions
   D. To orient new team members

6. The simulation educator is leading an interprofessional team in a meeting and is explaining the essence of interprofessional education (IPE). Which of the following would BEST describe the essence of IPE?

   A. Cooperation between different healthcare professions
   B. Meeting accreditation standards and criteria
   C. A licensure and/or certification requirement
   D. To learn from, with, and about other healthcare professions

7. In designing an interprofessional (IP) simulation case that will meet the core competency of "roles and responsibilities," which of the following cases would allow learners to meet that objective?

   A. A case where nurses, pharmacists, and doctors must form an ad hoc team to quickly provide care for an acutely decompensated patient
   B. A case with nurses and doctors who must communicate a complex care plan to a patient and their family
   C. A case with nurses and doctors who must resolve an IP conflict
   D. A case with nurses and nurse practitioners where they must develop a complex care plan for a dying patient

8. The simulation educator is observing an interprofessional education (IPE) case and notices the team asking for input from the patient and family for their wishes for end-of-life care, as well as checking with all professions in the room before developing a plan. This demonstrates the team meeting which of the following core competencies?

   A. Values and ethics
   B. Roles and responsibilities
   C. Communication
   D. Teamwork

9. The simulation educator is designing an interprofessional education (IPE) curriculum between nursing students and medical students on different academic calendars and wants to proactively address the MOST COMMON barrier, which is:

   A. Lack of awareness of IPE among faculty
   B. Scheduling different professions
   C. Misalignment with the schools' mission and values
   D. Conflict among interprofessional faculty

## 5. C) To increase communication across professions

Interprofessional education (IPE) simulation has been demonstrated to improve communication. The IOM report is about decreasing patient errors due to lack of inter- and intraprofessional communication. The report does not address efficiency, orientation, and attrition within the healthcare setting.

## 6. D) To learn from, with, and about other healthcare professions

Learning together is the core of IPE and is included in the World Health Organization's (WHO's) definition. IPE is not a current licensure, certification, or accreditation standard. While cooperation is an outcome of IPE, it is not the core; the essence is learning together so there is a team approach to patient care.

## 7. A) A case where nurses, pharmacists, and doctors must form an ad hoc team to quickly provide care for an acutely decompensated patient

This will allow an IP team to practice the core competency of roles and responsibilities. Communicating with patients, families, and conflict resolution would meet the core competency of communication. Nurses practicing with nurse practitioners is intraprofessional education.

## 8. A) Values and ethics

This demonstrates value and ethics 4—respect the unique cultures, values, roles/responsibilities, and expertise of other health professions and the impact these factors can have on health outcomes. Requesting patient and family preference is not highlighted under roles and responsibilities, communication, or teamwork, although there are components of them in the interaction. It is specifically identified under values and ethics.

## 9. B) Scheduling different professions

Scheduling is documented as a common barrier. Hopefully there is no lack of awareness in any health profession. The mission and values of healthcare professionals are usually aligned and deal with caring for people and populations. Conflicts must be overcome and cannot be justified as a barrier.

10. The simulation educator is evaluating outcome measures for an interprofessional education (IPE) program. Which of the following would be the BEST approach?

    A. Do not use any outcome measures as this is a new program
    B. Review the literature and use a previously designed tool that is appropriate
    C. Realizing their center is different, create a new tool without reviewing the literature
    D. Use uniprofessional outcome tools and evaluate each profession separately

**10. B) Review the literature and use a previously designed tool that is appropriate**

This approach uses a tool with prior reliability and validity data. Creating a new tool without the appropriate rigorous process can provide inaccurate data. Not collecting data is a missed opportunity to evaluate the impact of the program, and using a uniprofessional tool will result in data that DO NOT measure IPE outcomes.

# REFERENCES

Agency for Healthcare Research and Quality. (2003). *AHRQ's patient safety initiative: Building foundations, reducing risk* (Chapter 2). http://www.ahrq.gov/research/findings/final-reports/pscongrpt/psini2.html

Agency for Healthcare Research and Quality. (2012). *TeamSTEPPS: National implementation.* http://teamstepps.ahrq.gov

American Association of Colleges of Nursing. (2011). *Team-based competencies: Building a shared foundation for education and clinical practice.* Health Resources Service Administration. http://www.aacn.nche.edu/leading-initiatives/IPECProceedings.pdf

Capella, J., Smith, S., Philp, A., Putnam, T., Gilbert, C., Fry, W., & Remine, S. (2010). Teamwork training improves the clinical care of trauma patients. *Journal of Surgical Education, 67*(6), 439–443. https://doi.org/10.1016/j.jsurg.2010.06.006

Centre for the Advancement of Interprofessional Education. (2002). *About CAIPE.* https://www.caipe.org/about

Cochrane, H. J., Baker, G. A., & Meudell, P. R. (1998). Simulating a memory impairment: Can amnesics implicitly outperform simulators? *British Journal of Clinical Psychology, 37*(Pt 1), 31–48. https://doi.org/10.1111/j.2044-8260.1998.tb01277.x

Connolly, F., De Brun, A., & McAuliffe, E. (2021). A narrative synthesis of learners' experiences of barriers and facilitators related to effective interprofessional simulation. *Journal of Interprofessional Case (Online), 36*, 222–233. https://doi.org/10.1080/13561820.2021.1880381

D'Amour, D., & Oandasan, I. (2005). Interprofessionality as the field of interprofessional practice and interprofessional education: An emerging concept. *Journal of Interprofessional Care, 19*(Suppl. 1), 8–20. https://doi.org/10.1080/13561820500081604

Dieckmann, P., Molin Friis, S., Lippert, A., & Østergaard, D. (2009). The art and science of debriefing in simulation: Ideal and practice. *Medical Teacher, 31*(7), e287–e294.

Flexner, A. (1910). *Medical education in the United States and Canada: A report to the Carnegie Foundation for the Advancement of Teaching.* The Carnegie Foundation for the Advancement of Teaching.

Foronda, C., MacWilliams, B., & McArthur, E. (2016). Interprofessional communication in healthcare: An integrative review. *Nurse Education in Practice, 19*, 36–40. http://doi.org/10.1016/j.nepr.2016.04.005

Frenk, J., Chen, L., Bhutta, Z. A., Cohen, J., Crisp, N., Evans, T., Fineberg, H., Garcia, P., Ke, Y., Kelley, P., Kistnasamy, B., Meleis, A., Naylor, D., Pablos-Mendez, A., Reddy, S., Scrimshaw, S., Sepulveda, J., Serwadda, D., & Zurayk, H. (2010). Health professionals for a new century: Transforming education to strengthen health systems in an interdependent world. *Lancet, 376*(9756), 1923–1958. https://doi.org/10.1016/s0140-6736(10)61854-5

Greiner, A. C., & Knebel, E. (Eds.). (2003). *Health professions education: A bridge to quality.* Institute of Medicine of the National Academies.

Horsley, T. L., O'Rourke, J., Mariani, B., Doolen, J., & Pariseault, C. (2018). An integrative review of interprofessional simulation in nursing education. *Clinical Simulation in Nursing, 22*, 5–12. https://doi.org/10.1016/j.ecns.2018.06.001

Institute of Medicine. (1972). *Educating for the health team.* Institute of Medicine of the National Academies.

Institute of Medicine. (1999). *To err is human: Building a safer health system.* https://www.iom.edu

Institute of Medicine. (2011). *The future of nursing: Leading change, advancing health.* National Academies Press.

Institute of Medicine. (2015). *Measuring the impact of interprofessional education on collaborative practice and patient outcomes.* National Academies Press.

Institute of Medicine. (2001). *Crossing the quality chasm: A new health system for the 21st century.* National Academies Press. http://iom.edu/Reports/2001/Crossing-the-Quality-Chasm-A-New-Health-System-for-the-21st-Century.aspx

Interprofessional Education Collaborative. (2022). *IPEC core competency revisions, 2021-2023.* https://www.ipecollaborative.org/2021-2023-core-competencies-revision

Interprofessional Education Collaborative Expert Panel. (2011). *Core competencies for interprofessional collaborative practice: Report of an expert panel.* Interprofessional Education Collaborative.

Interprofessional Education Collaborative Expert Panel. (2016). *Core competencies for interprofessional collaborative practice.* Update. Interprofessional Education Collaborative.

Josiah Macy Jr. Foundation. (2011). *Team based competencies: Building a shared foundation for education and practice.* https://macyfoundation.org/publications/team-based-competencies-building-a-shared-foundation-for-education-and-clinicalpractice

Kohn, L. T., Corrigan, J. M., & Donaldson, M. S. (2000). *To err is human: Building a safer health system.* The National Academies Press. https://doi.org/10.17226/9728

Kolb, D. A. (1984). *Experiential learning: Experience as the source of learning and development* (Vol. 1). Prentice Hall.

Marion-Martins, A. D., & Pinho, D. L. M. (2020). Interprofessional simulation effects for healthcare students: A systematic review and meta-analysis. *Nurse Education Today, 94*, 104568. https://doi.org/10.1016/j.nedt.2020.104568

Marr, M., Hemmert, K., Nguyen, A. H., Combs, R., Annamalai, A., Miller, G., Pachter, H. L., Turner, J., Rifkind, K., & Cohen, S. M. (2012). Team play in surgical education: A simulation-based study. *Journal of Surgical Education, 69*(1), 63–69. https://doi.org/10.1016/j.jsurg.2011.07.002

Montgomery, K., Griswold-Theodorson, S., Morse, K., Montgomery, O., & Farabaugh, D. (2012). Transdisciplinary simulation: Learning and practicing together. *Nursing Clinics of North America, 47*(4), 493–502. https://doi.org/10.1016/j.cnur.2012.07.009

Montgomery, K., Morse, C., Smith-Glasgow, M. E., Posmontier, B., & Follen, M. (2012). Promoting quality and safety in women's health through the use of transdisciplinary clinical simulation educational modules: Methodology and a pilot trial. *Gender Medicine, 9*(Suppl. 1), S48–S54. https://doi.org/10.1016/j.genm.2011.11.001

National Center for Interprofessional Practice and Education. (2021). *Homepage.* https://nexusipe.org

Riley, W., Davis, S., Miller, K., Hansen, H., Sainfort, F., & Sweet, R. (2011). Didactic and simulation nontechnical skills team training to improve perinatal patient outcomes in a community hospital. *Joint Commission Journal on Quality and Patient Safety, 37*(8), 357–364. https://doi.org/10.1016/s1553-7250(11)37046-8

Society for Simulation in Healthcare. (2021). *Certified healthcare simulation educator handbook.* https://www.ssih.org/Portals/48/Certification/CHSE_Docs/CHSE%20Handbook.pdf

Starmer, A. J., Spector, N. D., Srivastava, R., West, D. C., Rosenbluth, G., Allen, A. D., Noble, E. L., Tse, L. L., Dalal, A. K., Keohane, C. A., Lipsitz, S. R., Rothschild, J. M., Wien, M. F., Yoon, C. S., Zigmont, K. R., Wilson, K. M., O'Toole, J. K., Solan, L. G., Aylor, M. … Landrigan, C. P. (2014). Changes in medical errors after implementation of a handoff program. *New England Journal of Medicine, 371*(19), 1803–1812. https://doi.org/10.1056/NEJMsa1405556

Steinemann, S., Berg, B., Skinner, A., DiTulio, A., Anzelon, K., Terada, K., Oliver, C., & Speck, C. (2011). In situ, multidisciplinary, simulation-based teamwork training improves early trauma care. *Journal of Surgical Education, 68*(6), 472–477. https://doi.org/10.1016/j.jsurg.2011.05.009

Theilen, U., Fraser, L., Jones, P., Leonard, P., & Simpson, D. (2017). Regular in-situ simulation training of paediatric medical emergency team leads to sustained improvements in hospital response to deteriorating patients, improved outcomes in intensive care and financial savings. *Resuscitation, 115*, 61–67. https://doi.org/10.1016/j.resuscitation.2017.03.031

Theilen, U., Leonard, P., Jones, P., Ardill, R., Weitz, J., Agrawal, D., & Simpson, D. (2013). Regular in situ simulation training of paediatric medical emergency team improves hospital response to deteriorating patients. *Resuscitation, 84*(2), 218–222. https://doi.org/10.1016/j.resuscitation.2012.06.027

West, C., Graham, L., Plamer, R. T., Fuqua Miller, M., Thayer, E. K., Studer, M. L., Awdishu, L., Umoren, R. A., Wamslet, M. A., Nelson, E. A., Joo, P. A., Tysinger, J. W., George, P., & Carney, P.A. (2016). Implementation of interprofessional education (IPE) in 16 U.S. medical schools: Common practices, barriers and facilitators. *Journal of Interprofessional Education & Practice, 4*, 41–49. https://doi.org/10.1016/j.xjep.2016.05.002

World Health Organization. (2010). *Framework for action on interprofessional education & collaborative practice.* Author. http://apps.who.int/iris/bitstream/handle/10665/70185/?sequence=1

# Ethical, Legal, and Regulatory Implications in Healthcare Simulation

**Bonnie A. Haupt and Colleen H. Meakim**

*Ethics is knowing the difference between what you have a right to do and what is right to do.*
*—Potter Stewart*

This chapter addresses Domain I: Professional Values and Capabilities (Society for Simulation in Healthcare [SSH], 2021).

## ▶ LEARNING OUTCOMES

- Discuss the regulatory requirements and issues that affect simulation practice.
- Identify the ethical and legal implications associated with healthcare simulation.
- Examine case studies and practice questions as they relate to legal, ethical, and regulatory issues that may arise during simulation scenarios.

## ▶ INTRODUCTION

As healthcare professionals, our teams are held accountable for ethical, professional, and organizational policies and processes to maintain a safe healthcare environment. Healthcare education teams have utilized simulation modalities to improve patient safety, enhance professional performance, reduce errors, and improve overall patient outcomes. Simulation education creates a safe "simulated" environment for learners to gain knowledge, skills, and abilities without causing harm to our patients. Simulation education must not only focus on creating a safe learning environment to protect patients from future harm, but should also protect our learners. Establishing trust in the learner–educator relationship is crucial to implementing successful simulation experiences. This chapter explores the importance of ethical, legal, and regulatory implications in healthcare simulation education, including the role of simulation in the development of learners' personal professional integrity.

## ▶ HISTORY

What thoughts come to mind when you hear the word "Coronavirus?" Do you think of the flu, a viral infection that infects our communities historically in winter months? Or do you think of "COVID-19," a worldwide pandemic that spread rapidly and has led to thousands of deaths? As the virus began to spread, researchers accelerated standard timelines and practices to develop an effective vaccine. According to Johns Hopkins University School of Medicine (2021), typical vaccine development can take 5 to 10 years or longer to assess the vaccine's safety and efficacy in clinical trials. The current vaccines for COVID-19 were developed and approved for emergency use authorization by the U.S. Food and Drug Administration (FDA) in less than a year. This response was necessitated by the need to speed up vaccine research, which was opposed by the need for protection of research subjects and which led some to ponder this ethical dilemma (Wibawa, 2021).

Are you familiar with the name Henrietta Lacks? In 1951, Ms. Lacks's cells were used without her permission or knowledge. The cells were used by the scientific community to develop cloning, gene mapping, and other historical research (Skloot, 2010). Ethical dilemmas created in the scientific community have led to changes in research involving human subjects to prevent ethical and moral harm. A code of ethics was developed by the American Educational Research Association (AERA) in 2011. This code governs the ethical standards and principles for researchers working in education (AERA, 2021). The importance of preparation for ethical issues that arise in healthcare cannot be underestimated. Without adequate ethical preparation, providers may not serve as adequate advocates for patients, become burnt out, or leave the profession (Rushton et al., 2021).

---

**Evidence-Based Simulation Practice 7.1**

Rushton et al. (2021) used simulation as one intervention in a repeated-measure study to assess healthcare students' ($N = 415$) skills in mindfulness, resilience, confidence, and competence in confronting ethical issues. The researchers found that resilience and mindfulness were positively correlated with moral competence and work engagement and that the use of experiential discovery learning practices and high-fidelity simulation was effective in enhancing skills in addressing moral adversity in clinical practice.

---

# ▶ CREATING A SAFE ENVIRONMENT

The Agency for Healthcare Research and Quality (AHRQ) recognizes simulation as an educational tool used to enhance skills and allow healthcare providers to test new clinical procedures in a safe learning environment (AHRQ, 2017). The *Healthcare Simulation Dictionary* defines a *safe learning environment* as a learning environment where it is verified that learners feel physically and psychologically safe to act, interact, and make decisions in a simulation environment (Lioce et al., 2020). Providing a safe environment fosters open communication, respect, and support for all participants. For simulation to be credible, it must be developed on a strong foundation of safety and trust between the learners and the educators (Hovland et al., 2021).

Globally, simulation centers are developing standards and guidelines to create a safe environment, focusing on protecting learners' ethical, legal, and regulatory rights. A review of simulation centers within universities and healthcare institutions found specific guidelines that address ethical standards, including the following:

- codes of conduct and confidentiality guidelines
- learner evaluation processes
- recording and photo-use consent forms in release contracts

## CODES OF CONDUCT AND CONFIDENTIAL GUIDELINES

Codes of conduct and confidential guidelines developed by simulation centers stress the importance of abiding by the Health Insurance Portability and Accountability Act of 1996 (HIPAA) regulations during simulation scenarios. Simulation experiences are to be considered as real-life events. Learners are expected:

- to act in a professional manner
- to be prepared to participate
- not to discuss the information outside of the simulation center

**Simulation Teaching Tip 7.1**

Many simulation centers ask learners to sign an agreement letter prior to beginning coursework, agreeing to the confidentiality of the simulation experience, thereby creating an ethical environment for all learners.

Sharing of information outside the simulation environment could impede participants' confidentiality or affect future participants' learning opportunities. The International Nursing Association for Clinical Simulation and Learning's (INACSL's) revised Healthcare Simulation Standards of Best Practice™: Professional Integrity highlights the need for professional integrity in simulation (INACSL Standards Committee, 2021a). *Professional integrity* refers to the conduct and ethical behaviors of all involved in the simulation experience. Mindfulness of each profession's code of ethics builds the foundation of respect for the interprofessional team and needs to be maintained by everyone who is involved in simulation-based experiences (INACSL Standards Committee, 2021a).

## LEARNER EVALUATIONS

How learners are evaluated has received a great deal of interest from simulation educators and learners alike. Formative evaluation occurs during the learning activity or program and focuses on the development and progression toward a goal of achieving specific outcomes (INACSL Standards Committee, 2021c). The purpose of formative evaluation is to promote self-assessment, identify gaps in knowledge, skills, and attitudes, and provide ongoing constructive feedback for individual and/or group improvement (INACSL Standards Committee, 2021c). Formative evaluation may be used at the end of a learning period or other defined time frame, or can be used for competency determination.

Summative evaluation focuses on meeting the final objectives or measurement of outcomes at a clear moment in time, such as at the end of a program of study (INACSL Standards Committee, 2021c). Summative evaluations are used to award a grade, or degree, or to certify competency, using a standardized criterion (INACSL Standards Committee, 2021c). Another evaluation is known as a high-stakes evaluation, which has consequences for the learner based on the outcome of the simulation (INACSL Standards Committee, 2021c). When evaluating learners, they must be informed as to whether they are participating in a formative, summative, or high-stakes simulation experience. When developing scenarios, healthcare simulation educators should determine the goals/purpose of the simulation and match them with the appropriate evaluation type. Simulation researchers are developing reliable and valid instruments to assist educators with student evaluations (Sweeney et al., 2020). The INACSL Healthcare Simulation Standards of Best Practice™: Evaluation of Learning and Performance outlines the details associated with participants' evaluation for formative, summative, and high-stakes evaluation (INACSL Standards Committee, 2021c).

## RECORDING AND PHOTO USE

One of the essential components of simulation activities is the implementation of prebriefing to establish educational standards and create psychologically safe environments for learners (INACSL Standards Committee, 2021d; Mohamed et al., 2021). Recording of simulation experiences is widely used in healthcare simulation education. In formative simulation scenarios, recording provides an opportunity for learners to watch the video to self-reflect on their performance or for the educators to highlight a particular noteworthy behavior following the simulation session during debriefing. Use of a recording recalls precise moments and interactions during the simulation to focus on what went well and what needs improvement, allowing for critical reflection. In summative cases, recording provides an opportunity to return to the scenario for accurate grading, allows additional reviewers to observe the scenario, and provides for a reevaluation in case of a grading discrepancy (Meakim & Rockstraw, 2018).

Recording consents and releases should emphasize the following:

- how long the material(s) will be stored
- purpose of the recording
- that participants have no right to compensation

---

### Simulation Teaching Tip 7.2

Developing a standard of practice or a policy about expectations regarding video recording and photography taking will allow learners, standardized patients, and healthcare simulation educators to decide whether they can meet the learning outcomes or expectations of the experience.

---

Simulation centers have been challenged with concerns regarding religious objections to being recorded, and in some instances standardized patients (SPs) who are members of the Screen Actors Guild who may decline to be recorded or photographed.

## ▶ PROFESSIONAL DEVELOPMENT THROUGH SIMULATION

Part of the simulation process includes the development of individual learners' understanding of their profession's value system. Therefore, initially, learners and the healthcare simulation educator must come to a common understanding of what the group's professional value system entails. In the broadest sense, professionalism includes requirements for practitioners to be honest and responsible, which ultimately can lead to a sense of professional integrity.

Together learners and educators share responsibility for the learning activities associated within the simulation environment. Both must participate in preparation for simulation, as well as in identifying knowledge gaps and strategizing to address these gaps. If these activities are integrated throughout the curriculum and constructed based on the profession's code of conduct, this process can lead to an enhanced moral reasoning process (Francis et al., 2018). If learners can develop their own personal and social responsibility within the simulated clinical environment, they should be more able to reflect and analyze situations to assist in clinical decision-making (INACSL Standards Committee, 2021a). A complicating factor associated with the development and defining of norms for ethical behavior is the globalization of cultures. As the world becomes more inclusive, clearly identified norms of professionalism become more difficult due to differences in cultural values and practices (Bennett, 2021).

Educators play a key role in the process of developing learners' moral and ethical reasoning processes. There are varieties of ways that moral and ethical situations can be woven into simulation activities, including simulations with overriding issues that have these components embedded in them. Scenarios focusing on specifically complex healthcare issues can include the following:

- care of vulnerable populations
- disclosure of adverse events
- "do not resuscitate" or "allow natural death" orders
- end-of-life care
- genetic and reproductive issues

■ informed consent
■ patient confidentiality

Such simulations can generate critical thinking, enhance communication, and allow for consideration of complex ethical issues from various participants. Participation in a mock ethics committee or in groups focusing on sensitive ethical experiences where learners assume various roles as committee, family members, or healthcare providers is another example of activities that can teach participants about communication-related issues for both medical personnel and families (Sedgwick & Yanicki, 2020). In addition, microethical situations (those involving decisions that are more routine and every day and include things such as poor infection control practices, unsafe or borderline medication administration practices, and/or breaches in confidentiality) can be embedded in a variety of simulation scenarios (Krautscheid, 2017). Discussion of these issues as part of other simulation scenarios can strengthen overall ethical decision-making.

## ▶ SUMMARY

Simulation experiences were created to improve patient safety, enhance professional performance, reduce errors, and improve overall patient outcomes. However, it is extremely important to remember that protection of human rights applies to learners as well. When developing simulation experiences, not only should there be an emphasis on objectives, methods, and outcomes, but healthcare simulation educators must also consider the importance of ethical, legal, and regulatory concerns when developing these experiences.

 ## CASE STUDY 7.1

Review the following case study and answer questions 1 and 2.

The healthcare simulation team is excited to have received funding and equipment and plans to activate a new simulation training center. The interprofessional team has worked tirelessly on developing and coordinating the first simulation scenario that will be piloted this fall with undergraduate students. The scenario's objectives, methods, and outcomes will focus on a failure-to-rescue case. The simulation environment consists of high-fidelity manikins, and learners will be recorded during each session. The team has decided *not* to inform the learners of the recording or that the findings of the scenario will be shared with administrators and could potentially cause the learners to be removed from the program.

1. Reflect on what major ethical, legal, and regulatory implications the simulation training center team has overlooked in their planning phases for the simulation experience.

2. The simulation team wants to try a new product during a simulation scenario. Would the team need to obtain learner consent to participate?

1. A student is participating in a summative simulation activity and has failed in an area that has been identified as a "critical element." It is clearly stated in the testing standards that if a student misses a "critical element," the student must fail the exam. The evaluator is rationalizing that the student's omission is an oversight and therefore the student should not be failed. What is the BEST action for the simulation leader/manager?

   A. Leave it alone as the faculty are the experts
   B. Call in an administrator to lead the discussion about the situation
   C. Inform the evaluator that their behavior will be reported to administration
   D. Discuss the situation, focusing on the potential ramifications if the standards are ignored

2. Participation in ethical simulation experiences is important for healthcare professionals because they can assist students in:

   A. Developing moral reasoning and recognizing professional values
   B. Learning to work out healthcare problems in a neutral way
   C. Focusing on the negative aspects of the healthcare professions
   D. Rationalizing behavior when making moral decisions

3. The simulation educator is completing a summative testing session with students in an educational program. The testing session is about to start, but one of the faculty evaluators is not present due to traffic issues. The faculty member has phoned in and will be at least 60 minutes late. The simulation center leader/manager's BEST decision is to:

   A. Have the students wait until the faculty evaluator arrives
   B. Step in as a substitute evaluator until the faculty member arrives
   C. Call in a substitute faculty evaluator with similar content expertise and training in testing
   D. Inform the students that they will have to return and be tested on a different day

4. A student is participating in a simulation scenario and must give a medication. The correct calculation to give the patient should have been 0.5 mL of the medication but the student drew up and administered 0.6 mL. During debriefing, the student's response is that it was not a big deal because it was only 0.1 more milliliters than the desired dose of the medication. The facilitator's BEST response should be which of the following?

   A. "Well, it was not a critical medication, but next time please be more cautious."
   B. "Any medication error with or without an adverse reaction is ethically important and should be considered serious."
   C. "All medications should be given using the 10 rights of medication administration."
   D. Ignore the student's response because they are embarrassed by the error.

## 1. D) Discuss the situation, focusing on the potential ramifications if the standards are ignored

Discussing the situation is the best alternative in order to understand if the learner and the evaluator know the severity of leaving out a critical element. Involving administrators is not the first step, and reciting and following the policy per se without investigation does not include due process. Ignoring it may not produce the student learning outcomes intended.

## 2. A) Developing moral reasoning and recognizing professional values

It is important to develop moral reasoning and professional values. It does not include rationalization, but does include reflection. It is not always possible to work things out in a neutral manner, and focusing on the negative may not build confidence in students.

## 3. C) Call in a substitute faculty evaluator with similar content expertise and training in testing

The evaluator should be a content expert. Respecting students' time is important and being free to manage the simulation center as the leader is also important. Waiting does not respect students' time and may increase their anxiety. Stepping in decreases the leader's availability to deal with other issues should they arise. Rescheduling should be a last resort because usually there is a lack of time and space.

## 4. B) "Any medication error with or without an adverse reaction is ethically important and should be considered serious."

Reinforcement of the ethical issue that accompanies a mistake is important for students to understand. The error should not be addressed in an embarrassing way, but also cannot be minimized. Using the 10 rights of medication administration should be done for every dose administered.

5. A group of educators is creating an end-of-life scenario. In addition to creating the details about the patient and the family, what other considerations related to designing the simulation are critical to make the scenario appropriate for the participants?

   A. Standards of care and culture of the region should be considered
   B. Skipping the prebrief, as to not disclose the simulation objectives
   C. The scenario must be based on a real-life situation
   D. The scenario must include all healthcare disciplines

6. A student is in the hall discussing the last simulation scenario with their peers. They state that the standardized patient had HIV and was being told for the first time about the disease. The healthcare simulation educator overhears the conversation. The appropriate action by the healthcare simulation educator would be to:

   A. Ask the students to take the conversation into a private room
   B. Call the student who was discussing the patient later and explain that the conversation breached confidentiality
   C. Stop the conversation and explain that it breaches confidentiality
   D. Explain to the students that if it were a real patient this would be a Health Insurance Portability and Accountability Act (HIPAA) violation

7. A healthcare student states that they had a bad day and does not want to participate in the scheduled simulation scenario. The healthcare simulation educator should:

   A. Remind the student of professional expectations
   B. Excuse the student for the day and reschedule
   C. Have the student observe the scenario from the window
   D. Tell the student they can make with a case study

8. The healthcare simulation educator wants to determine the intravenous administration competency level of junior healthcare students and then develop a module for remediation of identified weaknesses. This is an example of:

   A. Summative evaluation
   B. Ongoing assessment
   C. Competency-based simulation
   D. Formative evaluation

### 5. A) Standards of care and culture of the region should be considered

Standards of care and culture are always important in depicting emotionally charged situations. Prebriefing should never be skipped and basing scenarios on real life is good, as is including other disciplines, but both are not necessary.

### 6. C) Stop the conversation and explain that it breaches confidentiality

The conversations should not be allowed to continue. Taking it to a private room continues the HIPAA violation. Calling the student at a later point does not stop the violation. The students should already be aware of what HIPAA is so the faculty member should not have to reexplain the concept.

### 7. A) Remind the student of professional expectations

Professional code of conduct calls for healthcare learners to do their best as a team member. Rescheduling, observing, and completing a case study are not as effective as meeting the learning outcomes as participating with a team. If the student does not have a valid excuse, such as a documented healthcare issue, they should join the simulation scenario.

### 8. D) Formative evaluation

Since there is an option for students to learn to meet the competency, it is formative assessment. It is only ongoing if there are scheduled sessions, while competency-based education includes student-driven assessments. Summative assessments are final and usually provide a grade or a pass/fail designation.

9. Graduates from a healthcare educational program see an advertisement for the educational organization on a billboard with their pictures in it from a simulation experience. The students did not give consent for the pictures to be used as external advertisements. This is an example of:

   A. Fair trade
   B. Extended use of educational material
   C. Lack of consent
   D. Academic freedom

10. An example of a microethical situation embedded in a simulation scenario would be:

    A. Administering the wrong medication to a patient, causing an allergic reaction
    B. Forgetting to wash hands before assisting a patient to the bathroom
    C. Forgetting to identify the patient by two means and just asking their name
    D. Leaving a Foley in all night that was supposed to come out the evening before

### 9.  C) Lack of consent

There should be a written consent to use photographs of a simulation publicly. Using photos without consent is not fair trade, extended use of educational material, or academic freedom. Students usually consent to being videotaped or having their picture taken in a simulation scenario for learning purposes, not advertisements.

### 10.  B) Forgetting to wash hands before assisting a patient to the bathroom

Forgetting to wash hands, the basic of infection control, is a microethical violation. The other violations are more severe because administering the wrong medication produces harm, forgetting two identifiers can cause a wrong patient incident, and leaving a Foley catheter in place for an extended time is a known teratogen.

# REFERENCES

Agency for Healthcare Research and Quality. (2017). *Simulation research*. https://www.ahrq.gov/patient-safety/resources/simulation.html

American Educational Research Association. (2021). *Research ethics*. http://www.aera.net

Bennett, B. (2021). The impact of teaching culture online during COVID-19. *International Social Work, 64*(5), 739–741. https://doi.org/10.1177/00208728211017963

Francis, K. B., Gummerum, M., Ganis, G., Terbeck, S., & Howard, I. S. (2018). Virtual morality in the helping professions: Simulated action and resilience. *British Journal of Psychology, 109*(3), 442–465. https://doi.org/10.1111/bjop.12276

Hovland, C., Milliken, B., & Neiderriter, J. (2021). Interprofessional simulation education and nursing students: Assessing and understanding empathy. *Clinical Simulation in Nursing, 60*, 25–31. https://doi.org/10.1016/j.ecns.2021.07.002

International Nursing Association of Clinical and Simulation Learning Standards Committee, Bowler, F., Klein, M., & Wilford, A. (2021a). Healthcare Simulation Standards of Best Practice™ professional integrity. *Clinical Simulation in Nursing, 58*, 45–48. https://doi.org/10.1016/j.ecns.2021.08.014

International Nursing Association of Clinical and Simulation Learning Standards Committee, McDermott, D., Ludlow, J., Horsley, E., & Meakim, C. (2021b). Healthcare Simulation Standards of Best Practice™ prebriefing: Preparation and briefing. *Clinical Simulation in Nursing, 58*, 9–13. https://doi.org/10.1016/j.ecns.2021.08.008

International Nursing Association of Clinical and Simulation Learning Standards Committee, McMahon, E., Jimenez, F. A., Lawrence, K., & Victor, J. (2021c). Healthcare Simulation Standards of Best Practice™ evaluation of learning and performance. *Clinical Simulation in Nursing, 58*, 54–56. https://doi.org/10.1016/j.ecns.2021.08.016

Johns Hopkins University of Medicine. (2021). *Coronavirus resource center-vaccine research and development*. https://coronavirus.jhu.edu/vaccines/timeline

Krautscheid, L. C. (2017). Embedding microethical dilemmas in high-fidelity simulation scenarios: Preparing nursing students for ethical practice. *Journal of Nursing Education, 56*(1), 55–58. https://doi.org/10.3928/01484834-20161219-11

Lioce, L. (Ed.)., Lopreiato, J. (Founding Ed.)., Downing, D., Chang, T. P., Robertson, J. M., Anderson, M., Diaz, D. A., Spain, A. E. (Assoc. Eds.), & the Terminology and Concepts Working Group. (2020, September). Healthcare simulation dictionary. *Agency for Healthcare Research and Quality (AHRQ)* (2nd ed.). AHRQ. https://www.ssih.org/Portals/48/sim-dictionary-2_1.pdf

Meakim, C. H., & Rockstraw, L. J. (2018). Lights, camera, action! The process of evaluating, acquiring, and implementing an audiovisual capturing solution to enhance learning. In S. Hertzel Campbell & K. M. Daley (Eds.), *Simulation scenarios for nurse educators: Making it real* (3rd ed.; p. 61–78). Springer Publishing Company.

Mohamed, E., Harvey, G., & Kilfoil, L. (2021). Pre-brief in simulation-based experiences: A scoping review of the literature. *Clinical Simulation in Nursing, 61*, 86–95. https://doi.org/10.1016/j.ecns.2021.08.003

Rushton, C. H., Swoboda, S. M., Reller, N., Skarupski, K. A., Prizzi, M., Young, P. D., & Hanson, G. C. (2021). Mindful ethical practice and resilience academy: Equipping nurses to address ethical challenges. *American Journal of Critical Care: An Official Publication, American Association of Critical-Care Nurses, 30*(1), e1–e11. https://doi.org/10.4037/ajcc2021359

Sedgwick, M., & Yanicki, S. (2020). Teaching how to practice ethics during simulation: Exploring clinical nurse educators' experiences. *Clinical Simulation in Nursing, 47*, 57–59. http://doi.org/10.1016/j.ecns.2020.07.009

Skloot, R. (2010). *The immortal life of Henrietta Lacks*. Broadway Paperbacks, Random House.

Society for Simulation in Healthcare. (2021). *Certified healthcare simulation educator handbook.* https://www.ssih.org/Portals/48/Certification/CHSE_Docs/CHSE%20Handbook.pdf

Sweeney, N. L., Rollins, M. C., Gantt, L., Swanson, M., & Ravitz, J. (2020). Development and reliability testing of the Sweeney-Clark simulation evaluation rubric©. *Clinical Simulation in Nursing, 41,* 22–32. https://doi.org/10.1016/j.ecns.2019.04.002

Wibawa, T. (2021). COVID-19 vaccine research and development: Ethical issues. *Tropical Medicine & International Health: TM & IH, 26*(1), 14–19. https://doi.org/10.1111/tmi.13503

# PART III
## Healthcare and Simulation Knowledge/ Principles

# Human Patient Simulator Simulation

Carol Okupniak

*Simulation is fiction—your decisions are real.*

*—John Cornele*

This chapter addresses Domain II: Healthcare and Simulation Knowledge/Principles (Society for Simulation in Healthcare [SSH], 2021).

## ▶ LEARNING OUTCOMES

- Discuss the principles of human simulator simulation learning in healthcare education.
- Describe the variety of methodologies for the use of human simulator simulation.
- Integrate the principles of interprofessional teamwork.

## ▶ INTRODUCTION

When considering the incorporation of human simulator simulations in the education of healthcare professionals, it is important to understand the principles, practice, and methodologies necessary for a successful simulation experience. Included in this understanding is knowledge of the relationship between the learner and the environment and how healthcare decisions will be assessed and evaluated. When using human simulators as an educational tool, the designer of the simulation scenario incorporates learning methodologies into the process of planning, implementation, and evaluation of the learning that takes place with human simulator simulation experiences. There are many outcomes that can be measured using simulation. Among them are technical and nontechnical skills, as well as the ability to assess human behavior (Santomauro et al., 2020).

## ▶ SIMULATION PRINCIPLES

### SIMULATION-BASED LEARNING

Simulation-based learning (SBL) provides a real-life scenario in an accurate setting where participants respond as they would in an actual event. Many healthcare institutions and academic settings are using SBL to educate and evaluate healthcare professionals and those in educational programs to become future healthcare professionals. SBL includes three stages.

- In the first stage, the participant receives information from the facilitator about the scenario, discovers the objectives of the simulation, what their role will be, and other necessary information.

- In the second stage, the participant actively engages in the simulation.
- In the third stage, debriefing, participants share their experience, emotions, and actions (Kaldheim et al., 2021).

In addition to task and technical skills, SBL can also be used to identify problem-solving and decision-making skills. Sarfati et al. (2019) found that SBL can help prevent medication errors if the key elements of scenario design, debriefing, and assessment of perception are clearly identified. Team education, communication, and interpersonal skills are evaluated during SBL. To use simulation effectively, sound teaching–learning principles are needed. Without sound principles and planning, adverse consequences can easily occur during a simulation experience. Some common problems identified during simulation scenarios involving teams include:

- a group that does not understand that each team member has a unique role
- lack of clear role definition resulting in role confusion
- no plan in place to use when mistakes or errors occur
- no method to measure individual or team performance

The success of using simulator scenarios to educate healthcare professionals should be measured in relationship to the improvement in clinical competence and the potential or actual impact on patient safety and outcomes. It is important to evaluate team performance during simulations, not just individual demonstration of knowledge, skills, and attitudes (Son, 2021).

## DELIBERATE PRACTICE

Using human simulator experiences gives the learner an opportunity to practice and acquire clinical skills without causing patient harm (Hanshaw & Dickerson, 2020). A core principle of human simulator education is the concept of *deliberate practice* (*DP*). *DP* is defined as a learner's endeavor to practice for the purpose of improving a task or skill beyond the current level of proficiency (Gonzalez & Kardong-Edgren, 2017).

Using the concept of DP, simulation can improve the effectiveness of the learning experience. An integral component of DP is *critical reflection*. A student must recognize a deficit in knowledge in an effort to seek learning opportunities to narrow this gap in knowledge. With the assistance of a healthcare simulation educator, the learner becomes actively engaged in practicing and improving a task, skill, or decision-making process. When a learner engages in DP, feedback from the healthcare simulation educator is necessary to communicate improvement in learner' skill acquisition and retention (Johnson et al., 2020).

## TEAM TRAINING

Similar to a real clinical environment, human simulator scenarios often include a small group of participants rather than just an individual learner. Understanding the role of each member of the healthcare team and knowing when to delegate are the goals of building teams (Jones et al., 2020). Knowing how to incorporzate the principles of team education and crisis resource management (CRM) into a scenario involving more than one learner builds this competency. The first step in team education in simulation is to articulate the specific competencies targeted toward acquiring team-building skills. Once these competencies are recognized, a level of measurement can be calculated to guide the debriefing process.

Using simulation to educate healthcare teams can help replicate conditions where a mix of professionals can practice and learn from each other. Interprofessional simulation can facilitate interaction among members to develop teamworking and communication skills. By practicing together, each participant will have a better understanding of each other's roles and responsibilities. Learners can use this opportunity to develop a professional identity and participate in shared decision-making (Astbury et al., 2021).

### Evidence-Based Simulation Practice 8.1

Badowski and Oosterhouse (2017) completed a quasi-experimental pretest/posttest design where a simulation-based, peer-coached, deliberate practice clinical substitution was implemented to compare nursing students' knowledge, skills, and attitudes in promoting safety. The results demonstrated improved knowledge and skill acquisition in the intervention and control groups. There was a trend toward improved team communication attitudes and skill performance.

Team learning principles can be applied with a team of students from the same discipline or an interprofessional group using human simulator education. The Agency for Healthcare Research and Quality (AHRQ) developed a framework for building teams: Team Strategies and Tools to Enhance Performance and Patient Safety (TeamSTEPPS; AHRQ, 2019). This process of team training is designed for healthcare professionals to improve patient safety and achieve better patient outcomes. Simulation aids in the acquisition of team skills by allowing the learner to practice in a simulated, safe environment. Using TeamSTEPPS in simulation is one way to aid in the design, measurement of objectives, and evaluation of team training (Table 8.1).

**Table 8.1 Components of Team Training in Human Simulator Simulations**

| | |
|---|---|
| Leadership | Members delegate tasks to other team members, plan, organize, and motivate other team members. |
| Peer observation | Members have a shared understanding of group dynamics and team roles and are able to recognize errors and openly communicate ideas and suggestions for correction. |
| Flexibility | Members are able to adapt or change as the scenario unfolds or the group dynamics change. |
| Group membership | Members recognize that the work of the team is paramount and individual goals are secondary. |
| Balance | The workload of all team members should be balanced and match the knowledge and skills of each individual. |
| Trust | An atmosphere of mutual trust should exist in which individuals are able to share knowledge and speak about errors in judgment and action and accept constructive feedback. |
| Communication | All members of the team are able to openly communicate, confirm that their message was heard and understood, and clarify the message if necessary. |

### Simulation Teaching Tip 8.1

If at all possible, when assigning learners to teams, make every team diverse. Diversity in race, gender, as well as role should be considered for every interprofessional team in order to teach cultural awareness and sensitivity as well as group collaboration.

Within TeamSTEPPS training is a principle known as *CUS*, which stands for:

- "I am **c**oncerned!
- I am **u**ncomfortable!
- This is a **s**afety issue!" (AHRQ, 2019)

The purpose of CUS is to empower individuals to speak up if they are concerned about an actual or potential breach in safety. Included in the CUS course of action is a two-challenge rule (AHRQ, 2019). Under this rule, if individuals feel that their concern has not been recognized:

■ They should verbalize this concern at least twice. If, after the second exchange, the team member concludes that the response is not acceptable, the team member is expected to take a different, more assertive course.
■ This alternate course may include following the chain of command to ensure a safe environment.

The CUS rule can be employed during a simulation scenario and measured as part of the evaluation criteria.

## CRISIS RESOURCE MANAGEMENT

Another method of assessing teams is through the process of CRM. When CRM began in the aviation industry, it was originally called *crew resource management*. The principles of CRM have been incorporated into the training of healthcare professionals. Healthcare teams can be large, composed of members with diverse skill sets, responsibilities, and actions (Orasanu & Fischer, 2017). The key principles of CRM are:

■ Have a clear leader and well-defined roles.
■ Value input from all resources and personnel.
■ Have a plan and share and adapt the plan as needed.
■ Request help early.
■ Distribute the work and support all members of the team.
■ Prioritize and delegate tasks to others.
■ Give everyone the right to be assertive and to speak up.
■ Have timely, specific, and constructive communication. (Wakeman & Langham, 2018)

Using the principles of CRM within a simulation scenario will help the team perform in a coordinated and efficient manner during the care of a simulated patient.

## CLOSED-LOOP COMMUNICATION

When communicating to members of the team during simulations, it is imperative that each individual's message is heard and understood. *Closed-loop* communication is a method of communication in which there is a sender and a receiver of a specific message (Exhibit 8.1). Employing a closed-loop communication aids the coordination of care, confirming to the sender that the message was received (Helmig et al., 2020).

### EXHIBIT 8.1 CLOSED-LOOP COMMUNICATION

■ A sender delivers a message to a receiver.
■ The receiver of the message acknowledges that the message was received and ascribes meaning to the message.
■ The sender communicates with the receiver to ensure that the expected meaning was conferred through the message.
■ If the sender does not feel that the message was interpreted as intended, the conversation continues until the loop is closed.

## SBAR COMMUNICATION

The acronym SBAR stands for introduction, situation, background, assessment, and recommendation. SBAR communication is an organized, structured method of two-way communication in a healthcare setting. The person conferring the information provides the following:

- ▦ S: a short, but relevant summary of the current situation
- ▦ B: the patient's background relevant to the information exchange
- ▦ A: important assessment findings
- ▦ R: a recommendation for action on the part of the receiver of the information

Healthcare providers must effectively and accurately communicate patient information. Using SBAR to communicate during simulation scenarios can improve the clarity of communication and give the learner an opportunity to practice this important skill (Stevens et al., 2020).

## ▶ SIMULATION METHODOLOGY

### EXPERIENTIAL LEARNING

A methodology is the theoretical analysis of the body of methods and principles associated with a body of knowledge. Kolb's model of experiential learning is often applied to simulation learning (Kolb & Fry, 1975). Kolb's model places the learner into one of four steps: concrete experience, reflective observation, abstract conceptualization, and active experimentation (Secheresse et al., 2020).

- ▦ *Concrete experience:* The learner will experience the situation by doing.
- ▦ *Reflective observation:* The learner will review the experience on a personal basis by thinking about what they did.
- ▦ *Abstract conceptualization:* The learner will form abstract concepts that can be used in future experiences.
- ▦ *Active experimentation:* The learner can apply what was learned in the previous steps.

Experiential learning requires the learner to develop competence over time through the practice of experiential learning (Kuraoka, 2018). Inherent within the concept of experiential learning is how experience contributes to the process of learning. For learning to occur, it is imperative that there is active participation, with reflection on the decisions made. In simulations, experiences are artificially constructed with the purpose of eliciting defined outcomes. Learning takes place through the simulation experience, during the debriefing process, and when participants conceptualize events and become involved in decision-making (Koivisto et al., 2017).

Because the learners are living the experience during simulation, they are able to increase their engagement. Due to the reality of the setting, the learners are more engaged and interact more fully in the activity. The goal of experiential learning is to gain new knowledge and understanding of key concepts or principles. During experiential learning, learners are asked to perform within a defined role in an activity that has context and meaning for them.

### ADULT LEARNING

Simulation is a technique that uses guided experience to replicate the real world in a manner that is thoroughly interactive. Adult learners practice the concepts of andragogy (teaching of adults) in the simulation environment. Knowles (1950) developed the concept of andragogy.

Adult learners are self-directed and independent and consider that they are responsible for their own learning. Adult learners also have experience and previously learned knowledge that can be used as a resource for future learning (Sanchez, 2017). Ensuring a proper environment for learning is another principle of adult learning. This is also the basis of using simulation to educate healthcare professionals.

Because simulation allows adults to practice skills and behaviors in a team environment, it has the ability to motivate adults to learn (Sarikoc et al., 2017). Adult learners expect their performance is confidential after a simulation is concluded. This is especially challenging when both the simulation and the debriefing are group experiences. The simulation educator, while providing a safe, rich learning environment, must maintain respect and support for the adult learner during simulation and maintain the confidentiality of all involved. In addition, the participants of the simulation must also respect the need to maintain confidentiality of the actions during the simulation scenario and debriefing to protect the privacy of all participants.

There are additional concepts related to adult learners not originally considered by Knowles (1950). Not all adults learn in the same way. Learning is situation-specific and there are many factors that affect the adult learner. One important factor in adult learning is how a person's culture affects learning and professional growth (Bleich, 2017). It is also assumed that adults experience information overload and are not capable of additional learning. In addition to teaching tasks, simulation andragogy can also be used to develop interpersonal relationships such as empathy, which is linked to caring, compassion, kindness, and responsiveness (Simko et al., 2021). The challenge for educators using simulation is to convey the importance and value of the experience for the adult learner.

## SITUATIONAL AWARENESS

*Situational awareness* is comprised of three parts

- gathering information from the environment,
- synthesizing, interpreting, and prioritizing the current system, and
- predicting and planning for future events (Rosenman et al., 2018).

This shared cognizance helps each team member to see the larger picture during a simulation scenario rather than concentrating only on an individual task. When situational awareness is employed during a scenario, all team members are kept informed and updated on the plan of care and all new developments in patient status. Ensuring that the learner is oriented to the simulation environment will contribute to a successful encounter (Robertiello et al., 2021).

## RAPID-CYCLE DELIBERATE PRACTICE

A novel approach to simulation learning is a methodology termed *rapid-cycle deliberate practice*. This process allows the learner to complete a simulation, receive immediate feedback, and continue to practice until mastery is achieved (Ozkara, 2021). Rapid-cycle DP can also be used in simulation to practice increasingly more challenging skills, with the facilitator giving immediate feedback with short debriefing and a pause and rewind technique within the scenario (Chancey et al., 2019).

## ▶ LOW- TO HIGH-FIDELITY SIMULATION

The concept of simulation is not new in medical education. However, the use of high-fidelity simulators in healthcare provider education has been a relatively new phenomenon. *Fidelity* is the measure to which the simulator or the simulation matches the real environment the scenario is attempting to simulate. Fidelity in simulation can include an array of approaches, from role-play to complex manikins with advanced physiology (Roberts & Cooper, 2019). Task trainers and low-, medium-, and high-fidelity manikins all have an established place in medical education (Scott & Gartner, 2019). Due to significant advancements in simulator technology, it is now possible to create a simulated environment using many simulation strategies to construct a setting very close to the real world. Today's high-fidelity manikins are capable of a multitude of physiologic functions. In addition to manikin fidelity, there is also physical, functional, psychological, and task fidelity which adds to the realism for the learner. High-fidelity simulations can be more resource-intensive and costly (Diaz et al., 2021).

Current high-fidelity manikins are available in models representing different stages of the life span, from fetal and neonatal through adult. High-fidelity manikins can be used for specific tasks, such as central line placement, while whole-body manikins can be used to respond with complex, multisystem, physiologic adaptation to the learner's actions or inactions. Advancement in the science of designing high-fidelity human simulators continues as technology improves. What is available today may seem primitive in only a few years as advancements in computerization, robotics, and materials science improve our ability to create a more realistic human simulator.

## Evidence-Based Simulation Practice 8.2

Landy et al. (2019) conducted a qualitative study exploring caregivers' perceptions of simulation-based education (SBE) in the care of a child with tracheostomy. The study found that caregivers preferred high physical fidelity in SBE and believed it influenced engagement during the experience.

## FUNCTIONAL FIDELITY

*Functional fidelity* is the degree of accuracy in the operation of the simulated system. When operating a computerized, high-fidelity manikin, the physiologic manifestations should be as close as possible to how a real person would respond. Responses to medication administration, oxygen delivery, and other treatments should be manifested in the manikin as in a real human. An important consideration is the training of the simulator operator. Adequate training is imperative to be able to present a manikin with high-function fidelity to the learner. Participants initially perceive the manikin as a technically based nonhuman. As the simulation progresses, the reality of the scenario improves and the responses become more meaningful as the participants interact with other people and objects within the environment. Learners who are socially engaged during the simulation are more likely to perceive what is being represented as real (Schoenherr & Hamstra, 2017).

## TASK FIDELITY

*Task fidelity* is the measure of how authentic the simulated task is compared with the real task. It is important to match the task with the knowledge of the learner. During simulation, learners should not be expected to perform a task for which they have not been educated or that is outside of their scope of practice. Using complex high-fidelity simulators to educate a novice in basic skills is not necessary when a less complex simulator may be more appropriate (Alconero-Camarero et al., 2021). When using a simulator to learn a skill, task fidelity should be very close to what the learner will experience within a real setting to avoid transfer of negative motor skills and to promote transfer of positive motor skills.

## PHYSICAL FIDELITY

*Physical fidelity* refers to the environment where the simulation takes place. This includes the visual, auditory, kinesthetic or tactile, and spatial surroundings. When able, the setting should resemble real clinical structures as closely as possible. Equipment and furnishings within the setting should be fully functioning. Attention to detail is an important part of physical fidelity. Some simulation centers take every aspect of the physical environment into consideration when preparing for a simulation scenario. Changing the room temperature, changing time on the clocks, and adding authentic odors are some examples of increasing the physical fidelity of a simulation scenario.

## PSYCHOLOGICAL FIDELITY

*Psychological fidelity* is the degree to which the educational situation evokes the same psychological conditions that would be present in a real clinical setting (Fritúz et al., 2018). This aspect of simulation fidelity is not always easy to secure. Simulations ask the learner to forget temporarily that the scenario is not real and engage in the activity, believing in its authenticity. It can take great effort to plan the physical, functional, and task fidelity, but it is up to the learner to consider the psychological fidelity of the scenario.

 CASE STUDY 8.1

The healthcare simulation educator is running an interprofessional high-fidelity simulation experience that involves learners of medicine, nursing, respiratory therapy, and unlicensed assistive personnel (UAP). The scenario involves a patient with sepsis whose respiratory and circulatory status is declining to the point of circulatory collapse, and a "code" is initiated. During the code, the medical learner shouts orders to the other members and the nursing learners who are having difficulty finding the equipment in the "code cart" where it should be. The respiratory therapist is asking for guidance as to what they should be doing for the team effort. The UAP is recording the times of events. If you were the Certified Healthcare Simulation Educator™, how would you handle this situation? What aspects of team collaboration need to be emphasized? How would you prepare the next interprofessional team for the simulation experience?

1. Which of the following is the MOST common problem identified during simulation-based education involving teams?

   **A.** Active engagement by all team members
   **B.** Inexperienced simulation operators
   **C.** Limited physical fidelity
   **D.** Lack of clear role identification

2. Which student is participating in a rapid-cycle deliberate practice? A student who is:

   **A.** Reflecting on their mistakes and trying again
   **B.** Repeating chest compressions until the correct depth is achieved
   **C.** Reading up on the task that they are about to perform
   **D.** Discussing how to improve the task with the healthcare simulation educator

3. The student understands the goal of crisis resource management when they state:

   **A.** "I should keep trying to figure out the correct patient intervention."
   **B.** "The team members need to provide each other with direction, and I will do the intervention."
   **C.** "I should request help as soon as possible when a serious situation occurs."
   **D.** "I should flex my role during a serious situation and do what is needed."

4. The healthcare simulation educator realizes a student incorporated the Team Strategies and Tools to Enhance Performance and Patient Safety (TeamSTEPPS) during a simulation when they make which of the following statements after the simulation?

   **A.** "When I become uneasy about an intervention being done, I will say something."
   **B.** "My only role is to remain at the bedside and calm the patient and family members."
   **C.** "Patient safety includes both physical and psychological safety."
   **D.** "Understanding CUS provides me with more autonomy as a practitioner."

5. During a simulation scenario, a team member contacts the patient's provider, gives a summary of the patient's current condition, a brief healthcare history of the patient, pertinent evaluation, and requests a medication order. This is an example of:

   **A.** SBAR communication
   **B.** Reflective practice communication
   **C.** Team Strategies and Tools to Enhance Performance and Patient Safety (TeamSTEPPS) communication
   **D.** Closed-loop communication

## 1. D) Lack of clear role identification

Clear role identification is needed for teams to work well together and not overlap or exclude needed patient interventions; this is the most common problem and the one that team simulations are trying to overcome. All members should be actively engaged, there should be fidelity, and the simulation operator should have experience; however, lack of experience should not disrupt healthcare roles.

## 2. B) Repeating chest compressions until the correct depth is achieved

Rapid-cycle deliberate practice allows students to receive immediate feedback and practice until competency is achieved. Reflection, reading, and discussing do not provide the practice needed for competency mastery.

## 3. C) "I should request help as soon as possible when a serious situation occurs."

The goal of crisis resource management is to recognize serious situations and react. It is not trying to decide alone on the correct intervention or being provided with direction. Flexing roles is sometimes needed but not the goal and healthcare providers still must stay within their scope of practice.

## 4. D) "Understanding CUS provides me with more autonomy as a practitioner."

CUS (concerned, uncomfortable, safety issue) is used in TeamSTEPPS and is a method used to identify if something is wrong in a patient situation and speaking up about what is possibly wrong. Saying that you are uneasy in a situation and remaining calm are good attributes but not specific to TeamSTEPPS. Understanding the concept of patient safety is also important but not a concept specifically of TeamSTEPPS.

## 5. A) SBAR communication

This communication follows the SBAR pattern. It provides the summary, background, assessment, and recommendation. This example does not fit the modality of reflective practice, TeamSTEPPS, or closed-loop communication.

6. The student is demonstrating the proper method of using closed-loop communication in a simulation scenario when they state:

   A. "I know you can give me an order to help."
   B. "Let me repeat back what you ordered . . ."
   C. "The past health history of this patient includes all of the following . . ."
   D. "The referrals made so far for this patient's discharge are . . ."

7. A simulated arm with a tactile response that mirrors the actual insertion of an intravenous catheter is an example of which kind of fidelity?

   A. Physical fidelity
   B. Functional fidelity
   C. Task fidelity
   D. Psychological fidelity

8. According to Kolb, what step would a learner be at if they revealed to the simulation educator that they would do the intervention differently?

   A. Concrete experience
   B. Reflective observation
   C. Abstract conceptualization
   D. Active experimentation

9. The healthcare simulation educator allows a learner to repeat a procedure as many times as they would like until they feel as though they have mastered the skill. Studies demonstrate that deliberate practice assists students in:

   A. Memorizing procedures
   B. Providing efficient patient care
   C. Increasing self-confidence
   D. Decreasing healthcare errors

10. Adult learners have specific needs. One such need is:

    A. Professional growth
    B. Past experiences
    C. Sharing experiences
    D. Memorizing procedures

*(See answers next page.)*

## 6. B) "Let me repeat back what you ordered . . ."

Closed-loop communication provides a read or repeat back. Knowing that a practitioner is capable of providing an order to assist is not a closed-loop communication. Stating the history of a patient is just telling another something, as is telling another that referrals have been made.

## 7. A) Physical fidelity

Physical fidelity includes something that can be touched or manipulated, which simulates a real hands-on experience. Functional fidelity has to do with how a piece of equipment works and its durability. Task fidelity usually refers to a part-task trainer that is made so practitioners can become competent in a single noncomplex task. Psychological fidelity includes the environment, culture, and social awareness of the simulation event.

## 8. B) Reflective observation

The student has reflected on what they did during simulation and understands that they can change to improve; this would be reflective observation since they have reflected on what they did and what they can change. In concrete experiences, the learner will experience the situation by doing. In the abstract conceptualization step, the learner will form abstract concepts that can be used in future experiences. In the active experimentation step, the learner can apply what was learned in the previous steps.

## 9. C) Increasing self-confidence

Deliberate practice (DP) assists students in building confidence. Studies have not demonstrated that it is just memorization or that patient care outcomes are positively affected. DP does not promote memorization or efficient patient care as an outcome. DP has not yet been shown to reduce healthcare errors.

## 10. A) Professional growth

Adult learners need professional growth in their healthcare role. They do not need memorization of procedures because they prefer to know why they are learning or doing something and how it applies. Their past experiences are not their need because they already had them and are applying their knowledge to the new competencies they are learning. Sharing experiences may be helpful, but adult learners are focused on what they need to know.

# REFERENCES

Agency for Healthcare Research and Quality. (2019). *TeamSTEPPS®: About TeamSTEPPS*. https://www.ahrq.gov/teamstepps/about-teamstepps/index.html

Alconero-Camarero, A. R., Sarabia-Cobo, C. M., Catalán-Piris, M. J., González-Gómez, S., & González-Lopez, J. R. (2021). Nursing students' satisfaction: A comparison between medium-and high-fidelity simulation training. *International Journal of Environmental Research and Public Health, 18*(2), 1–11. https://doi.org/10.2290/ijerph18020804

Astbury, J., Ferguson, J., Silverthorne, J., Willis, S., & Schafheutle, E. (2021). High-fidelity simulation-based education in pre-registration healthcare programmes: A systematic review of reviews to inform collaborative and interprofessional best practice. *Journal of Interprofessional Care, 35*(4), 622–632. https://doi.org/10.1080/13561820.2020.1762551

Badowski, D. M., & Oosterhouse, K. J. (2017). Impact of a simulated clinical day with peer coaching and deliberate practice: Promoting a culture of safety. *Nursing Education Perspectives, 38*(2), 93–95. https://doi.org/10.1097/01.NEP.0000000000000108

Bleich, M. (2017). Reducing stereotyping when developing leaders. *Journal of Continuing Education in Nursing, 48*(11), 492–493. https://doi.org/10.3928/00220124-20171017-04

Chancey, R. J., Sampayo, E. M., Lemke, D. S., & Doughty, C. B. (2019). Learners' experience during rapid cycle deliberate practice simulations: A qualitative analysis. *Simulation in Healthcare: Journal of the Society for Medical Simulation, 14*(1), 18–28. https://doi.org/10.1097/SIH.0000000000000324

Diaz, D., Anderson, M., Hill, P., Quelly, S., Clark, K., & Lynn, M. (2021). Comparison of clinical options: High fidelity-based and virtual simulation. *Nurse Educator, 46*(3), 149–153. https://doi.org/10.1097/NNE.0000000000000906

Fritúz, G., Blaskó, Á., Kasos, K., Varga, K., Eke, C., & Gál, J. (2018). Comparison of psychological fidelity of drama and simulation based medical education (DSBME) and simulation based medical education (SBME)—A study design. *Resuscitation, 130*, e85–e85. https://doi.org/10.1016/j.resuscitation.2018.07.175

Gonzalez, L., & Kardong-Edgren, S. (2017). Deliberate practice for mastery learning in nursing. *Clinical Simulation in Nursing, 13*(1), 10–14. https://doi.org/10.1016/j.ecns.2016.10.005

Hanshaw, S. L., & Dickerson, S. S. (2020). High fidelity simulation evaluation studies in nursing education: A review of the literature. *Nurse Education in Practice, 46*, 102818–102818. https://doi.org/10.1016/j.nepr.2020.102818

Helmig, S., Cox, J., Mehta, B., Burlison, J., Morgan, J., & Russo, C. (2020). Handoff communication between remote healthcare facilities. *Pediatric Quality & Safety, 5*(2), e269. https://doi.org/10.1097%2Fpq9.0000000000000269

Johnson, C. E., Kimble, L. P., Gunby, S. S., & Davis, A. H. (2020). Using deliberate practice and simulation for psychomotor skill competency acquisition and retention: A mixed-methods study. *Nurse Educator, 45*(3), 150–154. https//doi.org/10.1097/NNE.0000000000000713

Jones, E. P., Brennen, E. A., & Davis, A. (2020). Evaluation of literature searching and article selection skills of an evidence-based practice team. *Journal of the Medical Library Association,* 1–17. https://doi.org/10.5195/jmla.2020.865

Kaldheim, H. K. A., Fossum, M., Munday, J., Johnsen, K. M. F., & Slettebø, Å. (2021). A qualitative study of perioperative nursing student's experiences of interprofessional simulation-based learning. *Journal of Clinical Nursing, 30*(1–2), 174–187. https://doi.org/10.1111/jocn.15535

Knowles, M. S. (1950). *Informal adult education: A guide for administrators, leaders, and teachers*. Association Press.

Koivisto, J. M., Niemi, H., Multisilta, J., & Eriksson, E. (2017). Nursing students' experiential learning process using an online 3D simulation game. *Education Information Technology, 22*, 383–398. https://doi.org/10.1007/s10639-015-9453-x

Kolb, D. A., & Fry, R. (1975). Toward an applied theory of experiential learning. In C. Cooper (Ed.), *Theories of group process*. John Wiley.

Kuraoka, Y. (2018). Effect of an experiential learning-based programme to foster competence among nurse managers. *Journal of Nursing Management, 26*(8), 1015–1023. https://doi.org/10.1111/jonm .12628

Landy, P., Ngo, Q., & Leung, J. (2019). 53 experiences and perceptions of fidelity in simulation-based education administered to caregivers. *Paediatrics & Child Health, 24*(Suppl. 2), e21. https://doi .org/10.1093/pch/pxz066.052

Orasanu, J., & Fisher, U. (2017). Improving healthcare communication: Lessons from the flightdeck. In C. P. Nemeth (Ed.), *Improving healthcare team communication: Building on lessons from aviation and aerospace* (1st ed.). Taylor and Francis.

Ozkara San, E., Maneval, R., & Myers, P. (2021). Incorporating rapid cycle deliberate practice cardiac arrest simulation program into nursing staff continuing professional development. *Journal of Continuing Education, 52*(6), 274–279. https;//doi.org/10.3928/00220124-20210514-06

Robertiello, G., Genee, J., & Marrera, A. (2021). Escape the sim! An escape room innovation to orient learners to the simulation environment. *Nursing Education Perspectives, 42*(3), 195–196. https://doi .org/10.1097/01.NEP.0000000000000585

Roberts, F., & Cooper, K. (2019). Effectiveness of high fidelity simulation versus low fidelity simulation on practical/clinical skill development in pre-registration physiotherapy students: A systematic review. *JBI Database of Systematic Reviews and Implementation Reports, 17*(6), 1229–1255. https://doi .org/10.11124/JBISRIR-2017-00931

Rosenman, E. D., Dixon, A. J., Webb, J. M., Brolliar, S., Golden, S. J., Jones, K. A., Shah, S., Grand, J. A., Kozlowski, S. W. J., Chao, G. T., Fernandez, R., & Cloutier, R. (2018). A simulation-based approach to measuring team situational awareness in emergency medicine: A multicenter, observational study. *Academic Emergency Medicine, 25*(2), 196–204. https://doi.org/10.1111/acem.13257

Sanchez, L. M. (2017). The power of 3: Using adult learning principles to facilitate patient education. *Nursing, 47*(2), 17–19. https://doi.org/10.1097/01.NURSE.0000511819.18774.85

Santomauro, C. M., Hill, A., McCurdie, T., & McGlashan, H. L. (2020). Improving the quality of evaluation data in simulation-based healthcare improvement projects. *Simulation in Healthcare: The Journal of the Society for Simulation in Healthcare, 15*(5), 341–355. https://doi.org/10.1097/SIH.00000000000 00442

Sarfati, L., Ranchon, F., Vantard, N., Schwiertz, V., Larbre, V., Parat, S., Faudel, A., & Rioufol, C. (2019). Human-simulation-based learning to prevent medication error: A systematic review. *Journal of Evaluation in Clinical Practice, 25*(1), 11–20. https://doi.org/10.1111/jep.12883

Sarikoc, G., Ozcan, C. T., & Elcin, M. (2017). The impact of using standardized patients in psychiatric cases on the levels of motivation and perceived learning of the nursing students. *Nurse Education Today, 51*, 15–22. https://doi.org/10.1016/j.nedt.2017.01.001

Schoenherr, J. R., & Hamstra, S. J. (2017). Beyond fidelity: Deconstructing the seductive simplicity of fidelity in simulator-based education in the health care professions. *Simulation in Healthcare: Journal of the Society for Medical Simulation, 12*(2), 117–123. https://doi.org/10.1097/SIH.0000000000000226

Scott, A., & Gartner, A. (2019). Low fidelity simulation in a high fidelity world. *Postgraduate Medical Journal, 95*(1130), 687–688. https://doi.org/10.1136/postgradmedj-2019-FPM.9

Secheresse, T., Pansu, P., & Lima, L. (2020). The impact of full-scale simulation training based on Kilb's learning cycle on medical prehospital emergency teams: A multilevel assessment study. *Simulation in Healthcare: The Journal of the Society for Simulation in Healthcare, 15*(5), 335–340. https://doi.org/ 10.1097/SIH.0000000000000461

Simko, L. C., Rhodes, D. C., Gumireddy, A., Schreiber, J., Booth, A., & Hawkins, M. (2021). Effects of a chronic pain simulation empathy training kit on the empathy of interprofessional healthcare students for chronic pain patients. *Clinical Simulation in Nursing, 56*, 66–75. https://doi.org/10.1016/ j.ecns.2021.04.003

Society for Simulation in Healthcare. (2021). *Certified healthcare simulation educator handbook*. https:// www.ssih.org/Portals/48/Certification/CHSE_Docs/CHSE%20Handbook.pdf

Son, H. K. (2021). The effects of simulation problem-based learning on the empathy, attitudes toward caring for the elderly, and team efficacy of undergraduate health profession students. *International Journal of Environmental Research and Public Health, 18*(18), 9658. https://doi.org/10.3390/ijerph181 8658

Stevens, N., McNiesh, S., & Goyal, D. (2020). Utilizing an SBAR workshop with baccalaureate nursing students to improve communication skills. *Nursing Education Perspectives*, *41*(2), 117–118. https://doi.org/10.1097/01.NEP.0000000000000518

Wakeman, D., & Langham, M. R. (2018). Creating a safer operating room: Groups, team dynamics and crew resource management principles. *Seminars in Pediatric Surgery*, *27*(2), 107–113. https://doi.org/10.1053/j.sempedsurg.2018.02.008

# Moulage in Simulation

John T. Cornele and Linda Wilson

*Start by doing what's necessary; then do what's possible; and suddenly you are doing the impossible.*

—*Saint Francis of Assisi*

This chapter addresses Domain II: Healthcare and Simulation Knowledge/Principles (Society for Simulation in Healthcare [SSH], 2021).

## ▶ LEARNING OUTCOMES

- Discuss the value of realism and the use of moulage in simulation.
- Discuss the relationship between fidelity, realism, and an effective learning environment.
- Describe the established methods of creating simulated injuries and medical conditions.
- Discuss the sources of moulage materials and the possibilities of adding moulage to simulation sessions.

## ▶ INTRODUCTION

*Moulage* is a French term that means casting or molding; today, it is the art of applying mock injuries for the purpose of training healthcare personnel. The formal practice dates back to the 18th century, when wax figures and castings of body parts were used for this purpose (Riva et al., 2010). The concept of using models in education can also be seen in early Greek culture. Thus, the use of simulated injuries and illnesses, or moulage, to educate healthcare practitioners is not new; however, its utilization in modern education is expanding.

This chapter provides an overview of moulage and its use in casualty and illness simulation. The chapter discusses makeup as well as an indication of the educational basis for its choice as a tool to use in simulation. Several broad areas are addressed, covering ideas involving the use of moulage in specific situations, with human patient simulators (HPS) or manikins and with standardized patients (SPs), setting the stage by adding props and standardized participants (confederates), and some of the specific techniques as well as the process of cleanup. The more advanced concepts of making your own moulage supplies and materials are also addressed. The chapter includes:

- educational basis for moulage
- basic moulage supplies
- actors and makeup: moulage for SPs
- manikins and makeup: moulage for HPS
- special effects basics: creating props and setting the stage
- striking the set: cleaning up and resetting the scenario

The use of moulage in a simulation scenario is limited only by the scenario developer's imagination and expertise. Care must be taken, however, to keep this imagination from running wild as excessive or inappropriate moulage or makeup can detract from the simulation or provide incorrect cues.

## ▶ EDUCATIONAL BASIS FOR THE USE OF MOULAGE IN SIMULATION

Although there has been a paucity of actual research on the use of moulage and makeup in educational simulation, this is beginning to change. Anecdotal reports are still plentiful and relate various degrees of success and failure. Some current studies are evaluating the degree of realism and its impact on the learner and are focusing the research agenda (Stokes-Parish et al., 2017). The use of moulage in simulation is covered in the International Nursing Association for Clinical Simulation and Learning (INACSL) standard on simulation design in criteria 6 (INACSL Standards Committee et al., 2021). It seems logical that when speaking of simulation as an experiential learning tool, anything that enhances the reality of the learning environment is supportive of the learner's experience. The appropriate level of authenticity and realism can contribute to the degree of the engagement of the learner in the simulation and that in turn can enhance the learning (INACSL Standards Committee et al., 2021; Stokes-Parish et al., 2017). Moulage, then, is one more tool that the educator can use to enhance the reality of the learning environment (Figure 9.1).

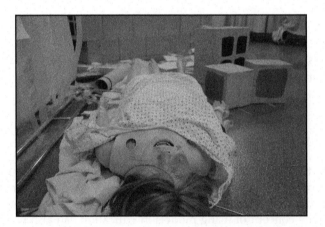

**Figure 9.1** The Drexel University simulation lab.
*Source:* Courtesy of Drexel University College of Nursing and Health Professions.

### Simulation Teaching Tip 9.1

Taylor et al. (2023) taught dermatologic conditions to nursing students using the nursing process, evidence-based treatments, transmission-based precautions, and teamwork. The conditions where simulated using moulage and the students had a positive active learning experience.

Caution should be exercised though, as improperly done moulage can detract from the experience. The choice to use or not use moulage should be driven by the objectives and design of the simulation and not solely by the expertise of the moulage artist. Makeup and props used for their own sake or to surprise or deliberately confuse or trick the learner will not support the learning outcomes and may send the learners down a false path by providing incorrect cues or information. This is not to say that moulage cannot be used as a distractor, increased noise, or distraction to add a higher level of difficulty to a scenario, but just that caution should be used. In fact, the use of varying complexities of moulage can quite nicely adjust the presentation to create several different versions of the same scenario, for example, altering the amount and consistency of wound drainage, leading the learners in one case to deal with an uncomplicated postoperative wound and in another with a grossly infected one. One must remember to match the need and type of moulage with the learning outcomes and design of the scenario.

## Simulation Teaching Tip 9.2

A word of caution: This is quite a captivating component of simulation and the more that you find yourself involved with moulage the more tricks you will collect and the larger your makeup kit will grow until you find yourself pushing it around on a cart.

## ▶ BASIC MOULAGE SUPPLIES

Assembling a good, basic moulage kit does not have to be time-consuming or expensive. It is best to start small and keep the kit consistent with the state of one's moulage skills (Figure 9.2). In the beginning, you may only be focusing on one or two items or appliances, such as:

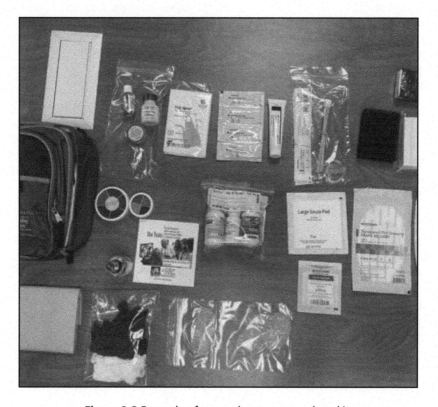

**Figure 9.2** Example of a sample starter moulage kit.

- a few application sponges, brushes, and a stipple sponge
- a color wheel or two of makeup bruises and burns color palettes, which are a good start
- some glycerin and water, the base materials for sweat
- a premolded commercial wound

In the beginning, some sweat, vomit, blood, and a wound or two may be all you need.

### Simulation Teaching Tip 9.3

An easy recipe for sweat or diaphoresis is to mix approximately one-third glycerin and two-thirds water by volume in a bottle with a spray attachment. This allows easy application on either standardized patient (SP) actors or manikins. The more glycerin used, the more the solution will bead on the skin. Some experimentation may be needed to get a mixture that works just the way you want it to. As a caution, glycerin does tend to build up and get gooey and sticky if not cleaned thoroughly at the end of the day. Soap and water are usually all that is necessary for cleanup. As always, care should be taken around the eyes when working with actors.

Table 9.1 contains a short list of some equipment you might need. As experience increases, the materials used to create injuries and illnesses become more varied.

#### Table 9.1 Suggested Basic Supplies for a Moulage Kit

| Supplies | Possible Sources |
|---|---|
| Makeup (a bruise wheel and burn wheel)<br>Sponges (application)<br>Sponges (stipple)<br>Cotton-tipped applicators (lots)<br>Makeup brushes (inexpensive to start)<br>Liquid latex<br>Spirit gum<br>Cold cream<br>Glycerin<br>Petroleum jelly<br>Tongue depressors (lots)<br>Stage blood, both thick and thin<br>Cleanup products<br>Baby wipes<br>Tissues | Halloween stores, theatrical supply stores, online stores, makeup counters, drugstores, etc. |

Advanced materials may include:

- *Liquid latex:* exercise caution regarding potential allergies
- *Silicone:* both as premade purchased wounds as well as silicone adhesive used to assist in application
- *Gel effects:* special effects-grade gelatin materials
- *Modeling wax:* soft sculpting wax to create three-dimensional wound representations

## ▶ PREPARING SUBSTANCES

When trying a new product, be sure to review its properties and characteristics before using it in an actual simulation. Working with a platinum silicone rubber compound is quite different when compared with a liquid latex preparation with regard to setting time and compatibility with plastics. Whatever you choose to work with, time should be set aside well in advance of the event to allow for familiarization with the product and the techniques needed to produce a realistic result. Substances that need time to dry or set may change your preparation timeline; moulage of the manikins may need to be started hours or even days ahead of the simulation event. If using actors, in addition to the need for more time for application, new materials require a reassessment of sensitivities and allergies. The time to find out that the blood does not "run" correctly or that the pus is the wrong color or that the adhesive you chose makes the actor itch and break out in a rash is not when students are in the scenario. Gauging the effect of moulage in a scenario is part of the testing process that should be done with any new or revised scenario design.

## ▶ MOULAGE FOR STANDARDIZED PATIENTS

Using moulage with an SP can produce a greatly enhanced learning experience. A natural conversational interaction with a person as a patient coupled with properly applied makeup or an appliance can produce a very realistic environment. As Garg (2009) noted in a study of second-year medical students, simulation education improved learners' ability to correctly recognize skin lesions as well as retain clinical skills longer. The quality of the makeup used can have an impact on this process; generally, the better the makeup or appliance (prosthetic), the better the result.

> ### Simulation Teaching Tip 9.4
>
> As you are learning moulage techniques, remember to take pictures of your work. This will show you your progression and, we hope, your improvement. At times, a static picture and quiet reflection by the moulage artist can reveal inconsistencies in technique as well as outright errors. In addition, this process will build a portfolio of your work as well as provide a reminder of past solutions to moulage challenges.

## ▶ MAKEUP

Although it is generally true that makeup used in simulations does not need to be expensive, a modest increase in investment can have a positive impact. A higher quality of theatrical-grade makeup from manufacturers, such as Ben Nye or Mehron to name but two, will produce more consistent results and be easier to work with. Frequently, companies such as these will package makeup in wheels or stacks that have colors grouped for specific purposes: bruise or burn wheels, for example. This makes the challenge of choosing the correct colors for the desired illness or injury easier. Makeup that is designed and tested to be used on people can also have a lower risk of allergic or sensitivity reactions. Quite a few of the commercial products are manufactured with this in mind, but it is always prudent to check using small amounts and allowing time for any reaction. Good-quality makeup can also be obtained from obvious sources of makeup counters and drugstores; however, at times, color selections for illness and injury can be a bit sparse. Although there are many good-quality sources of makeup available, determining what works best requires trial and error, and in the end choices are frequently made by personal preference. The application of moulage on a live person will produce more satisfactory results mostly because makeup blends better on the skin of the actor, and this process allows for more natural coloration and appearance. Materials that are designed for use on the skin work best in that environment. SPs are favorable to work with for several reasons:

- Generally, it is easier to produce more realistic results.
- Makeup blends more easily and consistently.
- Most human-approved adhesives work better.
- SPs can be taught to care for or refresh the makeup, shortening the reset time between encounters.
- They can assist with cleanup and removal of appliances.

The following are some drawbacks to working with live actors:

- They move (sometimes a lot).
- They must go to the restroom (sometimes a lot).
- They may have allergies.
- They are sometimes fussy.
- It is sometimes difficult to get them to sit still for hours.

It can be frustrating for the moulage artist if, after an hour of constructing a realistic wound, the patient returns from the restroom and states that the wound "just fell off." Patience is one other key ingredient that should be stocked in any makeup case (Figure 9.3).

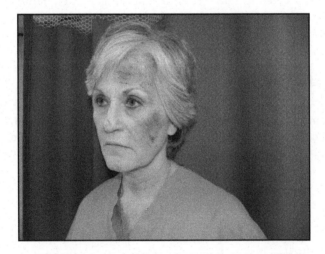

**Figure 9.3** The application of moulage to a live person will produce more satisfactory results. The makeup blends better on the skin of the actor, allowing for more natural coloration and appearance.

## ▶ MANIKINS AND MAKEUP: MOULAGE FOR HUMAN PATIENT SIMULATOR

Applying moulage to manikins can be quite a challenge and produce widely varied results, especially when one compares the results achieved with live actors. The variation of the types of plastics that are found in the construction of most manikins makes it difficult to have a standard approach to the application of makeup or appliances. Some of the issues encountered when working with manikins and makeup include:

■ Blending of the makeup is more difficult and the results look less realistic at times.

> ### Simulation Teaching Tip 9.5
>
> Recycling of old manikin arms, legs, and so on can produce parts with wounds that can be swapped out after the session. This can also help with the use of adhesives as well; if the limb will be reused to display similar wounds, permanently bonded appliances can be left in place.

■ Some types of makeup can stain easily; this calls for all newly used makeup to be tested on a sample manikin part or hidden area in advance. Generally, the softer and more porous the plastic, the greater the chance that staining may occur.
■ When attaching appliances, some may not fit well unless specifically made for use with the manikin in question.

A concern that many people have when using makeup on manikins is the fear that it will stain or permanently mark the manikin. Although this is a valid concern, much of the higher quality makeup is useable with manikins. Of course, the manikin's manufacturer recommendations should be followed to take the most care. Cautious testing in an area that would not be seen if there is staining can produce favorable results and show which makeup can best be used (Figure 9.4). Testing on the reverse of the manikin's chest skin or behind a removable leg pad or skin and then cleaning the area not only lets you know how the makeup behaves on the plastic, but also what is the best product to use for cleanup.

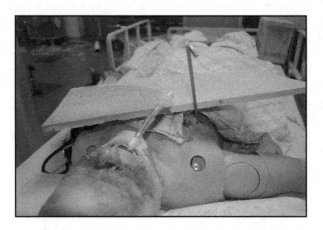

**Figure 9.4** The Drexel University simulation lab.
*Source:* Courtesy of Drexel University College of Nursing and Health Professions.

Another problem is the compatibility of the plastics with both the makeup that you are using as well as with the different types of plastics and adhesives that are used together. Care must be taken when combining plastics of different types, as some will inhibit the curing of some adhesives, leaving the appliance sliding off the manikin. In addition, not all adhesives are created equal and stick to all plastics. One solution is to use a sheet of plastic material as a base, especially if it has some adhesive properties; a clear occlusive dressing comes to mind. At times, the challenge is finding an adhesive that has good sticking ability to keep wound appliances in place, but not so good that it forms a permanent bond or else you may end up with an unintentionally dedicated trauma manikin.

Some manikin manufacturers will produce wound sets that will fit onto their manikins. These may not look as realistic as they should, and there is expense involved, but the ease of use may outweigh the investment. The realism can be enhanced with some makeup and a drizzle of blood. And if the part is repeatedly used in the same type of scenario, minimal staining may not be an issue. As with all moulage, some experimentation is needed to be sure what you implement is what you intended.

## ▶ SPECIAL EFFECTS BASICS: CREATING PROPS AND SETTING THE STAGE

Many items needed for a simulation may be created as well as purchased. One is only limited by resources and imagination. Sometimes simply changing the manikin's clothes, moving it from a bed to a stretcher, and adding a code cart will add the impression that care is being delivered in an ED. In the movie industry, this is called *setting the stage* or *dressing the set*. This should not be a daunting task or involve a great expense. Most often, the supplies that you need you can find in your environment or around you with only a bit of looking. A good source of wardrobe items for your manikins may be only as far away as the local thrift store or an email to your faculty and staff requesting old cast-off clothing. Perhaps a short trip to a local beauty supply store or a wig shop for some new hair will really change the characteristics of the patient: Add a pair of glasses, a sweater, and a purse, and Mrs. Jones begins to emerge.

Empty cardboard boxes painted gray and black can make passable cinder blocks that can be used for the wall that will fall on the SP at the end of the disaster, providing yet one more victim; the best part is that they fold flat for storage, ready for use in future scenarios. Foam blocks painted gray will work as well but are more challenging to store. Making props and scene decorations can be fun and creative. Using props to add realism to the scenario makes it a much richer experience for the learners. All components should support the story and be logical additions that reinforce the reality for the learners. Props, however, should not get in the way or cause distractions, causing the learners to commit errors due to the incorrect representation of the scene. Therefore, it would seem that we need to construct completely realistic environments that use only real equipment and materials. This is not necessarily true; a fabricated prop can be valuable and inexpensive if it gives the proper and correct clue or clues to the learners in the simulation. A cardboard box with the image of the front panel of a fetal monitor and actual monitoring strips pulled from the opening can assist the suspension of disbelief and provide information that the learner needs to navigate through the scenario. With props and set dressing, as with moulage, if the learner spends more time trying to guess what they are looking at than getting useful information to use in the scenario, you have missed the mark and quite possibly the intent of the scenario design.

### Simulation Teaching Tip 9.6

When designing the scenario, the characteristics of the room should not be forgotten; it is as important to moulage the room as it is to moulage the patient.

# ▶ STRIKING THE SET: CLEANING UP AND RESETTING

The session is not over until the cleanup is done, and this can be one of the more challenging aspects of using moulage. It is wise to check the materials used in moulage beforehand for ease of cleanup (Figure 9.5). Essentially, *striking the set* is a theater term that means to put the performance space back to the condition in which you found it. This means not only cleaning the manikin and the simulation space, but also putting all the appliances and props away. If a logical and protective system is designed to store these materials when not in use, it will extend the useful life of the items. For example, the useable life of silicone- or latex-molded wounds can be extended if they are cleaned properly, removing excess adhesive and makeup, and stored in an airtight container with a light dusting of talcum powder. Proper care of moulage supplies will ensure they will be available for many more uses. Props and wardrobes of both the manikin and the SP should be stored in a way that will make them easily accessible for the next session. One method is to create a scenario container to house all the essentials for that scenario; this will help keep all materials in one place, and if the storage container is portable, it may be taken to the location of the manikin or actor during setup.

Cleaning materials needed for after the sessions are not much different from those needed for daily cleanup in the simulation laboratory. Sponges and nonbleach-containing wipes are staples. Attention should be paid to items that can be used on humans, gentle cleansing wipes and makeup remover, cold cream, and the like. Manikins may need some additional help, adhesive removers and alcohol, for instance. Some common needs for cleanup are as follows:

- *Baby wipes:* These are particularly helpful when working with actors and for keeping your hands clean during the makeup process.
- *Alcohol:* Any strength is good, but if you are working with liquid silicone compounds you will need at least 90% as it does a better job of cleaning up the unreacted material.
- *Adhesive removers:* When using adhesive removers, start with the mildest form before using the acetone-based removers, as these may remove the coloring on the manikin.
- *Makeup remover or cold cream:* This does work best on SP actors and can help with the cleanup. Some products can be used on manikins as well.

It is important to follow the manikin manufacturer's guidelines on products used for cleanup, and it is always a good practice to test all cleaning materials on a small nonobvious

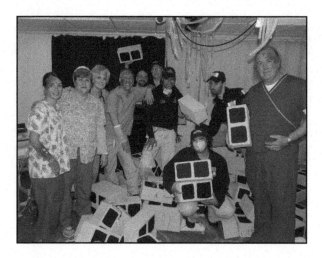

**Figure 9.5** Striking the set: cleaning up and resetting the scene.

area of the manikin before large-scale use. Sometimes it is a good idea to put a barrier material on the manikin to make cleanup of makeup easier. Plastic wraps or adhesive clear dressings work well. Some experimentation may be needed to see what method fits your expertise and budget.

## ▶ SUMMARY

Moulage is a great art to add to simulation and to encourage realism. Moulage is an art that calls for creativity, practice, and developing authenticity. Moulage can be applied to both the human simulation instrument and the environment to better assist healthcare learners in understanding patient care.

 ## CASE STUDY 9.1

You are setting up a trauma scene for interprofessional healthcare providers. You need to transform a large room into a car accident scene in which four teenagers are involved. One is thrown from the car and has a compound femur fracture. The driver has a head injury. The third has an abdominal wound and the fourth has a lacerated arm. What materials would you use to set the stage? How would you develop the wounds to produce realism? Where would you place the victims in the environment?

 ## CASE STUDY 9.2

You are asked to design a scenario involving patients and nurses in an ICU.
You are a team who has been called to an incident in the ICU of the hospital. A nearby incinerator chimney has fallen, landing on the ICU which is located on that corner of the building. The incident has interrupted the power to that part of the building so there are no lights except for emergency backup and no available power. The damage has also resulted in several small fires, causing the area of the rescue to be charged with smoke. The victims include six patients, three are on ventilators and need continued ventilation. There are also eight nurses who were working with the patients at the time of the incident.
What moulage challenges do you expect? What questions would you have for the content experts? What specialized equipment might be needed to enhance the fidelity of the simulation?

 ## CASE STUDY 9.3

You are asked to develop a scenario in which several patients have been exposed to irritating chemicals due to an explosion at a rail yard. Two workers who were close to the blast have traumatic wounds secondary to flying shrapnel, as well as the more severe chemical burns. Three workers who were walking near the railroad crossing had been in contact with airborne chemical particles. What materials would you use to set the stage? How would you develop the wounds to produce realism? Where would you place the victims in the environment? What wardrobe would you consider for the railroad workers?

1. When considering using moulage in a simulation scenario, which is the MOST effective use of time and effort when preparing the moulage for a simulation session?

    A. Concentrate principally on the wounds or representation of the illness to save time and reduce the cost of the simulation

    B. Strike the best balance between effort on the principal illness or wound wardrobe and the scene staging to provide the best authenticity

    C. Concentrate on the patient, clothing, and monitor settings as these are all the students will focus on

    D. Spend most of the time and effort on developing charting materials and wound characteristics that can be documented

2. The degree of authenticity of the moulage used in a simulation scenario is important to how the learner engages and performs because high authenticity will:

    A. Shock or jar the learner into paying attention to the simulation and give them reason for paying attention

    B. Resonate with the learner's sense of fun and playing along with the simulation

    C. Keep the learner on their toes and thinking ahead to the next realistic surprise

    D. Have an impact on the learner's conception and engagement in the learning activity

3. It is important to teach the standardized patient to protect/preserve the moulage because:

    A. It is extremely expensive

    B. It has to be perfect

    C. It is very time-consuming to apply

    D. It is a work of art

4. Two advantages of using moulage on standardized patients (SPs) are that:

    A. Most SPs see moulage as fun and make the day of simulation more enjoyable and they do not mind coming in early to prepare

    B. The SPs can be taught to care for and protect the moulage before and during the session as well as assist with cleanup after the session

    C. The anatomy of the SPs is very similar to the manikin so appliances fit well and the adhesives work better on the SPs

    D. SPs usually do not move much so the appliances tend not to fall off and the dyes in the moulage do not stain the SPs

**1. B) Strike the best balance between effort on the principal illness or wound wardrobe and the scene staging to provide the best authenticity**

Balancing the effort between the wounds and the environment will assist with authenticity and decrease extra energy expenditure that would be on just the wounds or the patient or the environment. Concentrating on the illness or wounds may not increase overall fidelity if nothing else is done to make the entire scenario realistic. Concentrating on just the patient and not the environment may decrease realism. Developing charting material may overlook the learning objectives of the scenario.

**2. D) Have an impact on the learner's conception and engagement in the learning activity**

Moulage has an impact on the way the student engages with the scenario because it adds to the authenticity of the situation. It should not shock the learner, its purpose is not fun, and it is not used to anticipate the next step or intervention. Moulage is used to increase realism and engagement.

**3. D) It is a work of art**

Moulage is a work of art and should not be haphazardly destroyed. It does not have to be expensive, perfect or time-consuming. What is done during a moulage session is important to the scenario and should remain intact.

**4. B) The SPs can be taught to care for and protect the moulage before and during the session as well as assist with cleanup after the session**

The SPs can assist and care for the work of art, moulage, and should not consider it fun. SPs should not be asked to come in early without pay, and the dye can stain. The anatomy of real people is not the same as a manikin. The SP should understand the importance and the time put into the moulage and can assist with the cleanup.

5. When starting out working with moulage, the BEST type of kit to begin with is:

   A. One that contains one of each of the most commonly used makeups as well as a varied assortment of application tools

   B. A professionally designed set with an organized case to carry and separate moulage used for manikins from supplies used on standardized patients

   C. A kit assembled from the sale items at the makeup shop to keep the cost down in spite of the quality

   D. One that matches the expertise of the user and provides enough variation to meet the objectives of the simulation while growing with the increased experience of the moulage artist

6. The MOST accurate statement regarding odors is:

   A. They are always required as they help to involve all the senses in a simulation

   B. They can be wild and uncontrollable and must be used with caution only as the scenario design dictates

   C. With increased numbers of manufacturers they are easy to find in the correct quantity and quality so that anyone can apply them during the scenario

   D. Involving multiple senses does not affect learner engagement so odors are not necessary

7. The MOST important concept when considering the recipe for vomit is that the moulage artist should:

   A. Include some real food products as they can increase the gag factor and do not have any cautions to worry about

   B. Choose the visual representation to match the simulation learning points and carefully clean up to minimize unwanted growth and contamination in the lab

   C. Pay attention to the liquid content so that the resulting mixture is soupy and will run easily down the manikin's face and neck

   D. Consider that it could possibly block the airway and choke the manikin

8. Which items and materials that are found in the kitchen may be problematic for moulage?

   A. Chocolate syrup

   B. Cherry pie filling

   C. Clear gelatin

   D. Honey

9. Which would be the BEST choice of material to make a bruise on a manikin?

   A. Oil-based makeup with high concentrations of red dye

   B. Wax crayons heated to soften them

   C. Cream-based theatrical makeup

   D. Blue and purple crushed grapes

10. What is the BEST source to acquire makeup for your kit?

   A. Local drugstore

   B. Local grocery store

   C. Local theater supply store

   D. National department store

**5.  D) One that matches the expertise of the user and provides enough variation to meet the objectives of the simulation while growing with the increased experience of the moulage artist**
The moulage kit should match the expertise of the applier and meet the student learning outcomes. It does not have to contain an assortment of tools, be professionally designed, or all be gathered from only sale items.

**6.  B) They can be wild and uncontrollable and must be used with caution only as the scenario design dictates**
Odors should be used with caution and meet the student learning outcomes for the scenario. They are not required, or easy to find, and elicit the sense of smell specifically, not multiple senses.

**7.  B) Choose the visual representation to match the simulation learning points and carefully clean up to minimize unwanted growth and contamination in the lab**
Cleanup is very important to keep the laboratory clean, and the vomit should look as real as possible. Vomit should not be used to promote gagging and does not have to be liquefied. Manikins do not always need to be programmed to choke.

**8.  D) Honey**
Honey may be difficult to clean due to its stickiness. Chocolate syrup, cherry pie filling, and clear gelatin are easier to use and can be cleaned up more easily.

**9.  C) Cream-based theatrical makeup**
Cream-based makeup can be removed more easily than oil-based makeup, wax, or dye substances like grapes. With moulage, removal must always be considered whether used on a manikin or a standardized patient.

**10.  C) Local theater supply store**
The local theater supply store contains makeup that is specific to moulage that can be removed easily. The grocery store, drugstore, and department store may not sell the variety of easy-to-remove makeup needed.

# REFERENCES

Garg, R. (2009). *Modeling and simulation of two-phase flows* (Paper 10657) [Doctoral dissertation, Iowa State University]. Iowa State University Digital Repository. http://lib.dr.iastate.edu/etd/10657

International Nursing Association of Clinical and Simulation Learning Standards Committee, Watts, P., McDermott, D., Alinier, G., Charnetski, M., Ludlow, J., Horsley, E., Meakim, C., & Nawathe, P. (2021). Healthcare simulation standards of best practice simulation design. *Clinical Simulation in Nursing, 58*, 14–21.

Riva, A., Conti, G., Solinas, P., & Loy, F. (2010). The evolution of anatomical illustration and wax modelling in Italy from the 16th to early 19th centuries. *Journal of Anatomy, 216*(2), 209–222. https://doi.org/10.1111/j.1469-7580.2009.01157

Society for Simulation in Healthcare. (2021). *SSH certified healthcare simulation educator handbook.* https://www.ssih.org/Portals/48/Certification/CHSE_Docs/CHSE%20Handbook.pdf

Stokes-Parish, J. B., Duvivier, R., & Jolly, B. (2017). Does appearance matter? Current issues and formulation of a research agenda for moulage in simulation. *Simulation in Healthcare, 12*(1), 47–50. https://doi.org/10.1097/sih.0000000000000211

Taylor, T., Kolcun, K., & Tornwell, J. (2023). Application of the nursing process using moulage as a problem-based approach to teaching dermatologic content. *Nursing Education Perspectives, 44*(1), 63–65. https://doi.org/10.1097/01.nep.0000000000000912

# Simulation Principles, Practice, and Methodologies for Standardized Patient Simulation

Linda Wilson, H. Lynn Kane, and John T. Cornele

*All we got is all we need.*

*—Philadelphia Eagles*

This chapter addresses Domain II: Healthcare and Simulation Knowledge/Principles (Society for Simulation in Healthcare [SSH], 2021).

## ▶ LEARNING OUTCOMES

- Discuss the history of standardized patient (SP) simulation.
- Describe the process for SP simulation case development, training, implementation, and evaluation.

## ▶ INTRODUCTION

Standardized patients (SPs) were introduced into medical training in a limited fashion in the 1960s, but it took almost 30 years for the concept to enter the fields of nursing education and research (Barrows, 1993; Bolstad et al., 2012). Initial objections toward using SPs included the high cost of implementation (hiring and training SPs, videotaping experiences), the so-called "Hollywoodization" of the hard sciences, and a skepticism that an actor, not a trained healthcare professional, could correctly help assess learners' skills (Bolstad et al., 2012; Wallace, 1997). Yet SPs are not necessarily all trained actors and they have been found to have lower levels of unreliability and bias than nursing instructor observation or preceptor input (Bolstad et al., 2012). Overcoming this original skepticism and proving their usefulness, reliability, and consistency in a healthcare education setting, SP experiences have greatly increased in popularity, and for good reason, because they offer a safe environment for learners.

The realism of the SP encounter relies on effective case writing by the Certified Healthcare Simulation Educator® (CHSE®) and precise training by either the CHSE or the specific SP trainer. The training is based around measurable learning outcomes, but not every single question or reaction that the SP might encounter during a day of work can be preemptively trained for; however, an SP can be given guidelines and direction and may even use their own personal background in some situations. A well-trained SP will react naturally, determined by the role they are playing that day. It is also important that the CHSE keeps the personality, attributes, and capabilities of the SP in mind when writing the scenario. It would not make much sense to write the case with a gender-specific problem if the available SPs are not all the same gender.

Flexibility is another benefit of working with SPs. During an SP experience, learners practice communication, history taking, and physical examination skills (Rutherford-Hemming & Jennrich, 2013). Different cases may emphasize certain illness manifestations, complications, or ethical challenges. The SP can even be instructed to emphasize their attitudes toward health professionals (Wallace, 2007). This attitude could range from a healthy skepticism to mild verbal aggression to contempt. The SP can be trained to propose a number of challenging situations that the learners might face with a real patient, and the entire group of learners can undergo the same experience due to the consistency and standardization provided by the SP.

According to the Society for Simulation in Healthcare's (SSH's) *Healthcare Simulation Dictionary*, SPs are also referred to as standardized participants or simulated participants (Lioce et al., 2020).

## ▶ STANDARDIZED PATIENT CASE DEVELOPMENT

The SP case development begins with identification of the simulation objectives or educational goals and the setting of the simulation scenario (Alexander et al., 2015; International Nursing Association for Clinical Simulation and Learning [INACSL] Standards Committee et al., 2021; Olive et al., 1997). It is very important to be clear on the setting of the scenario to help learners understand their role and what is expected of them during the simulation scenario. In an SP simulation scenario, the SP can have the role of a symptomatic patient, a nonsymptomatic patient, a psychiatric patient, an emotionally hysterical patient, a severely depressed patient, or any type of patient you need. The SP can also portray a family member. With the SP being a real person, the sky is the limit—anything is possible (Gorter et al., 2000; Wilson & Rockstraw, 2011). A well-written simulation scenario includes clear objectives; training materials, including a detailed script; and medical details that are clearly and appropriately described for the SP's use, along with enough background to describe the complexity of the patient (Wallace, 2007).

There are many different templates available to help develop your SP scenario and it is important to find which template works best for your simulation center or institution.

**Evidence-Based Simulation Practice 10.1**

Davies et al. (2021) investigated templates and protocols that enable standardized patients (SPs) to accurately and consistently adopt these roles. The researchers conducted a meta-analysis examining published templates and protocols used in medical, nursing, allied health, and veterinary medicine disciplines.

## ▶ TIMING OF THE SIMULATION SCENARIO

When planning the simulation scenario, you must consider the timing of the scenario. This is important for planning and scheduling the participants for the experience. The entire simulation encounter includes the following: (a) presimulation briefing; (b) total time the learner has to work with the patient; (c) time for the patient to complete the learner observation checklist; (d) time for the patient to provide feedback to the learner; (e) time after the encounter if you want the participant to do documentation, or a survey, or a posttest; and (f) time for the SP to prepare for the next learner. Many SP simulation scenarios do not include anything after the encounter. So, for example, if you are planning 15 minutes for the prebrief, planning for the learner to be with the patient for a maximum of 15 minutes, and you are going to allow 5 minutes for the SP to complete the checklist, 7 minutes for the feedback session, and 3 minutes for the patient to prepare for the next learner, each total encounter will take 45 minutes. The following (Exhibit 10.1) demonstrates an example of the time management needed for an SP scenario.

| EXHIBIT 10.1 TIME MANAGEMENT FOR A STANDARDIZED PATIENT SCENARIO | |
| --- | --- |
| Example 1 | Prebrief: 15 minutes |
| | Time with patient: 15 minutes |
| | Checklist time: 5 minutes |
| | Feedback time: 7 minutes |
| | Turnaround time: 3 minutes |
| | Total encounter time: 45 minutes |
| Example 2 | Prebrief: 15 minutes |
| | Time with patient: 30 minutes |
| | Checklist time: 10 minutes |
| | Feedback time: 15 minutes |
| | Turnaround time: 5 minutes |
| | Total encounter time: 75 minutes |

This will assist you with planning the schedule of the simulation experience, also taking into consideration the number of simulation rooms you have available and the number of learners who have to complete the simulation experience.

## ▶ IDENTIFY THE SETTING

The setting is a very important part of scenario planning. Where is your scenario taking place? Is it in a physician's office, in an ED, in a medical-surgical unit, in a critical care unit, in the community, in a patient's home, in a clinic, or in a surgical family waiting room? Ideally, the simulation room should depict this environment, or if this is not possible a sign should be clearly posted to remind the learner of the environment where the scenario is taking place.

## ▶ STANDARDIZED PATIENT ROLE

The role of the SP must be clearly identified. The SP can portray a patient, a family member, a learner, or any other role imagined.

## ▶ STANDARDIZED PATIENT POSITION AND ATTIRE

As part of the scenario development, you must also identify the position of the patient when the learner enters the room and the attire the patient should be wearing.

Position examples:

- sitting in the chair
- sitting on the exam table
- walking back and forth in the room
- pacing anxiously in the room

Attire examples:

- wearing a patient gown, with underwear on
- wearing a patient gown, no underwear on
- wearing regular clothes
- wearing a gown with pants on

---

**Evidence-Based Simulation Practice 10.2**

Bond et al. (2022) examined the influence of high value care and focused virtual standardized patients (SPs) on learner attitudes toward cost-conscious care, performance on subsequent SP encounters, and the correlation of virtual SP's performance with educational outcomes. The researchers found that high value care didactics combined with virtual SPs or SPs positively influences attitudes toward cost-conscious care.

---

## ▶ LEARNER'S ROLE

The role of the learner should also be very clear. Is the learner working in a new graduate nurse role, a physician role, a physician assistant role, or an advanced practice nurse role? The learners should be reminded of their roles in the simulation instructions and to observe the door sign so that they function within their scope of practice.

## ▶ IDENTIFY THE FOCUS, OBJECTIVES, OR OUTCOMES

The SP simulation scenario has to have a clear focus and objectives. Is the scenario going to be based on a specific medical diagnosis (asthma, congestive heart failure, shortness of breath, abdominal pain), a mental illness (psychosis, hearing voices), psychosocial challenges (depression, anxiety), ethical situations (do not resuscitate [DNR], organ donation, assisted suicide), or another scenario? This selection will be the basis for writing your case. It is important to include clear information about the selected condition/situation highlighted in the case for the education of the SPs.

Next, what are the objectives or educational goals for the learners completing the scenario? For example, if you are working with undergraduate nursing learners, the objectives could include the following:

- Obtain a complete history from the patient.
- Complete a focused physical exam based on the patient's diagnosis.
- Provide patient education based on the educational needs identified during the time with the patient.

If you are working with medical learners or advance practice nurses, the objectives could include the following:

- Obtain a complete history from the patient.
- Complete a focused physical exam based on the patient's diagnosis.
- Identify the patient's diagnosis.
- Order diagnostic tests as appropriate.
- Provide the patient with appropriate information and plan of care.

The objectives are also linked to the specific course, educational program, or clinical unit of the learner. It is important that the learner is aware of the required objectives or educational goals of the simulation experience.

## ▶ STANDARDIZED PATIENT QUESTIONS AND ANSWERS

The SP case should also include any questions the learner may ask during the scenario and the response the patient is supposed to provide to the learner. Any questions specific to the diagnosis or condition of the patient will need a specific answer, such as symptoms and medications. For other questions that do not have a direct impact on the direction of the scenario, you may have the patients use their own information and not require a specific answer. Depending on the complexity of the case, one must be realistic as to how many specific lines or questions the SP can memorize and portray.

## ▶ DOOR SIGN

The door sign is the sign that will be posted outside the simulation room to provide information to the learner (Exhibit 10.2). The door sign should include the following:

- information about the scenario
- what you expect the learner to do in the scenario
- how much time the learner has to complete the scenario
- reminder to refer to the patient chart if one is included as part of the scenario

### EXHIBIT 10.2 DOOR SIGN EXAMPLES

**Door Sign Example 1**

Mr./Mrs. Pat Foles came to the ED with complaints of increased thirst, increased urination, and hunger, and is now admitted to the medical-surgical unit. You have 45 minutes to complete a history, focused physical exam, and appropriate patient teaching.

**Door Sign Example 2**

Mr./Mrs. Pat Wentz came to the ED with complaints of a severe headache and is now admitted to the medical-surgical unit. You have 45 minutes to complete a history, focused physical exam, and appropriate patient teaching. Please refer to the patient chart for additional information.

**Door Sign Example 3**

Mr./Mrs. Fran Victorino has been in the hospital for the past week and was diagnosed with HIV. The patient is preparing to be discharged from the hospital. You are to give the patient discharge instructions, including the important steps to prevent transmission of HIV to others, such as measures for safe sex and so on. The discharge instructions have already been prepared for you by the doctor and are provided in the patient chart. You have 15 minutes to complete this encounter.

## ▶ EVALUATION CHECKLIST

The evaluation checklist is a detailed checklist of what you expect the learner to do during the scenario. In most institutions, this checklist is completed by the SP immediately after the completion of the scenario and before the patient provides feedback to the learner. Depending on how you decide to design your checklist, you can choose to separate the checklist items by categories, such as communication, physical exam, patient teaching, diagnostic tests, or other categories. If a checklist item is subjective, it can be helpful to put a descriptor to provide information on how to evaluate that checklist item. For example, in Table 10.1, you will see the checklist item "good eye contact," with the descriptor explaining that if the learner has good eye contact at least half of the time they will get credit for that checklist item. It is also important to remember that the longer the checklist, the more time you have to allow for the SP to complete it.

**Table 10.1 Example of Evaluation Checklist Items**

| Communication | Physical Exam |
|---|---|
| Introduced self (name and title) | Washed hands before the examination |
| Checked the patient's identification band | Explained what they were doing with each step of the exam |
| Good eye contact (50% of the time or greater) | |
| Spoke clearly in terms the patient can understand | Helped to position the patient |
| Active listener | Was professional in manner |
| Asked the patient's age or date of birth | Maintained modesty during exam |
| Asked about the patient's marital status | Checked blood pressure in both arms |
| Asked about the patient's work history | Checked blood pressure sitting or lying down |
| Asked about previous hospitalizations | Checked blood pressure standing |
| Asked about allergies | Counted the pulse |
| Asked about medical history | Counted the respiratory rate |
| Asked about current medications | Listened to the heart in at least four places on skin |
| Asked about history of chest pain | |
| Asked about history of palpitations | Listened to the lungs in at least four places (two pairs), anterior and posterior on skin |
| Asked about smoking history | |
| Asked about alcohol history | |
| Asked about diet | |
| Asked about exercise | |
| Asked about stresses in life | |
| Created an atmosphere that put the patient at ease | |

**Simulation Teaching Tip 10.1**

If there is a checklist item that has more than one part—where a learner could possibly do one part correctly and one part incorrectly, such as listening to the lungs—it is helpful to separate that into two separate checklist items, as you will see in the example checklist in the following text.

## ▶ LEARNER EVALUATION CRITERIA AND PASSING SCORE

There are many ways to evaluate the learner checklist items. Some of the common evaluation methods include:

- done/not done/NA
- done/not done/done but not correctly
- Likert scale rating

Your simulation program may select one way to evaluate all of your simulation experiences or may be different based on a specific program or course.

If the simulation is a "high-stakes testing" simulation in which the learner has to achieve a specific score to pass, you must also pick a passing score. Many programs will pick the lowest score for a full grade of "C" at their school. Or the specific score might be mandated by your licensing agency.

Another aspect to consider is the value of each checklist item. Are the checklist items of equal value, or are some checklist items worth more points than others? You can also identify specific patient safety checklist items that are critical—if the learner misses that checklist item, they automatically fail or have to repeat the experience, such as verifying the patient's identity or checking the identification band.

Exhibit 10.3 demonstrates three SP simulation cases, including the evaluation checklist. The first and third cases are ethical dilemma cases, while the second case is a hypertension case.

---

**EXHIBIT 10.3 STANDARDIZED PATIENT SIMULATION CASES AND LEARNER CHECKLISTS**

### Case 1

### DNR (Do Not Resuscitate) Ethical Dilemma—Mini Case—Passing Score 76%

**Length of time for the encounter:** 15 min
**Checklist time:** 5 min
**Feedback time:** 7 min
**Turnaround time:** 3 min

**NAME:** Mr./Mrs. Fran Victorino

**SETTING:** Inpatient room on a medical-surgical unit

**SCENARIO:** Your mother, Isabelle Victorino, is 86 years old, has metastatic liver cancer, and was found unconscious on the floor at home.

**DOOR SIGN:** The person in the room is the daughter/son of your patient. This family member is very upset by the information received from the other nurse, who told them their family member is a DNR. The family member wants to speak with you since you are the current nurse for the patient. Your assignment is to talk with this family member. You have 15 minutes for the encounter.

**OPENING LINE:** "I'm so glad you're here. I need to talk to you about my mother. What does 'DNR' mean? The other nurse just told me my mom has been made DNR. Exactly what does that mean?"

You have been out of town and your sister, who lives with your mother, called you this morning and told you your mother had to be taken to the hospital. You are now at the hospital in the ICU's waiting room after seeing your mother. You just found out from the other nurse that your mother has a DNR order, which was given by your sister. You do not understand what "DNR" means and want "everything done" for your mother. You are a little bit anxious, a little upset, and are pacing a bit in the room. When the nurse arrives, you ask the nurse, "What does 'DNR' mean anyway? Who made my mother a DNR?" You add, "My mother, if she could speak for herself, would want everything done . . . she wants to live!"

**CHALLENGE QUESTION:**

"Are you sure this DNR is for my mom? I can't imagine my sister would do something like that."

**TRAINING QUESTIONS:**

**What do you think "DNR" means?** It means you do not do anything. Right?
**Do you understand what it means to resuscitate someone in your mother's advanced age and deteriorated condition?** Not really.
**Do you understand what is involved in the resuscitation?** No.
**Have you ever discussed this topic (DNR) with your mother?** No, but I am sure she would want to live. I'm sure she would want everything done.

(continued)

**EXHIBIT 10.3 STANDARDIZED PATIENT SIMULATION CASES AND LEARNER CHECKLISTS** (*continued*)

**Do you know whether or not your mother has a living will?** I'm not sure.
**Do you understand what a "living will" is?** No.
**Do you have power of attorney over your mother's medical conditions?** No, my sister does.
**Have you spoken to your sister?** No.
**Do you think it would be wise to talk to your sister?** Yes, perhaps I need to.
**Would you like to speak to your mother's physician?** Yes.
**Would you like us to arrange a family meeting?** Yes.
**Would you like to speak to a hospital counselor or a clergy member?** Yes, could I see a clergy member?

### Evaluation Checklist (Done/Not Done/NA)

Introduced self (name and title)
Checked the patient's identification band
Good eye contact (50% of the time or greater)
Spoke clearly in terms the patient can understand
Active listener
Allowed the patient to speak without interruption
Explained DNR in a sensitive, informative way
Examined the patient's perceptions, for example, what the patient thinks DNR is
Acknowledged the patient's emotions
Has a professional manner
Exhibited comforting body language
Asked about the patient's support system
Explained what DNR means
Verified the DNR order in the chart
Explained how a DNR order is obtained
Suggested speaking to the sister or suggested a family meeting
Offered to call the primary doctor to discuss the situation
Offered to call someone for support
                    **\*\*\*SP will also provide feedback.\*\*\***

### Case 2

#### Hypertension—Passing Score 76%

**Length of time for the encounter:** 40 min
**Checklist time:** 7 min
**Feedback time:** 10 min
**Turnaround time:** 3 min

**NAME:** Mr./Mrs. Fran Jackson

**SETTING:** Medical-surgical unit (inpatient hospital room)

**SCENARIO:** The patient has a 2-day complaint of severe headache. On arrival to the ED, the patient was diagnosed with severe hypertension. The patient's initial blood pressure (BP) in the ED was 200/120. **BACKGROUND:** The patient had been to the ED about 6 months ago with a similar complaint and was diagnosed with hypertension at that time. The patient was given a prescription for a hypertension medication: Lopressor. The patient was taking the medication as prescribed until they went to a health fair at the church about 1 week ago. The BP at the health fair was "normal." Because the BP was normal and the patient was feeling great, the patient decided to just stop taking the medication. In addition, the medication was very expensive and the patient can certainly use that money for something else. The patient started getting a severe headache about 2 days ago and thought they should get checked at the ED. The patient is pleasant and talkative.

**DOOR SIGN:** Mr./Mrs. Fran Jackson was admitted to the medical-surgical unit from the ED that day. The patient has a 2-day complaint of severe headache. On arrival at the ED, the patient was diagnosed with severe hypertension. Do a complete history, focused physical exam, and appropriate patient teaching. You have 40 minutes for the encounter.

**OPENING LINE:** "I thought my blood pressure was fixed!"

**CHALLENGE QUESTIONS:**

"The BP medicine that the doctor had me on . . . can you tell me how that medication works? The medication acts on certain receptors in the body and decreases BP and heart rate."
"Why was my BP normal at the health fair? The medication was working or was in you system, so that made your BP within normal range when you went to the health fair."

**TRAINING QUESTIONS:**

**What is your date of birth?** Use your own.
**Are you married?** Use your own.
**Occupation?** Worked in a factory (or store, or office, etc.), left on disability due to back injury, currently under a lot of stress due to having a difficult time making "ends meet" on the income you are receiving.
**When did the severe headache start?** It began 2 days ago.
**Does anything make it worse?** No. I don't think so.
**Does anything make it better?** No. I tried the usual over-the-counter medication that I take for headache but it did not help at all.
**Have you had any fever or chills?** No, not that I know of, but I haven't taken my temperature.
**Have you ever had anything similar in the past?** Yes, I came to the ED about 6 months ago with a similar headache. At that time, they said I had high BP. They gave me a prescription for a BP medication called Lopressor.
**Have you ever used any recreational drugs?** No.
**Have you ever been hospitalized?** No (or use your own history if necessary but nothing related to current complaint).
**Have you ever had surgery?** Answer as for yourself.
**Have you ever been pregnant?** Answer as for yourself.
**Do you have any chronic illnesses?** Yes, I guess the high BP could be considered a chronic illness, but I did not think I had it anymore.
**Are you taking any medications?** Yes, I was taking a medication after my last visit to the ED. It was a medication for my high BP. I stopped taking the medication after I had my BP checked at the health fair at church. My pressure was normal when they took it there, so I knew I did not need the medication any longer. I also felt great! Plus that medication was very expensive!
**How is your father?** Died from a stroke a few years ago. Father also had hypertension.
**How is your mother?** Alive if appropriate, or answer as deceased.
**How is/are your sibling(s)?** Healthy.
**Health history:** (None or use your own)
Neurologic (none)

(continued)

**EXHIBIT 10.3 STANDARDIZED PATIENT SIMULATION CASES AND LEARNER CHECKLISTS** (*continued*)

Cardiovascular (high BP)
Respiratory (none)
Gastrointestinal (none)
Genitourinary (none)
Gynecologic (none)
Obstetric (use your own)
**Diet:** I eat anything I want. I love potato chips, dill pickles, I love anything that tastes salty.
**Medications:**
Prescription medications (I was taking Lopressor once a day when I had the high BP, but prior to coming to the ED today I was not taking any medications.)
Over-the-counter medications (none or use your own)
Medication allergies (none)
Seasonal allergies (use your own)
**Psychosocial history:**
Smoking history (Yes, I've smoked one pack a day for as long as I can remember.)
Alcohol history (I like to have a few beers with my friends on the weekend or sometimes a margarita with extra salt.)
Recreational drug history (none)
Sexual history (use your own)
Stressors (I am stressed about finances; it is difficult making ends meet on the disability salary.)
**You should be in a hospital gown (bra and underwear are okay), sitting on the edge of the table.**

## Learner Checklist (Done/Not Done/NA)

**COMMUNICATION:**

Introduced self (name and title)
Verified the patient's identity
Good eye contact (50% of the time or greater)
Spoke clearly in terms the patient could understand (use the three-strikes rule)
Active listener
Asked the patient's age or date of birth
Asked about the patient's marital status
Asked about the patient's work history
Asked about previous hospitalizations
Asked about allergies
Asked about the patient's medical history
Asked about the patient's family's medical history
Asked about current medications
Asked about history of chest pain
Asked about history of palpitations
Asked about smoking history
Asked about alcohol history
Asked about the patient's diet
Asked about exercise
Asked about stresses in life
Created an atmosphere that put the patient at ease
Answered the patient's question about BP medication: Lopressor
Answered the patient's question about why BP was normal at the health fair

**EXHIBIT 10.3 STANDARDIZED PATIENT SIMULATION CASES AND LEARNER CHECKLISTS** (*continued*)

## PHYSICAL EXAM:

Washed hands before examination
Explained to the patient what they were doing during each step of the exam
Helped to position the patient
Was professional in manner
Maintained modesty during exam
Checked BP in both arms
Checked BP sitting or lying down
Checked BP standing
Counted the patient's pulse
Counted the patient's respiratory rate
Took the patient's temperature
Listened to the patient's heart in at least four places, anterior on skin
Listened to the patient's lungs in at least four places (two pairs) bilateral, anterior on skin
Listened to the patient's lungs in at least four places (two pairs) bilateral, posterior on skin

## PATIENT TEACHING:

Discussed the importance of taking meds as prescribed
Discussed the importance of a low-salt diet
Discussed the importance of exercise
Offered information or suggested some options for stress management
Offered information or suggested some options for smoking cessation

***SP will also provide feedback.***

### Case 3

#### Organ Donation

**Length of time for the encounter:** 30 min
**Checklist time:** 5 min
**Feedback time:** 7 min
**Turnaround time:** 3 min

**NAME:** Mr./Mrs. Fran Foles (mother or father of the patient)

**SETTING:** ICU (family waiting room)

**SCENARIO:** Your daughter was in an automobile accident and has been in the ICU for a week. Earlier today the physician told you the daughter is "brain-dead" and wants you to consider donating her organs. The representative from Gift of Life (the agency that coordinates organ donations) has spoken to you, but you are still confused. You do not understand how your daughter can be dead when she still has a pulse and blood pressure.

**DOOR SIGN:** Mr./Mrs. Fran Foles, who is the father/mother of the patient, is in the room, waiting to speak to the nurse. The physician spoke to the parent earlier today and informed them that the patient is brain-dead and they would like them to consider donation of the patient's organs. Please speak to the patient's family member in this private waiting room. You have 30 minutes to complete the encounter.

*(continued)*

**EXHIBIT 10.3 STANDARDIZED PATIENT SIMULATION CASES AND LEARNER CHECKLISTS** (*continued*)

**OPENING LINE:** "I'm so glad you're here. I need to talk to you about my daughter. My daughter was in an automobile accident and has been in the ICU for the past week. Earlier today the physician told me my daughter is 'brain-dead'. The doctor also said I should consider donating her organs. The representative from Gift of Life (the agency that coordinates organ donations) spoke to me, but I am still confused. I do not understand how my daughter can be dead when she still has a pulse and blood pressure. I do not want anyone to take her organs when she is still alive! That is horrible!" (upset/anxious)

**CHALLENGE QUESTION:**

"Are you sure my daughter is brain-dead? I need to be absolutely sure."

**TRAINING QUESTIONS:**

**What do you think brain death means?** It means the brain is injured or not working?
**Do you understand what is involved in the process of organ donation?** No.
**Have you ever discussed this topic (organ donation) with your daughter?** No, but I remember her saying she had a presentation on it at school.
**Do you know whether or not your daughter said she wanted to be an organ donor on her driver's license?** I'm not sure.
**Would you like to speak to your daughter's physician again?** Yes.
**Would you like to speak to the representative from Gift of Life again?** Yes.
**Would you like us to arrange a family meeting?** Yes.
**Would you like to speak to a hospital counselor or a clergy member?** Yes, could I see a clergy member?
**Do you have any family to support you through this process?** Yes (and use your own).

**You should be in regular clothes, sitting in waiting room, anxious to see the nurse.**

**Learner Checklist (Done/Not Done/NA)**

**COMMUNICATION:**

Introduced self (name and title)
Good eye contact (50% of the time or greater)
Spoke clearly in terms you can understand (use the three-strikes rule)
Was the learner professional in manner?
Did the learner demonstrate empathy?
Did the learner allow you to speak without interruption after asking you a question?
Did the learner tell you about organ donation in a sensitive informative way?
Did the learner try to find out what you know or your perceptions of brain death (what do you think brain death is and the process of organ donation)?
Did the learner acknowledge your emotions?
Was the learner supportive?
Was the learner an attentive listener?
Did the learner exhibit comforting body language?
Did the learner use silence appropriately?
Did the learner determine what your support systems are?
Did the learner explain what brain death means?
Did the learner basically explain the process of organ donation?
Did the learner suggest speaking to your other family members or suggest a family meeting?
Did the learner offer to call the physician for you to speak to them again?
Did the learner offer to call someone for your support (clergy, social worker, etc.)?
Did the learner create an atmosphere that put you at ease?
**\*\*\*SP will also provide feedback\*\*\***

## ▶ STANDARDIZED PATIENT FEEDBACK

Another important aspect of case development is planning for the SP's feedback at the end of the simulation experience. A common type of feedback is for the patient to provide interpersonal feedback on how the learner made them feel as a patient. The feedback can either be very specific or general (see Chapter 18, "Standardized Patient Debriefing and Feedback," for extensive information on SP feedback).

Examples of an SP case template and a blank SP case template are provided in Exhibit 10.4.

---

**EXHIBIT 10.4 STANDARDIZED PATIENT CASE TEMPLATE**

**Title of case:**

**Patient name:**

**Length of time for the encounter** (the maximum time the learner can be in the room is 15 min/ 30 min/45 min):

**Checklist time:**

**Feedback time:**

**Turnaround time:**

**Setting:**

**Overview of scenario/scenario background for the patient:**


**Instructions/door sign** (information for the learner to see prior to experience that includes what is to be done during the experience and ends with how many minutes the learner has to complete the experience):

Mr./Mrs. . . . . . . came to the . . . . . . for . . . . . .
You have . . . . . . minutes to . . . . .

**Opening line** (what you want the patient to say at the beginning of the experience):


**Patient position at the start of the scenario** (sitting on table/sitting in chair):

**Patient dress at the start of the scenario** (regular clothes/patient gown):

**Challenge question** (the question the patient is to ask the learner during the experience plus the answer to the question):


**Questions during the experience (training questions**; Identify the questions the learner may ask during the experience that *require a specific answer*. List the question below and the answer to the question. For all other questions, the patient can use their information.):

**\*\*\*Please delete/change/add to the list below.\*\*\***

---

*(continued)*

## EXHIBIT 10.4 STANDARDIZED PATIENT CASE TEMPLATE (continued)

What is your age?
Are you married?
Occupation?
Have you ever had anything similar in the past?
Have you ever used any recreational drugs?
Have you ever been hospitalized?
Have you ever had surgery?
Have you ever been pregnant?
Do you have any chronic illnesses?
Are you taking any medications?
How is your father?
How is your mother?
How is/are your sibling(s)?
**Health history:**
Are immunizations up to date?
Diet/activity/exercise:
**Medications:**
Prescription medications:
Over-the-counter medications:
Medication allergies:
Seasonal allergies:
**Psychosocial history:**

**Checklist items** (items used to evaluate the learner during the experience; each of these items will be marked with one of the following: done/not done/NA):

**Passing score:**

**Communication:**
 1. Introduced self (name and title)
 2. Verified patient identity
 3. Good eye contact (at least 50% of the time)
 4. Was professional in manner
 5. Spoke clearly in terms I could understand (use the three-strikes rule)
 6. Active listener
 7. Asked about
 8. Asked about
 9.
10.

**Physical Exam:**
 1. Washed hands before the exam
 2. Explained to me what they were doing with each step of the exam
 3.
 4.
 5.
 6.
 7.
 8.
 9.
10.

**EXHIBIT 10.4 STANDARDIZED PATIENT CASE TEMPLATE** (*continued*)

**Patient Education:**
1. Discussed the importance of . . .
2. Discussed the danger signs of . . .
3. Offered information or suggested some options for . . .
4.
5.
6.
7.
8.
9.
10.

**\*\*\*SP will also provide feedback.\*\*\***

# ▶ ORIENTATION, EDUCATION, AND TRAINING OF STANDARDIZED PATIENTS

The SP case scenario written by the CHSE is explained to the SPs during the SP training session prior to the simulation experience, and ideally in advance of the day of the simulation experience. If the training is taking place on the day of the simulation experience, it is important that the learners do not interact with the SPs before the experience to keep the level of realism as high as possible.

Depending on the type of SP experience the instructor has crafted, "[t]raining for a standardized patient involves, for example, learning what history questions to listen for or how the physical examination should be done" (Errichetti et al., 2002, p. 627). Along with describing the direction that the case is supposed to take, the CHSE will also explain the objectives of the scenario.

## Simulation Teaching Tip 10.2

If you are new to writing standardized patient (SP) case scenarios, when you have finished your first case and start your next case, just do a "save as" and start with your original case as a baseline.

The training of the SP begins with the specifics of the simulation case, including the following:

- name of the patient
- role of the patient (patient, family member, etc.)
- setting of the scenario (e.g., medical-surgical unit, ED)
- background of the scenario (i.e., why the patient came in)
- the information the learner will know before beginning the scenario (such as the door sign)
- an opening line or lines to use to begin the scenario (if included in the scenario)
- challenge question (i.e., a specific question about the condition or chief complaint about the SP's condition if included in the scenario)
- training questions (questions the learners might ask and what answer is required)
- checklist items
- feedback

Along with the education about the case itself, the SP must also be clear on the learner checklist and how it should be completed. After the scenario, the SP will complete the learner checklist prior to the feedback session. Through observation, the SP's completion of the checklist contributes to the learner's evaluation, which is formally done by the CHSE. In some institutions, the faculty or simulation educators may complete the checklist.

### Simulation Teaching Tip 10.3

When using SPs for simulation learning experiences, it is best to use a consistent set of actors who work routinely at your institution because they become part of the "culture of learning" at your educational organization.

After reviewing the case and the checklist, the SP can ask questions, discuss strategies, or practice through role-playing. The goal of the SP's training and education on the case is that they enter the role "so carefully coached . . . that the simulation cannot be detected by a skilled clinician" (Barrows, 1993, p. 444).

## ▶ STANDARDIZED PATIENT'S ROLE IN LEARNER'S EVALUATION AND FEEDBACK

For an SP scenario, the SP can be clearly instructed on how to complete the learner checklist. The SP's training is directly related to the accuracy of the SP's completion of the checklist (Wallace, 2007). In addition, for the results of the checklists to be valid, how the checklist is created is crucial to its validity and reliability (Gorter et al., 2000). As mentioned previously, the SP's completion of the checklist contributes to the learner's evaluation, which is formally done by the CHSE.

SPs have a unique role in postscenario feedback. The feedback time can be a heightened time of awareness for the learner, and the information provided to the learner at that time can make a lasting impression. Many learners, after completing the SP simulation experience, state, "I will never forget what that patient told me!" or "The SP feedback was the best part of the experience." The role of SPs in healthcare simulation education is depicted in Figure 10.1.

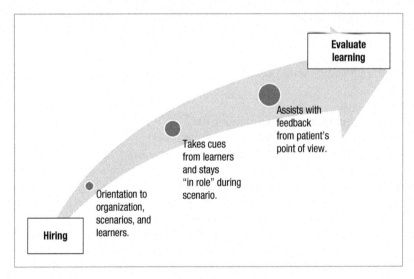

**Figure 10.1** The standardized patient's role in healthcare simulation education.

# ▶ HYBRID SIMULATION USING STANDARDIZED PATIENTS AS CONFEDERATES

Many simulation scenarios find it optimal to combine both the human patient simulator (HPS) and the SP in a simulation scenario. When SPs are used in this fashion, the simulation is referred to as *hybrid simulation,* or the SP can be referred to as a *confederate* in the simulation scenario (see Chapter 11, "Hybrid Simulation," for extensive information on hybrid simulation). The SSH's *Healthcare Simulation Dictionary* defines a *confederate* as "an individual(s) who during the course of the clinical scenario, provides assistance in locating/troubleshooting equipment or may provide support for participants in the form of 'help available'" (Lioce et al., 2020, p. 14).

# ▶ STANDARDIZED PATIENT SIMULATION DURING A PANDEMIC

During the pandemic, many organizations converted their SP simulation experiences to virtual experiences using one of the many available virtual software platforms, such as Zoom, Skype, GoTo Meeting, Microsoft Teams, and others. This format worked well for individual learners and groups of learners. If there was a group of learners, they could be moved into individual breakout rooms along with an SP for the simulation experience.

# ▶ SUMMARY

SPs are a very important aspect of healthcare simulation education. To have a successful SP simulation experience, the case development must be accurate and comprehensive. In addition to the carefully developed case scenario, SP training is equally important. The SP's completion of the checklist must be accurate and consistent. The SP's feedback has to be carefully structured because it can have a lasting impression on the learner. SP simulation provides the opportunity for the most realistic simulations in a safe environment. In the future, SP simulation will be an expected standard in every simulation program.

## ● CASE STUDY 10.1

A learner during an SP simulation scenario about suicide leaves the examination room upset without completing the experience. The learner is crying and tells the CHSE that a family member recently committed suicide and that they cannot continue with the experience. How would the CHSE best handle this specific situation?

1. A simulation educator is planning a simulation to practice therapeutic communication. What type of simulation would be MOST effective?

   A. Human patient simulator (HPS) simulation
   B. Computer-based simulation
   C. Standardized patient (SP) simulation
   D. Virtual reality (VR)

2. A simulation educator has hired a new group of standardized patients (SPs) who have minimal or no previous experience. During the training session, the majority of the SPs state they are not comfortable with providing feedback. The simulation educator should:

   A. Provide videos for the SPs to review from previous simulations
   B. Provide each SP with a book and feedback methods
   C. Provide the SPs extra time to practice and role-play
   D. Provide an education and training session on feedback methods

3. A role NOT usually associated with a standardized patient (SP) is a:

   A. Patient
   B. Family member
   C. Health professional
   D. Learner

4. What is the required length of time for the standardized patient (SP) training session?

   A. 1 hour if the case is simple with minimal technology
   B. 2 hours if there are multiple learners and technology involved
   C. 4 hours if the case is complex and there are many levels of learners
   D. The specific training time is based on the complexity of the case

5. During a simulation scenario, the learner, completing the assessment, proceeds to gag the patient with a tongue depressor. The patient should:

   A. Not do anything and allow the learner to continue
   B. Leave the exam room and state someone else needs to assess them
   C. Provide feedback during debriefing
   D. State, "Stop, I do not want you to do that to me."

### 1. C) Standardized patient (SP) simulation
Having a live person is the best method to teach therapeutic communication so that not only the verbalization can be heard but also the person's body language and expressions can be viewed. HPS, computers, and VR cannot provide the same reactions to questions, dialogues, and answers.

### 2. D) Provide an education and training session on feedback methods
A complete education and training session should be provided since feedback is very important to learners. Providing only a book, an example, and/or extra time to practice may not be as effective. The SP's feedback is important to the student's professional growth.

### 3. D) Learner
The SP is usually there to assist with learning and they are not the learner in a scenario. They can be a family member, a health professional, or a patient.

### 4. D) The specific training time is based on the complexity of the case
The time will be dictated by the learning needs of the SP and the complexity of the case. There is no specific time limit set on training SPs, such as 1, 2, or 4 hours.

### 5. D) State, "Stop, I do not want you to do that to me."
The SP should stop the learner while the procedure is going on to ensure safety and learning. Doing nothing or saving the comments for later does not ensure patient safety. Leaving the examination room does not assist with learning.

6. During a standardized patient (SP) scenario, the SP notices the learner chewing gum. The SP should:

   A. Do nothing since it is personal preference
   B. Make a note on the student checklist
   C. Ask the learner why they are chewing gum
   D. Notify the simulation educator

7. A new simulation educator is interested in learning how to write a standardized patient (SP) scenario. What is the BEST method for the expert simulation educator to use to provide this training?

   A. A book on SP simulation
   B. A simulation case they can copy
   C. Resources and meet with the new educator
   D. Resource websites on SP simulation

8. The standardized patient (SP) is reviewing the list of learners assigned to the room prior to the simulation experience. The SP notices that one of the names on the list is someone they may know personally. The SP should:

   A. Do nothing and stay in role
   B. Put a note on the checklist
   C. Notify the simulation educator after the simulation
   D. Notify the simulation educator immediately

9. At the completion of an assisted suicide simulation, the simulation educator notices several of the learners crying. The simulation educator should:

   A. Gather the learners together for a debriefing session
   B. Do nothing since they need to work through it themselves
   C. Notify the primary contacts for the learners
   D. Revise the scenario so the end is not traumatic

10. Following a simulation experience, a learner comes out of the room and appears very upset. The simulation educator should:

    A. Escort the learner out of the simulation lab
    B. Notify the primary contact for the learner
    C. Take the learner aside and speak with them privately
    D. Speak to the standardized patient (SP) about the reaction

## 6. B) Make a note on the student checklist

Chewing gum is not usually considered professional and it should be noted on the checklist and discussed during the feedback. It is a minor issue that should not disrupt the entire case. The SP should not ask the learner why they are chewing gum during the scenario since it is harmless to the patient. Notifying the simulation educator is not necessary; it is better to provide one-on-one feedback.

## 7. C) Resources and meet with the new educator

The training should be in person and tailored toward the needs of the new simulation educator. A book, example, copying, or website will not be as effective as face-to-face teaching and learning.

## 8. D) Notify the simulation educator immediately

The SP should have the learner reassigned to another SP to decrease familiarity and enhance objective learning. It may be difficult for the learner to assume a care provider role with an SP they are familiar with on a social level. The SP should not do nothing or just put a note on the checklist. Waiting until after the simulation does not assist in the objectivity needed for feedback.

## 9. A) Gather the learners together for a debriefing session

Emotional reactions need to be addressed during debriefing and can be addressed in a group. Doing nothing, notifying the primary contacts, or revising the scenario would not promote learning.

## 10. C) Take the learner aside and speak with them privately

The learner should be spoken to individually since it is not a group reaction. Notifying the primary contact, having the learner leave the scenario, and speaking to the SP will not provide the individual learning and reflection needed for professional growth.

## REFERENCES

Alexander, M., Durham, C. F., Hooper, J. I., Jeffries, P. R., Goldman, N., Kardong-Edgren, S., Kesten, K. S., Spector, N., Tagliareni, E., Radtk, B., & Tillman, C. (2015). NCSBN simulation guidelines for prelicensure nursing education programs. *Journal of Nursing Regulation, 6*(3), 39–42. https://doi.org/10.1016/S2155-8256(15)30783-3

Barrows, H. S. (1993). An overview of the uses of standardized patients for teaching and evaluating clinical skills. *Academic Medicine, 68*(6), 443–451. https://doi.org/10.1097/00001888-199306000-00002

Bolstad, A. L., Xu, Y., Shen, J. J., Covelli, M., & Torpey, M. (2012). Reliability of standardized patients used in a communication study on international nurses in the United States of America. *Nursing & Health Sciences, 14*(1), 67–73. https://doi.org/10.1111/j.1442-2018.2011.00667.x

Bond, W., Mischler, M., Lynch, T., Ebert-Allen, R., Mou, K., Aiyer, M., & Park, Y. (2022). The use of virtual standardized patients for practice in high value care. *Simulation in Healthcare, 00*, 1–8. https://doi.org/10.1097/sih.0000000000000659

Davies, E., Pelentsov, L., Montagu, A., Gordon, A., Hooper, K., & Esterman, A. (2021). "Who am I and why am I here?" A scoping review exploring the templates and protocols that direct actors in their roles as simulated (standardized) patients. *Simulation in Healthcare, 16*, 190–198.

Errichetti, A., Gimpel, J., & Boulet, J. (2002). State of the art in standardized patient programs: A survey of osteopathic medical schools. *Medical Education, 102*(11), 627–631.

Gorter, S., Rethans, J. J., Scherpbier, A., van der Heijde, D., Houben, H., van der Vleuten, C., & van der Linden, S. (2000). Developing case-specific checklists for standardized-patient-based assessments in internal medicine: A review of the literature. *Academic Medicine, 75*(11), 1130–1137. https://doi.org/10.1097/00001888-200011000-00022

International Nursing Association of Clinical and Simulation Learning Standards Committee, Watts, P., McDermott, D., Alinier, G., Charnetski, M., Ludlow, J., Horsley, E., Meakim, C., & Nawathe, P. (2021). Healthcare simulation standards of best practice simulation design. *Clinical Simulation in Nursing, 58*, 14–21.

Lioce, L. (Ed.)., Lopreiato, J. (Founding Ed.)., Downing, D., Chang, T. P., Robertson, J. M., Anderson, M., Diaz, D. A., Spain, A. E. (Assoc. Eds.) & the Terminology and Concepts Working Group. (2020, January). *Healthcare simulation dictionary–Second edition.* Agency for Healthcare Research and Quality. AHRQ Publication No. 20-0019. https://doi.org/10.23970/simulationv2

Olive, K. E., Elnicki, D. M., & Kelley, M. J. (1997). A practical approach to developing cases for standardized patients. *Advances in Health Sciences Education, 2*(1), 49–60. https://doi.org/10.1023/A:1009704030279

Rutherford-Hemming, T., & Jennrich, J. A. (2013). Using standardized patients to strengthen nurse practitioner competency in the clinical setting. *Nursing Education Perspectives, 34*(2), 118–121. https://doi.org/10.1097/00024776-201303000-00010

Society for Simulation in Healthcare. (2021). *SSH certified healthcare simulation educator handbook.* https://www.ssih.org/Portals/48/Certification/CHSE_Docs/CHSE%20Handbook.pdf

Wallace, P. (1997). Following the threads of an innovation: The history of standardized patients in medical education. *Caduceus, 13*(2), 5–26.

Wallace, P. (2007). *Coaching standardized patients: For use in the assessment of clinical competence.* Springer Publishing Company.

Wilson, L., & Rockstraw, L. (2011). *Human simulation for nursing and health professions.* Springer Publishing Company.

# Hybrid Simulation

Anthony Errichetti and Matthew Charnetski

*The whole is greater than the sum of its parts.*

*—Aristotle*

This chapter addresses Domain II: Healthcare and Simulation Knowledge/Principles (Society for Simulation in Healthcare [SSH], 2021).

## ▶ LEARNING OUTCOMES

- Provide an overview of patient simulation modalities.
- Compare hybrid patient simulations—varieties and possibilities.
- Describe how to develop manikin-based and human hybrid simulations.
- Evaluate documents to create manikin-simulated participant hybrid scenarios.
- Prepare the standardized patient/simulated participant for hybrid simulations.
- Identify issues of simulation fidelity.

## ▶ INTRODUCTION

Aristotle's maxim about how complexity is created from simplicity holds true for hybrid patient simulations, the use of two or more patient simulation modalities simultaneously or sequentially to enhance the fidelity of the experience (Lioce et al., 2020). For example, when manikin-based simulators are combined with simulated participants, there is an advantage gained that neither of the two could offer alone. Hybrid patient simulations combine two or more simulation modalities, learning strategies, and professionals into a powerful platform for teaching and assessing clinical competencies. This hybridization allows for a mixing of levels of technology and fidelity while also considering the cost and accessibility of modalities and other resources (Charnetski, 2019). However, the complexity of combining multiple simulation modalities—from the artificial to the human—requires planning and cooperation.

Simulation is an aid to the imagination for both the simulationist and the learner. "It allows us to create, populate and activate possible futures, and explore ramifications of these developed scenarios" (Vincenzi et al., 2009, p. ix). The "willful suspension of disbelief," a concept described by poet Samuel Taylor Coleridge (1817), is directly applicable to simulation learning. If writers could combine "human interest with a semblance of truth" (Coleridge, 1817, p. 2), then readers could overlook a story's implausibility (Barth, 2001). Indeed, the first task for simulationists is to get learners to "buy into" a scenario even though all learners know it is a construction, a representation of reality. Hybrid patient simulation is an approach that combines various elements of "constructed reality"—live, computerized, and mechanical—used in an environment that looks and sounds real. Live participants can be incorporated into a scenario and be given distinct roles to create that "semblance of truth" (Coleridge, 1817, p. 2), which makes learning compelling.

# ▶ FOUNDATIONS OF PATIENT SIMULATIONS

The use of simulation to teach essential skills is widespread and deeply embedded into human culture. We seem to be "hardwired" to substitute the authentic with constructed reality. From infancy, we practice sucking and rooting reflexes through a pacifier, essentially a part-task trainer that simulates a mother's nipple (Moroney & Lilienthal, 2009).

The military has used war simulation for millennia. The ancient Hindu game *Chaturanga* and the Chinese *Go* were used to practice strategic thinking, and large-scale "war games" replicated battlefield conditions (Allen, 1987). Roman Jewish historian Flavius Josephus (1981) notes that Roman general Tiberius conducted war games that were "bloodless battles" to prepare for actual battles that were "bloody drills" (Josephus, 1981, book 3.5.1).

Aviation has long been at the forefront of using simulation to teach core competencies in our era, and its use has been a model for healthcare simulation (Baily, 2019; Friedrich, 2002; Gaba & DeAnda, 1988). The Wright brothers used a "kiwi bird" simulator in 1910 to teach flight control using a defunct Wright Type B Flyer (Bernstein, 2000). The Antoinette trainer (*ca.* 1910; Figure 11.1) was a barrel split in half with short wings, allowing students to practice banking and turning, while an instructor pushing or pulling on the wings simulated turbulence. Such simulators were hybrids combining task trainers with an instructor acting as a "simulated participant," that is, an individual who plays a role in a simulation to add realism and to move critical action forward.

Human patient simulation today has two roots: computerized manikins and simulated participants. SimOne, the first computer-controlled mechanical patient simulator, was developed at the University of Southern California in 1967 by a team led by Stephen Abrahamson and Judson Denson (Abrahamson, 1997). In the late 1960s, the Harvey simulator, a hybrid between a cardiac task trainer and a computer-enhanced manikin-based simulator, integrated the bedside findings and realistically reproduced both common and rare cardiac diseases (Gordon, 1974).

Simulated participants, introduced by Howard Barrows in 1963 at the University of Southern California, have long been used to teach clinical skills and are the foundation of performance-based assessment (Harden & Gleeson, 1979).

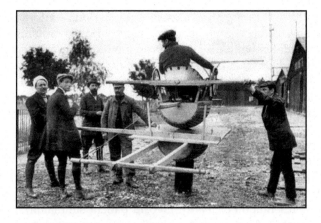

**Figure 11.1** Antoinette trainer.
*Source:* Owen, H. (2017). *Early flight simulators.* A History of Simulation. https://www.historyofsimulation.com/early-flight-simulators-2/

**Evidence-Based Simulation Practice 11.1**

Downar et al. (2017) studied the effects of using standardized patient simulation compared with didactic learning in improving the skills and patient comfort among medical students ($N = 94$) using a single-blind, randomized, controlled design. The findings supported simulation improved communication skills and empathy when compared with didactic learning alone.

# ▶ TYPOLOGY AND MODES OF SIMULATION

Simulations can be divided into four types (Andrews et al., 1998):

- *Live:* Learners interact with real systems or people, for example, evaluating the patients as simulated participants, or customer exercises in which actors, playing patients, assess the reception of office staff.
- *Virtual:* Learners interact with simulated systems, for example, training on a computer-based virtual reality (VR) surgical simulation (Gallagher et al., 2005).
- *Constructive:* Learners interact with simulated systems and simulated people, for example, operating room team training using VR in which simulated participants substitute for actual participants (Baydogan et al., 2009).
- *Hybrid:* This type of simulation combines live, virtual, and constructive modes of simulation in different combinations.

There are many modalities available to simulationists that may be combined to create hybrid simulation-based educational experiences (Charnetski, 2019; Watts et al., 2021). The types of simulated patients used by healthcare simulationists for teaching and skills evaluation include:

- part-task trainers
- humans (standardized patients and simulated participants)
- computerized manikins
- virtual (computer-based, mixed/extended reality, etc.) patients

**Evidence-Based Simulation Practice 11.2**

Bennett et al. (2017) completed a literature review ($N = 57$) about the use of different types of simulation for occupational therapy (OT) education and found that within the OT curricula simulationists have used the full scope of simulation modalities, including written case studies (22), standardized patients (13), video case studies (15), computer-based and VR cases (7), role-play (8), and (manikins) part-task trainers (4). Ten studies used hybrid simulation learning experiences. The review indicated that simulation was being used effectively in OT education.

The following summarizes their utilization and features, with examples of combining the modes into hybrid simulations.

## PART-TASK TRAINERS

Resusci Anne, a plastic manikin, was introduced in 1960 to teach CPR (Grenvik & Schaefer, 2004) and thus began the advent of commercially available part-task trainers. Today, a wide variety of trainers are available to practice airway management, vascular access, echocardiography, cardiovascular assessment, and many other tasks (Schaff & Russell, 2020).

**Simulation Teaching Tip 11.1**

Part-task procedures can also be practiced using common objects, for example, using an orange to practice injection or using a pig's foot to practice suturing. Additionally, increased access and ease of use of silicone-molding techniques and three-dimensional printing have significantly increased options for low-cost and readily available part-task trainers and other do-it-yourself simulation solutions.

Part-task trainers replicate the anatomy, for example, the skin, head, upper and lower extremities, esophagus, and thorax, and in some cases the physiology of a part of the human body. This allows learners and professionals to practice specific tasks or technical procedures (Aggarwal et al., 2004) without harming or hurting an actual patient. Parts of the whole task are used to prepare the learner for the whole task (Sinz, 2004). Part-task procedures can improve learning efficiency because a specific skill can be practiced multiple times until mastered. They can also reduce training costs because the learner would not participate in a full simulation exercise until a particular skill is mastered. Examples of part-task trainers, which are hybrids, include:

- starting an IV line on an arm attached to a simulated participant
- suturing a leg wound attached to a simulated participant
- using a pelvic trainer with a simulated participant
- performing a urinary catheterization on a part-task trainer with a simulated participant
- doing a rectal exam on a part-task trainer with a simulated participant

## HUMAN PATIENT SIMULATIONS

SP is a commonly seen abbreviation in the healthcare simulation world. Depending on context, this may refer to standardized patients, simulated patients, or simulated participants (Charnetski, 2019; Lioce et al., 2020). Commonly, standardized patients refer to individuals who have been specifically and particularly trained to portray a specific patient reliably and reproducibly with a standard presentation, often for assessment purposes. Simulated patients are often given more leeway in their portrayal, with specific elements required to simulate a specific situation or condition. Finally, simulated participants are nonpatient actors within a simulation-based experience. These may be any number of other people needed to enhance the fidelity and continuity of the simulation.

Although standardized patients are used mostly to teach and assess individual clinician competencies, they can be combined with simulated participants who portray nonpatient roles (Charnetski, 2019). Also, simulated participants are increasingly incorporated into manikin-based hybrid scenarios. They are scripted into a simulation to add realism and provide additional challenges and information to learners. They can portray, for example, a patient's (manikin) family member, a healthcare team member, or any other role required by the scenario. They can be "programmed" to portray distinct personality "types" and emotionally complex and nuanced roles that correspond to the learning objectives of a learning module. Simulated participants can also be used to assess skills (e.g., to determine whether procedures are used in a correct and timely manner, assess team communication) and provide feedback during the postencounter debriefing. Simulated participants, like standardized patients, require training for whatever roles they take on. The following are examples of how to use simulated participants with hybrid simulation:

- Learner interacts with a standardized patient, and a simulated participant is a healthcare team member.
- Learner must provide "bad news" to a distraught family member after examining a standardized patient who portrays an end-of-life patient.

## MANIKIN-BASED SIMULATIONS

Manikin-based simulations are often used for training and assessing healthcare teams. The advantage of using manikin-based simulators is when the patient condition is dynamic, particularly critical, or requires significant and often invasive interventions (Charnetski, 2019). Depending on the model, these computerized, mechanical, often high-technology and high-fidelity manikins represent patients at various developmental stages (infant, child, adult) and are used for different purposes (e.g., anesthesia training; birthing simulations; and with programmable cardiovascular, respiratory, and neurologic responses to clinical interventions). Depending on the model, the ingenuity of the simulation operations specialist, and the condition of the patient, all manikins can have a "voice." Talking through a microphone and listening through headphones, the patient's voice is sometimes that of a standardized participant placed at a distance, for example, behind a one-way mirror, and whose role is to answer questions as a patient would. Examples of hybrid simulations with standardized patients or simulated participants with manikins include but are not limited to:

- Learners interact with both the standardized patient and the manikin because they are portraying the same patient at different stages of the scenario and states of patient acuity.
- Simulated participants may be used as:
  - a manikin's voice
  - a family member
  - a healthcare team member
  - other bystander

## EXTENDED/MIXED REALITY AND COMPUTER-BASED SIMULATIONS

Computer-based simulations using videos, drawings, and animation to represent a patient have shown promise in developing clinical reasoning skills (Bracq et al., 2019; Cook & Triola, 2009). Learners interact with the patient by asking questions (typing or speaking); by viewing data from monitors, labs, or x-rays; and by performing diagnostic or therapeutic actions (typically by making choices with the mouse).

At a much higher technology level, VR systems allow learners to become immersed in a computer-generated environment with individuals or groups of individuals (Schmorrow et al., 2009). One purpose of VR is to immerse the user in a computer-generated environment (Pimentel & Teixeria, 1992). Recently, extended/mixed/augmented/VR systems have become much more reasonable in terms of financial and other resource costs. While not yet ubiquitous, their use is far more widespread than even a few years ago. Below are examples of hybrid VR; Chapter 13, "Virtual Reality," provides in-depth information on VR.

- a computer program that simulates the living conditions of a patient before the learner interacts with the simulated participant or manikin in the simulation laboratory
- use of real-time VR with a group of learners and multiple simulated participants
- augmented reality headset that creates a high-fidelity environment surrounding a simulated participant or manikin used for specific verbal and hands-on interaction
- any form of extended reality being used to teach and assess clinical decision-making or scene management in a complex scenario

# ▶ THE ROLE OF THE SIMULATIONIST IN HYBRID SIMULATION

Arguably, the most common hybrid simulation involves manikins and simulated participants. Such hybrids may involve several simulation education roles. However, there is a great deal of overlap in the following functions that may be performed by one or more people with multiple responsibilities:

- *Healthcare simulation operations specialist:* Often, this is an individual with advanced skill and/or knowledge in technology, clinical patient interaction, and simulation-based education, and typically an individual with a clinical background, for example, a physician, nurse, or paramedic. These individuals design healthcare team educational and assessment programs, construct manikin-based simulation scenarios, and participate in debriefing and feedback (Charnetski & Jarvill, 2021).
- *Healthcare simulation technician:* An individual with both mechanical and computer skills is desirable. The technician works with the specialist to prepare the manikin for the encounter, troubleshoots the manikin's technical/mechanical problems, keeps the manikin in good repair, and occasionally functions as the manikin's voice or simulated participant. Often, the specialist doubles as the technician.
- *Simulated participant educator:* Working with the simulation specialist, the simulated participant educator advises how to use people effectively in a scenario, writes simulated participant training notes, and trains them for the scenario.
- *Psychometrician:* This is an individual who designs assessment rubrics and collects, analyzes, and reports performance data.
- *Subject matter expert:* This is often an individual with specific experience and clinical expertise related to the learner and simulation scenario being designed and implemented.

Simulationists have several functions in this resource-intensive process, which are outlined here.

## STAKEHOLDER EDUCATION

One of the most important roles is to educate stakeholders (e.g., learners, clinical faculty, and subject matter experts) about how patient simulations are used as an educational strategy. Learning topics include:

- simulation as an educational strategy
- adult learning principles
- simulator capabilities
- logistics and implementation
- developing scenarios
- matching learning objectives and modalities
- assessing performance validly and reliably
- debriefing and feedback

Faculty and professional development can take many forms, for example, seminars, webinars, and discussion of articles (Hallmark et al., 2021). One of the most powerful ways to educate the faculty about how simulation works is to take them through actual encounters, experiencing the simulation, assessment, and debriefing process as the learner would. This step helps the faculty understand the needs of the learners and the strengths and limitations of simulation learning. The faculty need to understand the curricular, technical, and logistical issues involved in developing and implementing simulations to facilitate effective educational programs. These issues become more complicated when developing hybrid scenarios.

## SIMULATION VENUES

Where patient simulation takes place may dictate different processes and expectations. Simulation venues are often separated into "in situ" and "in silico" (Lioce et al., 2020). Simulation-based experiences that take place in the actual patient care setting/environment are considered "in situ," while simulations that occur in a more controlled lab environment are "in silico." In situ simulation often requires additional resources and planning.

Individuals working in their actual practice environment (in situ) often experience higher engagement due to the higher environmental and conceptual fidelity of the simulation. However, working in this environment often creates a few logistical challenges to the implementation of the experience. Working clinicians in an active environment may be called away suddenly or the space may be needed for actual patient care. In these instances, training may need to be cut short or canceled suddenly. In situ training is particularly useful for "just-in-time" training and systems testing.

In silico training allows for greater control of the environment and more deliberate scheduling of the space for simulation-based experiences. Depending on the resources available, lab spaces can be made very similar to actual patient care areas, but will always have some element of separation from those environments. This can be useful for training interprofessional groups or more generic and foundational training for early learners, as in medical or nursing schools. The lab environment also allows for training and testing in scenarios that would be very disruptive to actual patient care, such as power outages. In silico training can be more reliably scheduled and reserved with simulation-based experiences specifically built into the curriculum and more reliable assessment or gatekeeping to different levels of training.

## CURRICULUM DEVELOPMENT

Development of the educational curriculum with its various goals, objectives, methods, and intended outcomes is the first step in developing a program (Watts et al., 2021). Done in conjunction with clinical faculty and/or subject matter experts, simulationists determine what skills are best taught and practiced through simulations and at the appropriate learner level (Miller et al., 2021). They must decide what simulation modalities are best suited to the educational plan and be creative when the desired modality is not available, lacks fidelity, or is in short supply (Charnetski, 2019).

## SCENARIO DEVELOPMENT

Simulation scenarios are vehicles for assessing skills. All simulations are an opportunity to provide learners a formative or summative assessment and help the faculty self-assess the quality of their clinical education. The patient simulation scenario is a plan indicating how a program will unfold, how the manikin will be programmed or operated remotely, and how simulated participants will be part of the scenario (Kaneko & Lopes, 2019, Watts et al., 2021). An example of information provided to a simulated participant to prepare for role portrayal is shown in Table 11.1.

**Table 11.1 Hybrid Manikin With Simulated Participant Scenario Template**

| |
|---|
| **Scenario Summary**<br>■ Scenario name<br>■ Patient's name, age, and gender (manikin)<br>■ Scenario setting<br>■ Condition of the patient at scenario start<br>■ Educational plan<br>   ● Learner level<br>   ● Program goals<br>   ● Program learning objectives<br>   ● Modalities—e.g., types of simulators used<br>   ● Intended outcomes<br>   ● Challenges to the learner |
| **Simulated Participant Information**<br>■ Simulated participant's name(s) and relationship to the patient<br>■ Narrative—Describe the scenario, what the simulated participant will know about the patient's condition at the start of the scenario, how the simulated participant will interact with the healthcare team, and how the simulated participant will act. |
| **Patient Information (Manikin)**<br>List information the family member(s) will be able to give team members if requested.<br>NOTE: Write the answers to the following information as the family member would give it. Avoid jargon.<br>■ Patient's overall health<br>■ Medical history<br>■ Patient's medications and why taken<br>■ Surgical history<br>■ Health risk behaviors<br>   ● Exercise<br>   ● Diet<br>   ● Tobacco use<br>   ● Alcohol use<br>   ● Substance use<br>   ● Other pertinent information |

## SIMULATED PARTICIPANT TRAINING

Simulated participants can have several functions that require preparation, training, and rehearsal. Scenario notes that guide role portrayal, like simulated participant cases, must be written down and modified as needed. Training "on the fly" should be avoided, especially when assessing and comparing the performance of groups. All simulation scenarios may have the ability to be "standardized" (as in standardized test) if the conditions of testing are standardized to varying degrees.

■ training objectives
■ setting, scenario (the vehicle for assessing skills)
■ modality used
■ timing
■ equipment
■ performance assessment and debriefing/feedback

The following list is an outline of required training for simulated participants, depending on how extensive their role will be in the simulation:

- *Portraying a nonclinical role:* Simulated participants can be trained for a number of roles, such as a patient (as part of a two-part sequential simulation [e.g., a live patient who "becomes" a manikin patient]), a family member, or other auxiliary role required of the scenario (e.g., a bystander in a simulation taking place in the field).
- *Portraying a clinical role:* A clinician can enter a simulation as a simulated participant playing a clinical role they can perform with credibility. This adds verisimilitude to the simulation because the clinician can realistically participate and further the action from the inside out. Simulated participants can also "fill in" as simulated team members or clinicians, but their participation will be limited to whatever part they can play realistically.
- *Skills assessment:* Simulated participants, both clinical and nonclinical, can be trained to document when procedures are done in a timely and correct manner (e.g., correctly intubating a manikin patient or part-task trainer). It is recommended that all charged with this task practice the skill being assessed until mastered, and practice observing, assessing the skill, and remembering it for later documentation during practice encounters. Clinical experience and performance assessment experience are two separate skill domains.
- *Skills/communication teaching assistant:* Simulated participants, both clinical and nonclinical, can be trained in specific skills related to patient care. In these roles, the simulated participant may act as a "teaching assistant" providing directive feedback in the moment and assisting learners in very specific skills. These simulated participants may or may not have specific clinical backgrounds, but often receive additional training to enhance their ability to assess and guide performance of these specific skills. Most commonly, these are physical exam teaching assistants (PETAs) or genitourinary teaching assistants (GUTAs; Weaks et al., 2020).
- *Assessing team communication skills:* Simulated participants are arguably in the best position to assess team communication because they are participating from within. Their roles may also require them to challenge learners, for example, to be a demanding family member or an incompetent team member. Such challenges are dictated by the training objectives. They are therefore part of their training notes and they can then judge how well the learners respond to their challenges. Team communication is best assessed using an assessment rubric.
- *Debriefing and feedback:* Simulated participants who are clinicians as well as simulation specialists/facilitators are in the best position to explore clinical decision-making issues and identify "performance gaps" during debriefing (Rudolph et al., 2007). Their clinical knowledge and understanding of the teaching objectives can create a climate of trust and learner engagement. Both clinical and nonclinical simulated participants who have been charged with assessing communication have a role in debriefing communication. Their role may be to challenge learners to maintain both interpersonal and team communication throughout the encounter.

## ISSUES OF HYBRID SIMULATION AND PATIENT FIDELITY

*Simulation fidelity* refers to the extent to which a simulation or device replicates the environment or a patient's physiologic condition (Alessi, 1988; Lioce et al., 2020). Fidelity can be broken into several different categories (Charnetski, 2019; Lioce et al., 2020), most commonly conceptual, environmental, or psychological. Each type of fidelity may be reproduced with varying degrees of success. All simulation modalities have "fidelity issues," that is, they are more or less realistic, possessing a "degree of similarity" to the patient, the environment, the concept of the case, and psychologically to the scenario (Hays & Singer, 1989). In general, the more "standardized" or replicable the simulation is, the less realistic it may seem because of the need to standardize testing conditions for all. One advantage of hybrid simulations is that high- and low-fidelity elements can be balanced to create the most realistic simulation-based experience with consideration of resource availability, cost, and objective/learner level need. Hybrid simulation provides the best of all worlds to truly bring the simulation-based experience to life.

For instance, a simulated participant may provide very high conceptual and psychological fidelity in that they are a live person who can interact with the learner as a human might and who can evoke a level of cognitive processing similar to that experienced in an actual patient encounter. However, they may have lower conceptual fidelity in the sense that they may not reproduce very specific pathology or may not allow for the performance of certain assessments or interventions. Hybrid simulation allows for the judgment of the simulationists to determine what elements of fidelity are crucial to creating an appropriately engaging scenario for the specific learner population.

---

### Simulation Teaching Tip 11.2

Combining simulators and manipulating the environment, when done well, have the potential to add realism to a scenario and deflect artificiality.

---

One goal of simulation training, regardless of the simulators used, is to achieve the highest level of fidelity necessary for the learners to achieve their objectives, engage meaningfully with the scenario, "suspend their disbelief," and have the best chance of transferring their learning in the simulation experience to actual patient care. Different types of fidelity must be considered to achieve the best results with the most responsible use of resources available. This can only be achieved with the expertise of a simulationist who has the ability to construct a realistic work setting from simulation devices, humans, hybrids, environmental cues, and the judicious use of imagination.

## ▶ SUMMARY

Hybrid simulation is limited only by the imagination. It requires the simulationist to be proficient in human and manikin-based simulations and practices. Combining the best methods of simulation to achieve the learning outcomes is the goal of simulationists. Assessment of learners from within, that is, by utilizing simulated participants, has distinct advantages over assessment done by external or remote simulationists. Hybrid simulation methods provide flexibility and realism to help learners achieve the learning outcomes.

## ● CASE STUDY 11.1

As an experienced simulationist, you would like to teach fourth-year healthcare students the following learning objectives:
- Discuss the methods of attaining sobriety with the patient and the family.
- Recognize the symptoms of alcohol withdrawal.
- Implement treatment measures to minimize the effect of alcohol withdrawal.
- Communicate the prognosis of esophageal cancer that has metastasized to other organs.

Choose two different hybrid methods that could be used to accomplish these learning outcomes and explain how to do it.

1. An advantage of using hybrid simulation is:

   A. Combining interprofessional groups in a single training program
   B. Delivering formative versus summative feedback
   C. Using a trained simulated participant to provide feedback
   D. Skipping debriefing because scores are given by the simulated participant

2. It is important for the simulation educator to consider the simulation venue because it:

   A. Is the best place to conduct debriefing
   B. Can generate different processes and expectations
   C. Can dictate the types of scenario used
   D. Can incorporate simulated participants

3. Psychological fidelity occurs when:

   A. Students experience a high level of cognitive processing
   B. Patient safety measures are ensured through practice
   C. The learners experience positive emotions
   D. The simulationist adheres to the training objectives

4. A simulated participant:

   A. Can be a faculty member who plays the clinician
   B. Can be a high-fidelity manikin
   C. Can be a student who is learning the scenario
   D. Is always a hired actor who is trained in simulation

5. Fidelity is compromised when:

   A. The simulation assessors are not adequately trained
   B. The simulation includes hybrid modalities
   C. The learners are required to take excessive risks
   D. A patient condition cannot be realistically simulated

## 1. C) Using a trained simulated participant to provide feedback

Trained simulated participants can provide valuable feedback to students during a hybrid simulation. Hybrid simulation can combine interprofessional groups, but this can also be done with other types of simulation. Both formative and summative assessments can be done with hybrid simulation, and debriefing should always be completed.

## 2. C) Can dictate the types of scenario used

The simulation environment needs to be considered when choosing the type of simulation. It may not be the best place to debrief and the environment does not generate the processes. Many simulation venues can incorporate simulated participants.

## 3. A) Students experience a high level of cognitive processing

Psychological fidelity occurs when the student learning outcomes are being met with the correct content and at the correct level for knowledge acquisition. It is about the student experience, not the patient, and not about just following procedures. Learners' emotions are not an attribute of psychological fidelity.

## 4. A) Can be a faculty member who plays the clinician

It is someone (even a faculty member) who plays a role in the scenario other than the patient. It is not the student and it does not have to be a hired actor. Manikins are not considered a participant; they are usually the patient.

## 5. D) A patient condition cannot be realistically simulated

Fidelity has to do with realism and suspending disbelief; therefore, the scenario has to be of a nature that is possible in the patient care environment. It does not have to do with the simulation assessors, modality, or asking the learners to take risks. Healthcare professionals often take risks in the patient care environment to ensure patient safety.

6. To rate skills, it is recommended that the simulation assessors:

   A. Develop the clinical skills checklists to be used
   B. Always participate in the scenarios being assessed
   C. Know how to perform the skill being assessed
   D. Develop quality assurance practices

7. Which one of the following is NOT a role of standardized participants?

   A. Standardized patient
   B. Standardized family member
   C. Simulation assessor
   D. Simulated clinician

8. Hybrid simulation requires the simulationist to:

   A. Be proficient in multiple modes of simulation
   B. Understand the principles of test development
   C. Debrief the learners after each task practiced
   D. Manage technical problems that may arise

9. A simulated participant educator:

   A. Manages the simulation scenario
   B. Services the manikins when needed
   C. Trains simulated participants to participate in simulation
   D. Analyzes performance assessment data

10. Educating stakeholders and faculty should include:

   A. Conducting ongoing educational webinars
   B. Showing videos of actual simulation sessions
   C. Observing different types of simulations
   D. Participating in simulations as a participant

### 6. D) Develop quality assurance practices

There needs to be assessor validity and reliability. Establishing consistency in rating takes a quality assurance process. Assessors should not participate in the scenario and do not need to know how to perform the skill. A clinical checklist is important, but the assessor still needs to establish consistency in rating.

### 7. C) Simulation assessor

Standardized participants are not observing how others perform during the simulation. Standardized participants are involved in the scenario as the patient, family member, or clinician.

### 8. A) Be proficient in multiple modes of simulation

Hybrid simulation uses more than one modality; therefore, the simulationist needs to be proficient in multiple methodologies. The simulationist does not need to develop testing, debrief after each task, or troubleshoot mechanical issues.

### 9. C) Trains simulated participants to participate in simulation

The simulation participant educator trains the simulated participant on the role needed in the simulation scenario. Educators do not need to maintain manikins, manage the scenario, or conduct data collection and analysis.

### 10. A) Conducting ongoing educational webinars

Conducting ongoing educational webinars and informational sessions is a good way to educate stakeholders and faculty about simulation learning. Showing videos, observing, or participating may be enlightening and/or entertaining but may not explain the principles of simulation learning.

## ⬤ REFERENCES

Abrahamson, S. (1997). SimOne: A patient simulator ahead of its time. *Caduceus, 13*(2), 29–41.

Aggarwal, R., Moorthy, K., & Darzi, A. (2004). Laparoscopic skills training and assessment. *British Journal of Surgery, 91*, 1549–1580. https://doi.org/10.1002/bjs.4816

Alessi, S. M. (1988). Fidelity in the design of instructional simulations. *Journal of Computer-Based Instruction, 15*(2), 40–47.

Allen, T. B. (1987). *War games*. McGraw-Hill.

Andrews, D. H., Brown, J., Byrnes, J., Chang, J., & Hartman, R. (1998). *Enabling technology: Analysis of categories with potential to support the use of modelling and simulation in the United States air force.* Human Effectiveness Directorate, Air Force Research Lab.

Baily, L. W. (2019). History of simulation. In S. Crawford, L. Baily, & S. Monks (Eds.), *Comprehensive healthcare simulation: Operations, technology, and innovative practice* (pp. 3–11). Springer International Publishing.

Barth, J. (2001). *The symbolic imagination*. Fordham.

Baydogan, E., Belfore, L. E., Scerbo, M., & Mazumdar, S. (2009). Virtual operating room team training via computer-based agents. *International Journal of Intelligent Control and Systems, 14*(1), 115–122.

Bennett, S., Rodger, S., Fitzgerald, C., & Gibson, L. (2017). Simulation in occupational therapy curricula: A literature review. *Australian Occupational Therapy Journal, 64*(4), 314–327. https://doi.org/10.1111/1440-1630.12372

Bernstein, M. (2000). *Grand eccentrics: Turning the century: Dayton and the inventing of America*. Orange Frazer Press.

Bracq, M. S., Michinov, E., & Jannin, P. (2019). Virtual reality simulation in nontechnical skills training for healthcare professionals: A systematic review. *Simulation in Healthcare, 14*(3), 188–194. https://doi.org/10.1097/SIH.0000000000000347

Charnetski, M., & Jarvill, M. (2021). Healthcare simulation standards of best practice™ operations. *Clinical Simulation in Nursing, 58*, 33–39. https://doi.org/10.1016/j.ecns.2021.08.012

Charnetski, M. D. (2019). Simulation methodologies. In S. B. Crawford, L. W. Baily, & S. M. Monks (Eds.), *Comprehensive healthcare simulation: Operations, technology, and innovative practice* (pp. 27–45). Springer International Publishing.

Coleridge, S. T. (1817). *Biographia literaria*. Princeton University Press.

Cook, D. A., & Triola, M. M. (2009). Virtual patients: A critical literature review and proposed next steps. *Medical Education, 43*(4), 303–311. https://doi.org/10.1111/j.1365-2923.2008.03286.x

Downar, J., McNaughton, N., Abdelhalim, T., Wong, N., Lapointe-Shaw, L., Seccareccia, D., Miller, L., Dev, S., Ridley, J., Lee, C., Richardson, L., McDonald-Blumer, H., & Knickle, K. (2017). Standardized patient simulation versus didactic teaching alone for improving residents' communication skills when discussing goals of care and resuscitation: A randomized controlled trial. *Palliative Medicine, 31*(2), 130–139. https://doi.org/10.1177/0269216316652278

Friedrich, M. J. (2002). Practice makes perfect: Risk-free medical training with patient simulators. *Journal of the American Medical Association, 288*(22), 2808, 2811–2812. https://doi.org/10.1001/jama.288.22.2808

Gaba, D., & DeAnda, A. (1988). A comprehensive anesthesia simulation environment: Re-creating the operating room for research and training. *Anesthesiology, 69*(3), 387–394. https://doi.org/10.1097/00000542-198809000-00017

Gallagher, A. G., Ritte, E. M., Champion, H., Higgins, G., Fried, M. P., Moses, G., Smith, C. D., & Satava, R. M. (2005). Virtual reality simulation for the operating room: Proficiency-based training as a paradigm shift in surgical skills training. *Annals of Surgery, 241*(2), 364–372. https://doi.org/10.1097/01.sla.0000151982.85062.80

Gordon, M. S. (1974). Cardiology patient simulator. Development of an animated manikin to teach cardiovascular disease. *American Journal of Cardiology, 34*, 350–355. https://doi.org/10.1016/0002-9149(74)90038-1

Grenvik, A., & Schaefer, J. J. (2004). From Resusci-Anne to Sim-Man: The evolution of simulators in medicine. *Critical Care Medicine, 32*, S56–S57. https://doi.org/10.1097/00003246-200402001-00010

Hallmark, B., Brown, M., Peterson, D. T., Fey, M., Decker, S., Wells-Beede, E., Britt, T., Hardie, L., Shum, C., Arantes, H. P., Charnetski, M., & Morse, C. (2021). Healthcare simulation standards of best Practice™ professional development. *Clinical Simulation in Nursing, 58*, 5–8. https://doi.org/10.1016/j.ecns.2021.08.007

Harden, R. M., & Gleeson, F. A. (1979). Assessment of clinical competence using an objective structured clinical examination (OSCE). *Medical Education, 13*, 41–54. https://doi.org/10.1111/j.1365-2923.1979.tb00918.x

Hays, R., & Singer, M. (1989). *Simulation fidelity in training system design: Bridging the gap between reality and training.* Springer-Verlag.

Josephus, F. (1981). *The Jewish war* (G. A. Williamson, Trans.). Penguin.

Kaneko, R. M. U., & Lopes, M. H. B. D. M. (2019). Realistic health care simulation scenario: What is relevant for its design? *Revista da Escola de Enfermagem da USP, 53*, 1–8. http://doi.org/10.1590/S1980-220X2018015703453

Lioce, L. (Ed.)., Lopreiato, J. (Founding Ed.)., Downing, D., Chang, T. P., Robertson, J. M., Anderson, M., Diaz, D. A., & Spain, A. E. (Assoc. Eds.) and the Terminology and Concepts Working Group. (2020, September). Healthcare simulation dictionary. *Agency for Healthcare Research and Quality (AHRQ)* AHRQ Publication No. 20-0019 (2nd ed.), AHRQ. https://doi.org/10.23970/simulationv2

Miller, C., Deckers, C., Jones, M., Wells-Beede, E., & McGee, E. (2021). Healthcare simulation standards of best practice™ outcomes and objectives. *Clinical Simulation in Nursing, 58*, 40–44. https://doi.org/10.1016/j.ecns.2021.08.013

Moroney, W. F., & Lilienthal, M. G. (2009). Human factors in simulation and training: An overview. In D. Vincenzi, J. Wise, M. Mouloua, & P. A. Hancock (Eds.), *Human factors in simulation and training.* Taylor and Francis CRC Press.

Owen, H. (2017). *Early flight simulators.* A History of Simulation. https://www.historyofsimulation.com/early-flight-simulators-2/

Pimentel, K., & Teixeria, K. (1992). *Virtual reality: Through the new looking glass.* McGraw-Hill.

Rudolph, J. W., Simon, R., Rivard, P., Dufresne, R. L., & Raemer, D. B. (2007). Debriefing with good judgment. *Anesthesiology Clinics, 15*, 361–376. https://doi.org/10.1016/j.anclin.2007.03.007

Schaff, J., & Russell, C. (2020). Mannequin-based simulators and part-task trainers. In B. Mahoney, R. D. Minehart, & M. C. M. Pian-Smith (Eds.), *Comprehensive healthcare simulation: Anesthesiology* (pp. 107–115). Springer International Company.

Schmorrow, D., Nicholson, D., Lackey, S. J., Allen, R. C., Norman, K., & Cohn, J. (2009). Virtual reality in the training environment. In D. A. Vincenzi, J. A. Wise, M. Mouloua, & P. A. Hancock (Eds.), *Human factors in simulation and training.* (pp. 201–230). Taylor and Francis CRC Press.

Sinz, E. (2004). Partial-task-trainers and simulation in critical care medicine. In W. F. Dunn (Ed.), *Simulators in critical care and beyond* (pp. 33–41). Society of Critical Care Medicine.

Society for Simulation in Healthcare. (2021). *Certified healthcare simulation educator handbook.* https://www.ssih.org/Portals/48/Certification/CHSE_Docs/CHSE%20Handbook.pdf

Vincenzi, D. A., Wise, J. A., Moulana, M., & Hanock, P. A. (2009). *Human factors in simulation and training.* Taylor and Francis CRC Press.

Watts, P. I., McDermott, D. S., Alinier, G., Charnetski, M., Ludlow, J., Horsley, E., Meakim, C., & Nawathe, P. A. (2021). Healthcare simulation standards of best practice™ simulation design. *Clinical Simulation in Nursing, 58*, 14–21. https://doi.org/10.1016/j.ecns.2021.08.006

Weaks, C., Hopkins, H., Lyman, L., & George, S. W. (2020). Broader applications of communication: Using the human body for teaching and assessment. In G. Gliva-McConvey, C. F. Nicholas, & L. Clark (Eds.), *Comprehensive healthcare simulation: Implementing best practices in standardized patient methodology* (pp. 221–240). Springer International Company.

# Part-Task Trainers

Ruth A. Wittmann-Price and Stephanie Blumenfeld

*Practice does not make perfect. Only perfect practice makes perfect.*

—*Vince Lombardi*

This chapter addresses Domain II: Healthcare and Simulation Knowledge/Principles (Society for Simulation in Healthcare [SSH], 2021).

## ▶ LEARNING OUTCOMES

- Identify the principles behind choosing an appropriate part-task trainer (PTT).
- Compare the different types of PTTs.
- Review practice questions as they relate to PTTs.

## ▶ INTRODUCTION

Part-task trainers (PTTs) are probably among the oldest types of healthcare simulations known to professions besides practicing skills on one another. PTTs have been used successfully for years to teach "healthcare skills" and are still a valuable part of simulation education.

Simulation education using PTTs allows learners to obtain and/or enhance clinical skills and processes in a safe learning environment. PTTs can be incorporated into all levels of education, from novice to expert. The protected environment and the sense of security enhance students' self-esteem and confidence, thus promoting learning. In this way, the gap between theory and practice is substantially reduced (Koukourikos et al., 2021). Practicing skills deliberately helps learners know how to respond when a complex emergency occurs (Issenberg et al., 1999). The comprehensive use and worth of PTT cannot be understated. Spooner et al. (2012) state: "Task trainers are fundamental in the teaching of anatomic landmarks and in enabling learners to acquire, develop, and maintain the necessary motor skills required to perform specific tasks" (p. 59).

Their vital impact on quality patient care and safety is likely to become more prominent as learners are able to demonstrate enhanced psychomotor and cognitive thinking skills to reach a competency designated as an entrustable professional activity (EPA) for their profession. Choosing to use a PTT allows the faculty to validate a skill prior to practicing a competency on a real patient. PTTs are affordable, easy to move, skill-specific, and allow for standardization of a process.

## ▶ SIMULATORS, FIDELITY, PART-TASK TRAINERS, AND COMPLEX TASK TRAINERS

The *Healthcare Simulation Dictionary* defines *simulation* as an educational technique that replaces or amplifies real experiences with guided experiences that evoke or replicate substantial aspects of the real world in a fully interactive manner (Lioce et al., 2020). The dictionary goes on to define the term *simulator* as a device that duplicates the essential features of a task situation. A simulator generally has three elements: a modeled process which represents, emulates, or otherwise simulates a real-world system; a control system; and a human–machine interface which is representative of the inputs found in the real-world system. Examples include manikins and PTTs (Lioce et al., 2020).

*Fidelity* means that a simulator is able to realistically imitate true physiologic realism. *Fidelity* can be defined as the degree to which the appearance and capabilities of the simulator resemble the appearance and function of the simulated system. Low fidelity is the farthest from realism, showing no physiologic change, movement, animation, or progression. High fidelity is the closest to realism, showing physiologic change, movement, animation, and progression. The anatomic fidelity of PTTs assists students in mastering skills (Woo et al., 2017).

PTTs are devices designed to train in just the key elements of the procedure or the skill being learned, such as lumbar puncture, chest tube insertion, central line insertion, or part of a total system, for example, an EKG simulator (Levine et al., 2013).

Examples of PTTs are provided in Exhibit 12.1.

### EXHIBIT 12.1 EXAMPLES OF PART-TASK TRAINERS

- Intubation manikins
- IV arms
- Female pelvises
- CPR manikins

PTTs are used in healthcare education and include the anatomic segment relevant to a particular procedural skill. The cost, size, and risk of simulation equipment are considered when selecting resources. They are used to teach novices the basics of psychomotor skills and allow for maintenance and fine-tuning of expert skills. PTTs can be used in situ in a real clinical environment or set up in a simulated learning environment. The benefit of portability adds value to just-in-time education, education that takes place in relation to a decrease in census and downtime. PTTs minimize the wear and tear of high-fidelity manikins and are more cost-effective when used to acquire skills leading to an EPA.

PTTs range in complexity, from using a piece of fruit to teach injections to using a torso to teach central line placement and care. They typically do not include patient feedback. An important trend is the combination of PTTs with either standardized simulated patients (live actors) or full-manikin simulators to allow for task completion in a more fully immersive environment (Brown, 2017).

It is often difficult to *suspend disbelief* with PTTs, but they are often used in hybrid formats to increase realism if that is essential to the learning outcomes (Muckler, 2017). An example is placing a task-trainer arm for an IV line in the shirt sleeve of a standardized patient while the actual arm is concealed under a hospital gown. This can prevent pain while the learner is practicing an IV procedure on the task trainer. Chapter 11, "Hybrid Simulation," explains the hybrid concept more completely.

Complex PTTs increase the fidelity in the learning experience by allowing the learner to use a PTT along with a computer-simulated environment or different evaluative or technological techniques (Oussi et al., 2018). Examples are provided in Exhibit 12.2.

## EXHIBIT 12.2 EXAMPLES OF COMPLEX PART-TASK TRAINERS

- Surgical skills
- Central line catheterization
- Scopes, such as bronchoscopes
- Chest tube insertion
- Ultrasound techniques
- Lumbar puncture trainers

Complex task trainers represent both virtual reality and haptic technology in healthcare education using computer-based technology. This equipment tends to be more expensive. Complex task trainers work better in a simulated learning environment related to portability. *Haptic* refers to the sense of touch and the meaning of touch (Orledge et al., 2012). Favier et al. (2021) go on to describe the following levels of haptic fidelity: Simulators with a low haptic accuracy level could be used to learn basic manipulations of surgical materials or instruments and to increase hand–eye coordination. Simulators with a medium haptic accuracy level could be used to become familiar with surgical procedures (e.g., learning procedure steps). Finally, high haptic accuracy simulators may help in the acquisition of fine technical skills, such as with tumor dissection.

This type of trainer allows the faculty to clearly see where the learner is applying touch and the amount of pressure applied, as well as to assess whether a thorough exam has been done (Hagelsteen et al., 2017). Complex PTTs are used in combination with web-enhanced simulation programs so that physical interaction can occur within the virtual reality environment. This may be referred to as box-type simulation trainers. They can be used for surgical techniques, such as laparoscopic surgery.

### Simulation Teaching Tip 12.1

Learners can often practice on part-task and complex task trainers independently if the protocol for the procedure has been taught and is written out. This assists learners in providing self-directed deliberate practice and in being accountable for learning before it is time for evaluation of knowledge.

An example used commonly is an IV PTT that is attached to a computer program. The learner must demonstrate knowledge of the correct procedure on the computer for the PTT to respond to the tourniquet and the arm vein to protrude to accommodate an IV insertion. This may also provide haptic simulation.

## ▶ CURRICULUM DEVELOPMENT USING PART-TASK TRAINERS

Educational goals and simulation tools go hand in hand when thinking about the type of simulator equipment to use. The educator needs to have the end in mind. What will the learner achieve at the end of this learning encounter? The educator needs to identify whether there is financial value in using a high-fidelity manikin for placement of an IV line or practice of chest tube insertion when the consumable costs are much higher with higher fidelity simulation equipment. The faculty should weigh the benefits of using a PTT for individual educational encounters against the benefits of using a high-fidelity simulator to place a second line during a critical event in immersive team simulation training. Using technology to provide hands-on experience guided by proven educational principles, we can provide the very best evidence-based learning environment for our future caregivers (Brown, 2017).

### Simulation Teaching Tip 12.2

Part-task trainers (PTTs) are easy to transport to a classroom for in situ demonstrations.

PTTs are an invaluable asset when setting up a simulation experience for a group of learners. PTTs can be used as an "unmanned station" for learners to practice as long as they are properly prepared. Chapter 16, "Planning Simulation Activities," discusses setting up stations for learner practice in depth.

Additional studies are needed that focus on the evaluation of a learned skill on a PTT and the performance of that competency in actual practice, as well as the effect on communication and empathy (Bauchat et al., 2016).

### Evidence-Based Simulation Practice 12.1

Foronda et al. (2020) quantitatively studied the diversity in simulation centers internationally and found a lack of racial diversity in manikins, body parts/task trainers, standardized patients, and simulation facilitators. This study emphasizes the need for diversity and inclusion in simulation learning.

## ▶ ADVANTAGES OF PART-TASK TRAINERS

Of all the simulation methods, PTTs are probably the least expensive. Once the equipment is bought, it can usually be used over and over with very little maintenance.

### Simulation Teaching Tip 12.3

Care of part-task trainers (PTTs) is important. Follow the manufacturer's instructions on cleaning and storing PTTs to increase their usability and shelf life.

Table 12.1 provides examples of PTTs developed as cost-effective teaching tools to assist healthcare learners in reaching their learning goals.

### Table 12.1 Examples of PTT Use

| Authors | Use of PTTs |
|---|---|
| Komasawa et al. (2017) | Used problem-based learning and task trainer for central venous catheter insertion training successfully with medical students |
| Ng et al. (2018) | Developed a PTT to teach medical students safe aspiration of peritonsillar abscesses, a common condition that presents in EDs |
| Dedmon et al. (2017) | Used a PTT to improve the fine motor control of surgical residents for endoscopic ear surgery |

PTT, part-task trainer.

## ▶ SUMMARY

PTTs are among the first to be used as simulation modalities and are still very effective for student learners when used alone and in a hybrid format. PTTs are cost-effective and can be used by learners independently as well as with the guidance of a simulation educator.

When working in simulation, it is important to understand the use of PTTs in teaching the learner a specific skill. Where high-fidelity simulators are invaluable in practicing an entire patient encounter, task trainers allow for the refining of psychomotor skills in isolation; task trainers allow learners to familiarize themselves with various procedures that require repetitive practice in a safe environment before they are expected to perform the procedure on a real patient (Singh & Restivo, 2021). PTTs assist learners in reaching milestones or benchmarks leading to an EPA or competency (Wittmann-Price & Gitings, 2021).

## ● CASE STUDY 12.1

A learner is using a hybrid IV task trainer and uses a computer to run through the procedure (Figure 12.1). The learner does well on the IV insertion on the part-task trainer (PTT), but states, "I know this is not how it is really going to be with patients." As the simulation educator, how would you respond?

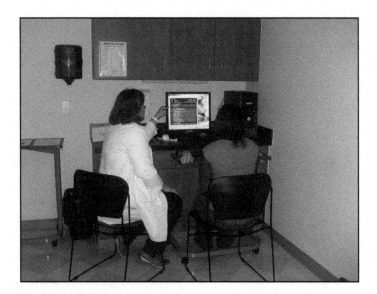

Figure 12.1 Hybrid task trainer.

1. The simulation educator is deciding on simulation fidelity to use to present a set of skills to interprofessional healthcare learners. The priority consideration should be:

   A. The cost of the equipment needed
   B. The learning level of the students
   C. The learning outcomes addressed
   D. The learners' experience with simulation

2. A simulation educator would like to teach the rate and depth of compressions for cardiac arrest response. The BEST simulation method to accomplish this would be:

   A. Using a part-task trainer (PTT) of a torso
   B. Using a standardized simulated patient
   C. Using a computer program in "real life"
   D. Using a high-fidelity manikin

3. The novice simulation educator understands the use of part-task trainers (PTT) when they state:

   A. "A part-task trainer (PTT) can only be used for simple procedures."
   B. "A part-task trainer (PTT) cannot be used in hybrid form."
   C. "A part-task trainer (PTT) is at times more durable."
   D. "A part-task trainer (PTT) jeopardizes suspending disbelief."

4. A simulation educator understands that a haptic experience should include:

   A. A part-task trainer (PTT) and a manikin
   B. Two different PTTs
   C. A PTT and a computer
   D. A PPT with the texture of skin

5. An asset of part-task trainers for deliberate practice is that they are:

   A. Movable
   B. Less expensive
   C. Easily replaced
   D. Durable

6. A method to increase realism of part-task trainers (PTT) would be to:

   A. Hire a standardized patient (SP) to use along with the PTT
   B. Add another PTT during the deliberate practice session
   C. Include a high-fidelity manikin in the skills environment
   D. Have a virtual environment prebrief session

### 1.  C) The learning outcomes addressed
The fidelity should be dependent on the learning outcomes that need to be accomplished. The level and experience of the student should be considered when developing the scenario once the learning outcomes are addressed. The cost of simulation is a consideration but not the priority. Learners' experience with simulation is important but also not the priority.

### 2.  A) Using a part-task trainer (PTT) of a torso
A PTT is durable and can be used for prolonged periods of practice. This cannot be done on a real person. Chest compression may harm a high-fidelity manikin. Real life may not produce the opportunity to practice.

### 3.  C) "A part-task trainer (PTT) is at times more durable."
PTTs are many times more durable and can be used for more complex procedures, in hybrid form, and they may not jeopardize disbelief used in hybrid methodology. Therefore, they are not always just used for simple procedures.

### 4.  D) A PPT with the texture of skin
Haptic simulation has a tactile realism because of the texture of the skin. Haptic experiences may not occur with any two PTTs if they do not have the haptic attribute. Not all PTTs or manikins are haptic. A computer program does not have haptic ability.

### 5.  D) Durable
Yes, durability is needed for deliberate practice. Students need a PTT that can endure being used multiple times. PTTs are many times more movable, less expensive, and may be more readily replaced, but it is their durability that makes them ideal for deliberate practice.

### 6.  A) Hire a standardized patient (SP) to use along with the PTT
Using an SP with a PTT can increase the realism because the SP can demonstrate the emotions of a patient. Virtual environments used as a prebrief will not add to the realism while the PTT is being used, and having a manikin in the environment or another PTT will not ensure realism.

7. A simulation educator would like students to meet the following student learning outcome: "Use sterile technique when placing an epidural catheter in a laboring patient." The BEST modality to use to accomplish the learning outcome would be:

A. A high-fidelity manikin in a simulated labor and delivery room
B. A low-fidelity torso in a laboratory environment
C. A mid-fidelity hybrid modality using a part-task trainer (PTT) and a standardized patient
D. Anatomic objects that demonstrate the vertebrae and the muscles in the lower back

8. Simulation educators understand the priority for using part-task trainers (PTTs) is:

A. Ease of use
B. Anatomic correctness
C. Portability
D. Outcome attainment

9. Using part-task trainers (PTTs) decreases the risk of:

A. Financing equipment
B. Mistakes in procedures
C. Simulation burnout
D. Assessment anxiety

10. A part-task trainer (PTT), which is a haptic intravenous arm, has a covering that is loose to touch. The simulation coordinator should:

A. Use special chemical to clean it well
B. Order a new one if budget allows
C. Take it apart and check functionality
D. Read the manufacturer's instructions

### 7. B) A low-fidelity torso in a laboratory environment

The learning outcome is using sterile technique and this can be done easily with a PTT. This cannot be practiced on a simulated patient. High fidelity should not be used for a competency that can be accomplished on a PTT. Anatomic objects are not as effective as a PTT torso because some realism is needed to identify appropriate techniques on the skin surface, not on the bone and muscle.

### 8. D) Outcome attainment

Outcomes attainment is the priority, and if they are aligned with the modality that is the best way to teach. Many skills/competencies are taught well with PTTs. PTTs are easy to use, transportable, and simulate anatomic portions of the body. The teaching goal of reaching students' learning outcomes is the priority.

### 9. A) Financing equipment

PTTs are durable and therefore do not have to be replaced as often. There is no evidence that PTTs decrease mistakes, burnout, or anxiety compared with other modalities.

### 10. B) Order a new one if budget allows

If the PTT is overused and is deteriorating, it should be replaced. Reading the manufacturer's instructions to troubleshoot the issue only helps if the PTT is in good shape. Cleaning and taking it apart will not solve the problem which is overuse.

# REFERENCES

Bauchat, J. R., Seropian, M., & Jeffries, P. R. (2016). Communication and empathy in the patient-centered care model—Why simulation-based training is not optional. *Clinical Simulation in Nursing, 12*(8), 356–359. https://doi.org/10.1016/j.ecns.2016.04.003

Brown, D. K. (2017). Simulation before clinical practice: The educational advantages. *Audiology Today, 29*(5), 16–24.

Dedmon, M. M., O'Connell, B. P., Kozin, E. D., Remenschneider, A. K., Barber, S. R., Lee, D., Labadie, R. F., & Rivas, A. (2017). Development and validation of a modular endoscopic ear surgery skills trainer. *Otology & Neurotology, 38*(8), 1193–1197. https://doi.org/10.1097/MAO.0000000000001485

Favier, V., Subsol, G., Duraes, M., Captier, G., & Gallet, P. (2021). Haptic fidelity: The game changer in surgical simulators for the next decade? *Frontiers in Oncology, 11*, 713343. https://doi.org/10.3389/fonc.2021.713343

Foronda, C., Prather, S. L., Baptiste, D., Toownsend-Chambers, C., Mays, L., & Graham, C. (2020). Underrepresentation of racial diversity in simulation: An international study. *Spectives, 41*(3), 152–156. http://doi.org/10.1097/01.NEP0000000000000511

Hagelsteen, K., Langegard, A., Lantz, A., Eklund, M., Anderberh, M., & Bergenfelz, A. (2017). Faster acquisition of laparoscopic skills in virtual reality with haptic feedback and 3D vision. *Minimally Invasive Therapy & Allied Technologies, 26*(5), 269–277. https://doi.org/10.1080/13645706.2017.1305970

Issenberg, S. B., McGaghie, W. C., Hart, I. R., Mayer, J. W., Felner, J. M., Petrusa, E. R., Waugh, R. A., Brown, D. D., Safford, R. R., Gessner, I. H., Gordon, D. L.., & Ewy, G. A. (1999). Simulation technology for healthcare professional skills training and assessment. *Journal of the American Medical Association, 282*, 861–866. https://doi.org/10.1001/jama.282.9.861

Komasawa, N., Berg, B. W., & Minami, T. (2017). Hybrid simulation utilizing problem-based learning and task trainer for central venous catheter insertion training. *American Journal of Emergency Medicine, 35*(9), 1379–1379. https://doi.org/10.1016/j.ajem.2017.03.068

Koukourikos, K., Tsaloglidou, A., Kourkouta, L., Papathanasiou, I. V., Iliadis, C., Fratzana, A., & Panagiotou, A. (2021). Simulation in clinical nursing education. *Acta Informatica Medica: AIM: Journal of the Society for Medical Informatics of Bosnia & Herzegovina: Casopis Drustva za Medicinsku Informatiku BiH, 29*(1), 15–20. https://doi.org/10.5455/aim.2021.29

Levine, A. I., DeMaria, Jr. S., Schwartz, A. D., & Sim, A. J. (2013). *The comprehensive textbook of healthcare simulation.* Springer Science & Business Media. https://doi.org/10.1007/978-1-4614-5993-4

Lioce, L. (Ed.)., Lopreiato, J. (Founding Ed.)., Downing, D., Chang, T. P., Robertson, J. M., Anderson, M., Diaz, D. A., Spain, A. E. (Assoc. Eds.)., & the Terminology and Concepts Working Group. (2020, September). Healthcare simulation dictionary. *Agency for Healthcare Research and Quality (AHRQ).* AHRQ Publication No. 20-0019 (2nd ed.), AHRQ. https://doi.org/10.23970/simulationv2

Muckler, V. C. (2017). Exploring suspension of disbelief during simulation-based learning. *Clinical Simulation in Nursing, 13*(1), 3–9. https://doi.org/10.1016/j.ecns.2016.09.004

Ng, V., Plitt, J., & Biffar, D. (2018). Development of a novel ultrasound-guided peritonsillar abscess model for simulation training. *Western Journal of Emergency Medicine: Integrating Emergency Care with Population Health, 19*(1), 172–176. https://doi.org/10.5811/westjem.2017.11.36427

Orledge, J., Phillips, W. J., Murray, W. B., & Lerant, A. (2012). The use of simulation in healthcare: From systems issues, to team building, to task training, to education and high stakes examinations. *Current Opinion in Critical Care, 18*(4), 326–332. https://doi.org/10.1097/MCC.0b013e328353fb49

Oussi, N., Loukas, C., Kjellin, A., Lahanas, V., Georgiou, K., Henningsohn, L., Felländer-Tsai, L., Georgiou, E., & Enochsson, L. (2018). Video analysis in basic skills training: A way to expand the value and use of BlackBox training? *Surgical Endoscopy, 32*(1), 87–95. https://doi.org/10.1007/s00464-017-5641-7

Singh, M., & Restivo, A. (2021). Task trainers in procedural skills acquisition in medical simulation. In *StatPearls.* StatPearls Publishing. https://www.ncbi.nlm.nih.gov/books/NBK558925/

Society for Simulation in Healthcare. (2021). *Certified healthcare simulation educator handbook.* https://www.ssih.org/Portals/48/Certification/CHSE_Docs/CHSE%20Handbook.pdf

Spooner, N., Hurst, S., & Khadra, M. (2012). Medical simulation technology: Educational overview, industry leaders, and what's missing. *Hospital Topics, 90*(3), 57–64. https://doi.org/10.1080/001858 68.2012.714685

Wittmann-Price, R. A., & Gittings, K. K. (2021). *Fast facts about competency-based education in nursing: How to teach competency mastery.* Springer Publishing Company.

Woo, J. A., Malekzadeh, S., Malloy, K. M., & Deutsch, E. S. (2017). Are all manikins created equal? A pilot study of simulator upper airway anatomic fidelity. *Otolaryngology—Head & Neck Surgery, 156*(6), 1154–1157. https://doi.org/10.1177/019459981667465

# Virtual Reality

**Arun Ramakrishnan and Carol Okupniak**

*Unless you try to do something beyond what you have already mastered, you will never grow.*
—*Ralph Waldo Emerson*

This chapter addresses Domain II: Healthcare and Simulation Knowledge/Principles (Society for Simulation in Healthcare [SSH], 2021).

## ▶ LEARNING OUTCOMES

- ▪ Discuss the basic components of virtual reality (VR).
- ▪ Identify ways in which VR can be used to facilitate learning.
- ▪ Discuss the platforms used to design virtual learning (VL) activities.
- ▪ Evaluate the feasibility of using VL and virtual simulation in designing classroom and clinical activities.

## ▶ INTRODUCTION

Today's healthcare environment is fast-paced and, with advancements in technology, is moving rapidly in the provision of patient care and learning environments. There is a large demand for clinical sites within the nursing field alone, and acute care facilities are not able to accommodate the large numbers of students seeking clinical placements. Simulation is increasingly becoming a cornerstone of clinical training, and although effective, it is resource-intensive (Pottle, 2019). In addition, the complexity of healthcare in today's world is moving toward interprofessional collaboration among healthcare providers, increased teamwork, enhanced critical thinking skills and clinical judgment, and time for skill practice. There has also been a proliferation of distance education programs that traditionally have been delivered in a two-dimensional (2D) environment with limited interaction between the learners and the faculty member. Another pressing need in today's classroom is the ability to host remote learning activities while providing students an effective way to practice their clinical skills. Due to the COVID-19 pandemic lockdowns, healthcare educators needed an alternative approach to teaching in physical classrooms and specialized simulation labs that can be delivered remotely. Changes are needed in the way learners are educated to meet the demands of complex healthcare settings.

Virtual learning (VL) technologies are evolving to meet the demands of this changing environment, thereby changing the way healthcare education is delivered (Bracq et al., 2019b; Chen et al., 2020; Farra et al., 2015). VL encompasses a wide range of technologies. Virtual reality (VR) in healthcare simulation is where a user enters a computer-generated (CG), three-dimensional (3D) simulated virtual world (VW) that simulates reality and allows learners to interact, practice skills, learn teamwork and collaboration, and manipulate medical equipment. The previous edition of this book explored screen-based VL such as Second Life (Tiffany & Hoglund, 2014) and Laerdal's vSim and Voki avatars, which are nonimmersive, single and multiplayer online environments where the user experiences the world as an avatar on a 2D screen. Simulation-based education is meant to replicate aspects of the real world in an interactive manner that allows learners to be immersed in the learning environment (Gaba, 2004; Jeffries, 2012). Immersive virtual reality (I-VR) using head-mounted displays (HMD or headsets) is an emergent technology that is poised to bridge this divide. This chapter begins with a description of VL environments, with a special focus on I-VR and its applications in medical virtual reality simulations (VRSs). This chapter also provides understanding of the various components of I-VR; the strengths, weaknesses, and current barriers to its adoption in healthcare simulation; and a quick primer to building effective I-VR simulations, along with examples of I-VR use in healthcare simulation.

## ▶ IMMERSIVE VIRTUAL LEARNING ENVIRONMENTS

Immersive VL environments, unlike screen-based VWs, completely envelope the user within an artificial environment, allowing them to fully engage with the surrounding in all directions. A well-designed I-VR presents the virtual learner with a realistic simulation of a healthcare environment that replaces their real world, convincingly enough that they can suspend disbelief. This has been achieved through technologies like VR headsets or multiple-projection systems like the Cave Automatic Virtual Environment (CAVE). While VR replaces the user's real world (Biocca, 1992), augmented reality (AR) superimposes digital information over the existing physical world. There are a variety of healthcare education tools that use semi-immersive AR using mobile devices (Dhar et al., 2021), as well as fully immersive AR (sometimes referred to as mixed reality) where virtual objects coexist along with the physical world, like the Microsoft's HoloLens (Moro et al., 2021). *XR* or *extended reality* has become an umbrella term encompassing augmented, mixed, and virtual realities (Lee et al., 2021). The term *metaverse* gained notoriety when Facebook (now Meta) used it to describe 3D spaces that allow users to socialize, learn, collaborate, and play. Although several other elements are attached to the metaverse, like the blockchain, non-fungible tokens (NFTs), and Web3, for the scope of this chapter, we will adopt Meta's definition. Most XR offerings are single-use and single-user applications. Multiuser virtual environments (MUVE) like AltspaceVR, VRChat, Engage, Virbela, and Horizons allow users to interact with others using avatars, while providing a familiar portal to enter the metaverse (Kye et al., 2021; Liaw et al., 2018). Many of these I-VR experiences are packaged in the form of single-use applications. Simulation learning systems (SLSs), on the other hand, combine the I-VR experience with a learning management system (LMS), enabling learner login, progress tracking, assessments, and an interface to interact with the instructor and peers.

I-VR has been used since the 1960s for activities such as gaming, therapeutics, training, and more recently teleconferencing. Its efficacy as a vital teaching tool has already been demonstrated in multiple fields, including aviation, oil, shipping, and the military, where real-world training is either prohibitively expensive or extremely dangerous or both. Healthcare training also addresses dangerous life-threatening scenarios where learners gain a certain level of competency in simulated environments before they are allowed to work on real patients. However, it was not until the release of reliable, low-cost portable consumer HMDs, like the Oculus Quest, that healthcare educators' institutions have found it financially feasible to incorporate I-VR into their curriculum (Hamilton et al., 2021; Pottle, 2019). The key features of the I-VR environment include the following:

- enhanced immersion and presence (Jensen & Konradsen, 2018)
- replicates authentic real-world spaces and activities
- allows users to interact with the virtual environment through embodied avatars
- allows users to communicate and collaborate with other users in the same environment
- haptics, rich multisensory feedback, and biosignal integration

The use of I-VR as an educational tool is grounded in the theory of situated cognition (Farra et al., 2015). The sense of self-location, the sense of agency, and the sense of body ownership are critical to learning. Although I-VR gives students a safe, realistic environment to help healthcare programs provide simulation virtually, determining if I-VR is the right technology for the learning objectives takes careful consideration. In the next section, we will explore the various elements that make up an I-VR.

> ### Simulation Teaching Tip 13.1
>
> Presence improves memory encoding. For meaningful learning to occur within immersive virtual reality (I-VR), learners must apply their knowledge to practice and learn from mistakes in *realistic environments*.

## ▶ VIRTUAL REALITY HEADSET

A VR headset uses digital screens placed in front of the eyes to completely replace the visual field with an artificial environment. Some have adjustments to match the facial characteristics of the wearer to effectively render binocular vision. Before designing VRS modules, it is important that every educator experiences I-VR firsthand on a VR headset. The choice of the headset vastly changes the fidelity of the simulation as well as its accessibility to the learners. There are two broad categories of VR headsets. PC-based VR headsets like the Oculus Rift, HTC Vive, Valve Index, Varjo XR-3, and Microsoft HoloLens offer a high-fidelity VR experience with high-quality graphics and precision motion tracking. However, these setups are expensive and require dedicated high-performance gaming computer and a precalibrated room space. Portable VR headsets like Meta Quest, PICO, Varjo Aero, and Samsung Gear VR (smartphone-based VR) can be set up anywhere. These are battery-powered, lightweight, stand-alone units with cloud connectivity and moderate amount of internal processing power for offline use. VR can deliver the clinical scenario in a small space (2 × 2 m), with under 5 minutes of setup (Pottle, 2019). VR headsets have built-in head tracking and are usually paired with handheld controllers, which are the primary user input devices in VR. Newer headsets come with fully articulated hand and eye tracking, eliminating the need for controllers.

## ▶ ENVIRONMENT

Creating a realistic learning environment is an important part of immersion. I-VR can transport the user to any VW, including abstract ones (like in the "Dreams of Dali"). In healthcare simulations, fidelity in representing the environment increases learner engagement, an essential component of learning (Choi et al., 2017). CG-VRS, like the ones offered by SimXVR, UbiSim, Oxford Medical Simulation, and Health Scholars, incorporate interactive 3D objects (like flashlights and medical instruments) and virtual patients (VPs). CG-VRS can also be used in MUVE by incorporating distance learning and telepresence (Lerner et al., 2020). Educators have also developed custom CG-VRS using software platforms like Unreal and Unity. Ultra-realism in these environments is still only possible on very sophisticated and expensive VR systems, making these inaccessible to many learners. On the other hand, Embodied Labs makes use of 360° or immersive videos in their VL program. Live capture of real environments and real people using 360° cameras gives much more visual fidelity and leads to a more realistic decision-making (Kittel et al., 2020). This allows for more accurate representations of facial expressions, movement, speech, and subtle body language cues, which are essential for good soft-skills training. For healthcare educators with expertise in staging and filming simulations, it is likely faster to create content using 360° VR than developing a full CG immersive environment (Ramakrishnan et al., 2020).

Interactive elements like clickable hotspots, branching logic, and quizzes can be added to 360° VR content using video authoring software like CenarioVR, Uptale, and 3DVista, thereby keeping the learners engaged. For these reasons and for its low cost of entry, immersive video-based I-VR is the most common medium in VR education. It has several benefits over screen-based learning, from increased student acceptance and higher engagement, to fewer distractions (Singh et al., 2020; Sultan et al., 2019). Unlike in person simulation, with 360° VR all learners get the best vantage point from which to watch the simulation. This could be the patient's view, the healthcare worker's view, a bystander's view, or a drone view, or learners could switch between views based on the content narrative. One limitation of 360° VR content is that the viewer can only experience the world from the camera's point of view. This restricts freedom of movement by the user, which is sometimes beneficial for new users who tend to wander off in an I-VR. Also, to minimize motion sickness, these experiences are best viewed while seated and are ideal for implementation in existing classrooms.

## ▶ AVATARS

Avatars are the digital representation of users in a virtual environment and the most common way of embodiment and interaction within the metaverse. Other users and nonplayer characters that occupy a virtual environment are also commonly referred to as avatars. The faculty and learners enter the VW by creating an avatar. The participant creates the characteristics of the avatar, including eye and hair color, clothing, age, race, ethnicity, and gender. However, it is highly recommended that the learners create an avatar that mimics their own features and appearance. Avatars interact with each other through talk, text, and gestures (Billings, 2009), as well as move around, perform skills, role-play, and even play "in-world" games. In most current I-VR systems, avatars are represented by a head and two hands connected to a floating torso, since these systems use head and hand tracking only. Most users have been able to embody such avatars and use them as extensions of their real self, although realistic full-body avatars were rated significantly more human-like and evoked a stronger acceptance in terms of virtual body ownership (Waltemate et al., 2018).

> ### Simulation Teaching Tip 13.2
>
> Personalized avatars significantly increase virtual body ownership, virtual presence, and dominance compared with generic counterparts. Hence, avatars representing the individuals embodying them should be as realistic as possible.

## ▶ VIRTUAL PATIENTS

A VP is an interactive computer- or video-based simulation of a real-life patient within a clinical scenario. Learners will either observe the VP or assume the role of the healthcare professional in the scene. Some computer-based VRSs allow the learner to create an avatar that will represent them within the scene. The role of the learner can be any healthcare professional, depending on the design of the VRS. Within their role, the learner can make judgments and clinical decisions based on the assessment of the VP (Guise et al., 2012; Patel et al., 2013). Participants learn the role of the professionals they represent through their assessment, clinical diagnosis, treatment, and care of the patient, just as they would if interacting with a real-life patient. The VP should have the same medical presentation for the learner as a real person with the same diagnosis. Depending on the program used to view the VP in VR, the learner may be able to speak with or interact with the VP, and in certain advanced simulations the VP can employ artificial intelligence (AI) to process and respond to the learner based on its character setting.

VP simulations are case-based computer simulations in which the user observes or makes choices as they progress through various steps (Guise et al., 2012). The pathway for clinical decision-making may be preprogramed or may have a branching algorithm, which allows for several alternative pathways depending on each action taken by the learner.

## ▶ SERIOUS GAMES

Gamification is the application of typical elements of game playing (e.g., points scoring, leaderboards, team activities, meaningful stories) in nongame environments (Sailer et al., 2017). The term *serious games* has loosely been defined in several contexts, including technology for professional use, interactive video simulation, avatars, and watching videos (Petit dit Dariel et al., 2013). The serious game has as its primary purpose educational and professional goals and not entertainment (Hogan et al., 2011). Serious games are computer-based simulations and combine knowledge and skills development with video game-playing aspects, thereby enabling active, experiential, situated, and problem-based learning (Petit dit Dariel et al., 2013). Serious games have been used to enhance the clinical reasoning, decision-making skills, and collaborative work of nursing students in a realistic, safe environment (Lerner et al., 2020; Sankaranarayanan et al., 2018).

Students enter the VW on a computer and can interact in a realistic environment to practice skills and develop different competencies. One of the major limitations of screen-based learning is that interactions are limited to the mouse and keyboard on a 2D interface. Interactions in VR could still use point-and-click mechanics, but also add a layer of spatial as well as gesture-based interactions to mimic interactions in the real world. This added level of motor planning and interacting with VR elements is key to making an engaging learning environment. Fully articulated hand tracking, eye tracking, electromyography (EMG), and other biosignals have been used in VRS to increase fidelity and learner engagement. Haptics is another essential component that uses robotics and other physical means to allow users to experience realistic interactions. Although studies have found that I-VR is not yet a viable replacement for in person training, it does show benefits in reducing anxiety among vocational and early learners and engaging remote learners.

The learner-centered approach is when the player controls the learning through interactivity (Ricciardi & De Paolis, 2014). The game can be designed so that as the student makes a choice with regard to an action or intervention, it leads to another step based on the previous decision. This design fits nicely with Kolb's (1984) experiential learning theory. Serious games may be designed as a means of summative evaluation based on specific outcomes or provide a means for formative evaluation to determine whether learning is occurring.

### Simulation Teaching Tip 13.3

The simulation or scenario must be appropriate for the level of the learner to minimize frustration and maximize engagement.

## ▶ SOFT SKILLS

I-VR simulations have been used in a variety of learning scenarios, including training clinical and procedural skills (Bracq et al., 2019a; Butt et al., 2018; Samosorn et al., 2020), cognitive decision-making and situational awareness (Farra et al., 2015; Sankaranarayanan et al., 2018), staff orientation, and lab safety orientation. However, the major transformative power of I-VR is in the psychological effect it has on the user in the way of altering consciousness.

VR is even touted as "the ultimate empathy machine," an essential behavioral competency required of healthcare providers (Brydon et al., 2021). This is often expressed when the learner experiences I-VR through the point of view (often referred to as first-person point of view) of another individual, a form of "to walk a mile in someone else's shoes." Some examples of these experiences include aging-related symptoms, blindness, hearing impairment, and racial bias. Although clinical skills are the most critical element of their practice, communication breakdowns are the most common cause of medical errors. Communication, collaboration, and delegation are frequently thought to be "soft skills." I-VR can not only improve communication and delegation in critical situations like the advanced cardiac life support (ACLS) training, but has also been used to improve communications with patients by having the caregiver experience patient-specific symptoms themselves as well as through interactive communications with a VP. With the rise of multidisciplinary and sometimes international team-based approach to healthcare, I-VR can facilitate quality interprofessional education at scale and without geographic limitations not only among healthcare learners but also related tracks like biomedical engineers, for whom clinical simulation training is cost-prohibitive or unavailable (Singh et al., 2018).

# ▶ THEORETICAL FRAMEWORKS

Serious games should be designed based on the objectives of the game, outcomes to be met by students, and processes that have a theoretical basis. The three main theoretical approaches are the constructivist theory, Kolb's experiential learning theory, and Knowles's adult learning theory.

The constructivist learning theory states that learners construct knowledge based on their experiences in relation to an event (Tran et al., 2020). The constructivist theory supports the movement of the learner from the novice to the advanced beginner level and recognizes that actions by the learner may be determined by previous exposure to a situation as well as the knowledge base of the learner.

Epp et al. (2021) describe the constructivist theory as a collaborative practice that assists the learner in developing their knowledge, skills, and attitudes by adding new knowledge to previous learning to build deep understanding of a concept. Scaffolding, associated with the constructivist theory, has faculty facilitating learners as they move through simple to complex concepts as they reach new potentials and independence (Epp et al., 2021).

When designing a serious game using the constructivist theory, it is important to formulate objectives and outcomes prior to the development of the scenario for the game. The level of the learner must also be taken into consideration; for example, a scenario designed for a beginning nursing student may require the instructor to be more actively involved in the game based on the learner's limited knowledge. As the student moves through the curriculum, there is less involvement from the instructor, and eventually the student assumes total control of the decision-making in the scenario. This type of design is termed *instructional scaffolding* (Keating, 2010).

Kolb's (1984) experiential learning theory provides a solid platform for the design of VL activities. Kolb describes learning "as the process whereby knowledge is created through transformation of experience" (p. 41). Kolb suggests that a person learns through concrete experience, which provides a basis for observation and reflection on the experience in the virtual simulated environment, and discovers new knowledge (Rogers, 2011). Kolb further proposes that reflections are then assimilated into abstract concepts and can be applied to a new experience. This in turn suggests that learning which has occurred from a simulation in a virtual environment can be applied to situations encountered in the real world (Rogers, 2011).

Green et al. (2014) postulate that Vygotsky's (1978) activity theory is important in the relationship of engagement in VWs. Vygotsky espoused that learning is a social experience and learners should be actively involved in their learning. Vygotsky proposed that social interactions are fundamental to the process of cognitive development, and that connections between people and how learners interact in shared experiences are essential to collaborative learning. The VW is ideal for social interaction with simulated environments (Green et al., 2014).

> ### Simulation Teaching Tip 13.4
>
> The development of a serious game should be based on sound theoretical principles and designed around the purpose, objectives, and outcomes of the learning exercise.

Knowles's adult learning theory (1978) can also be applied to the VR environment and development of serious games. Knowles proposed that adults learn differently from children, and their learning is dependent on autonomy, life experiences, personal goals, and relevance of the experience. He termed this *andragogy*. This theory is applicable to the VR environment as the learners can apply theoretical principles to the situation and receive immediate feedback on their decisions and actions. Virtual environments can stimulate adult learners to apply their knowledge and experiences to concrete situations in a controlled environment, then consider the consequences of their actions and make changes to future choices. Learners are actively engaged in the learning process through simulated activities and can apply what is learned to real-life situations.

## ▶ ADVANTAGES AND DISADVANTAGES OF IMMERSIVE VIRTUAL REALITY SIMULATIONS

The integration of VR learning is important in the learning environment in order to allow the learners an opportunity to immerse themselves in environments where they can practice skills; interact and collaborate with peers or other professionals; make decisions related to care and interventions; and manipulate equipment without fear of harming an individual. VL simulations can be used in any area of clinical practice, but are especially useful in environments where there is limited access to the experience, such as disaster or perioperative nursing. Some benefits and limitations are described in Table 13.1.

**Table 13.1 Advantages and Disadvantages of an Immersive Virtual Reality Simulation**

| Advantages/Benefits | Disadvantages/Challenges |
|---|---|
| It allows learners to repeatedly practice complex and demanding tasks in a safe environment and improves learning retention. | The initial cost of setting up a VR facility with necessary hardware and software is high. |
| It provides a rich, interactive, and engaging educational context that supports full immersion and better training effectiveness. | It lacks existing educational content. Creating custom VRS is expensive and time-consuming. |
| Body-tracked avatars allow for self-expression and realistic interaction, thereby increasing embodiment and engagement. | Educators and learners must be oriented on how to use VRS to minimize learner confusion. |
| It offers a student-centered approach by reducing real-world distractions and promotes active learning. | Technological support must be available to users and designers. |

*(continued)*

**Table 13.1** Advantages and Disadvantages of an Immersive Virtual Reality Simulation (*continued*)

| Advantages/Benefits | Disadvantages/Challenges |
|---|---|
| Spatial telepresence and MUVE foster collaboration with peers and users from other disciplines, both locally and globally. | Cybersickness and technical challenges break immersion and cause learner frustration. |
| Serious games are much more effective in immersive environments that use gestures to interact. | Educators and learners must keep an open mind and be willing to experiment with VRS. |
| Increasing immersion and presence are necessary for the suspension of disbelief, leading to better training effectiveness. | There is a lack of empirical evidence on the impact of VL over traditional teaching methods. |
| It is very effective in improving soft skills such as communication, collaboration, and delegation. | Unlike standardized patients, virtual characters are not yet suitable for certain learning objectives. |
| Cost per learner for VR training gets cheaper over time when compared with manikins or live exercise training. | Lack of interoperability between headsets and software limits VL offered to learners. |
| It lowers learner anxiety and in some instances cognitive load, while improving creativity, positive affect, and confidence. | Changes in VR market are swayed by other industries like gaming, therapeutics, and industry training. |

MUVE, multiuser virtual environments; VL, virtual learning; VR, virtual reality; VRS, virtual reality simulations.

## ▶ HEALTH AND SAFETY RISKS ASSOCIATED WITH VIRTUAL REALITY

VR is an innovative technology that is becoming more ubiquitous in the realm of healthcare simulation. This technology has great potential in informing learners in the health sciences. However, there are also potential risks to learners' health and safety. These risks can be mitigated by careful planning, management, and monitoring of learners' VR experience.

Cybersickness is one potential issue in certain users of VR. Cybersickness occurs when there is a divergence between what is seen and the vestibular system in the inner ear and brain controlling balance and eye movement. Cybersickness is similar to motion sickness and can cause the wearer of an HMD nausea, dizziness, and general disorientation. This can be mitigated by teaching the learner to move their head slowly, briefly close their eyes, or lift the headset away from their face until the sensation passes. However, even with these interventions, some people who are very sensitive to the sensations caused by the VR display may not be able to participate. If this occurs, a 2D version of the simulation should be available (Luo et al., 2021).

Another risk is immersion injury. When donning the immersive HMD, participants experience sensory deprivation of the real world around them. Although immersion, the hallmark of the VR, transports the participant into the VW, it also exposes the wearer to potential injury from collision with persons or objects, or the potential for falls when wearing the HMD. This factor can be eliminated by having the wearer remain seated during the scenario. It is also helpful to have the learner seated in a chair that can rotate 360°. A chair that can rotate allows the viewer to observe all of the actions within the scene. If the VRS does not permit the wearer to remain seated during the simulation, adequate room without obstacles that can cause potential injury or contribute to a fall should be the setting where the experience takes place.

Another potential for harm is the transmission of disease from the HMD and controllers. This has become a prevalent issue in education since the outbreak of COVID-19. Meticulous cleaning and sanitizing of the HMD and controllers must be employed between use of the VR equipment. Consider the construction of the equipment when determining the best method for cleaning and sanitizing. Electronic components should not be exposed to moisture. Lenses within the HMD may become scratched or clouded by harsh chemicals. Lens-cleaning wipes designed specifically for optics will protect the lenses. Using UV light is one consideration for sanitizing the HMD and controllers. Sanitizing wipes should also be utilized in order to kill the bacteria and viruses on parts of the HMD and controllers that are in contact with the skin.

## ▶ DESIGNING AN IMMERSIVE VIRTUAL REALITY SIMULATION

There are several steps involved in designing and implementing an effective VRS learning module. As with any course, the first step is to identify the content of the lesson and map out the learning objectives. Based on the strengths and weaknesses discussed earlier, and keeping in mind current institutional readiness, funding, infrastructure support, and class size, educators can decide if I-VR is the right medium. Here are some considerations for I-VRS educators.

### COST AND AVAILABILITY

VR headsets are expensive, ranging from a few hundred to a few thousand U.S. dollars. From an institution's perspective, there are other infrastructure needs that add to this cost, such as mobile charging stations, UV cleanbox, desktops, and VR-compatible rooms. Although in the case of healthcare simulation, where the cost of live training is much higher, the larger initial investment in VR can be spread across a large number of trainees and longer period of time (Farra et al., 2019). There is also hesitancy among institutions in investing in these technologies due to changes in market offerings. An example would be the unexpected demise of the Oculus Go production when several institutions have invested on these headsets. However, these have been replaced by a more capable Oculus Quest. Also, the ideal would be one headset per student; however, for big class sizes, institutions have managed with one headset for every 10 students.

### CONTENT AND INTEGRATION

The lack of relevant content has been the main reason cited by educators who want to adopt I-VR as a learning tool. Educators who have been developing custom teaching videos and learning materials for their simulation laboratory and screen-based courses will find 360° VR an effective way to create immersive content. CG-VRS typically require working with a software development team and would take a few months to create. It would be worthwhile to check the marketplace for preexisting VRS content that is both effective and relevant to the learning objectives.

### INTEROPERABILITY AND TECH SUPPORT

As the marketplace for I-VR expands, new and proprietary hardware and software products emerge. When educators purchase a specific device for their I-VR curriculum, the gear they ultimately choose sets up a trajectory of subsequent decisions dependent on the implications of that headset selection (Lee et al., 2021). The XR community recognizes the importance of interoperability, and several standards have been projected as viable pathways for hosting XR content, agnostic to the delivery device. WebXR is a new standard for XR running through web browsers. It supports both VR and AR content and can be viewed on any web browser, including computers, smartphones, tablets, and VR headsets. The fact that WebXR-based content can be written to work out of the box in simple consumer devices makes this technology widely available and accessible, as virtually any user with an internet connection and a capable device can benefit from it (Rodríguez et al., 2021). Similar steps are being taken to standardize SLS and education applications developed to run on VR headsets, including concurrent nonimmersive offerings and LMS integration.

## INSTITUTIONAL SUPPORT

Institutional support for training educators on developing XR modules is also an important consideration. Guides developed by instructional support, information technology (IT), and peers help set the stage for newcomers to quickly bring their vision to the classroom. Like any modern electronics device, VR devices, even the plug-and-play ones, require periodic maintenance (like software updates and recharging the batteries); if overlooked, it can pose major delays, especially in synchronous sessions. ThinkReality by Lenovo is a device management platform that can remotely monitor the charge level and update the status of their VR headsets. University initiatives in establishing immersive learning centers like the XR initiative at the University of Michigan or the VR pilot projects at Georgian College have shown high degree of success in student engagement, remote learning, improved outcomes, as well as serving as a training hub for the rest of the XR community. Several leading universities are now offering online courses on XR module development for education.

Once the VR content is ready for the learners, the next step is setting the VR classroom. There are several ways of conducting a VR course: synchronous or asynchronous, in person or remote, self-guided or instructor-led, and individual or in groups. A VR session can be broken down into the following phases: orientation, briefing, action, and debriefing.

## ORIENTATION

Most learners and educators are new to I-VR and must be properly oriented to the technology prior to actual VL. Learner confusion can be induced through various factors, including complex instructions, insufficient orientation, and ill-developed learning modules. Because I-VR can be extremely immersive, complicated button presses, motion sickness, disorientation, and technical issues increase frustration and break immersion. Educators should aim to design their course to find the right balance between engagement and frustration (Arguel et al., 2017). However, even with all these provisions, some learners may not be able to benefit from I-VR either due to physiologic incompatibilities with technology or by choice. Such learners should be provided with viable alternative learning tools.

## BRIEFING

During the briefing stage, learners create their avatar and familiarize themselves with the platform interface. Unlike screen-based learning, I-VR learners cannot interact with the real world once they are immersed in the VRS. Educators should incorporate adequate instructions in the briefing or incorporate them within the VL so that learners should not have to break immersion within the VRS. Educators must be cognizant of the learner's physical safety in VRS that require them to look and move around. This may be a quick check to clear the physical surroundings to avoid serious injury or falls.

## ACTION PHASE

Learners enter the VW scenario created for them. Instructors and teaching assistants must be cognizant of the learner's inability to see their real world. Some VRS have companion apps through which the educator can monitor in real time their learners' progress and engage with them live in the VRS. Learners interact in the environment based on the design of the simulation, which may be acting alone or working in teams and collaborating with others. Some learners may feel a sense of shock due to the sudden change in environment when they remove the headset.

## DEBRIEFING

In healthcare simulation, debriefing is where most of the learning occurs. It is a key feature in designing VWs and should be done after each VL experience (Billings, 2009). Educators facilitate the reflection (reflective observation) of learners' experiences during the simulation. Meaning (abstract conceptualization) is derived from the experience. Further application of the meaning may be initiated. Debriefing after VRS can be done either in the traditional classroom, within an MUVE, or even with AI avatars (Verkuyl et al., 2018). Educators should also consider including VR-specific questionnaires (Somrak et al., 2021) for items like presence, simulator sickness, and user experience to better understand their learners' needs.

## ▶ COMMUNITY RESOURCES

The VR education community is small but very active and is a great resource for VL educators and learners. Several professional organizations such as the Immersive Learning Research Network (iLRN), VR/AR Association (VRARA), International Society for Virtual Rehabilitation, and Institute of Electrical and Electronics Engineers (IEEE) VR have incorporated VL as a key vertical in their organization. Since I-VR is an area heavily influenced by industries like gaming, therapeutics, industrial training, and many others, these membership organizations play a pivotal role in bringing together educators, hardware manufacturers, software developers, and solution integrators to share ideas and solutions to further the implementation of VR in education. Attending online workshops and conferences is a great way to interface and collaborate. Several publishers, including Frontiers, Springer, and Elsevier, have dedicated journals and special topics on VL. In keeping up with times, social media and podcasts provide up-to-date information from educators, content creators, and researchers, as well as industry experts and market trend analysts. Podcasts focusing on VL include Voices of VR, VR in Education, and Everything VR & AR.

---

### Evidence-Based Simulation Practice 13.1

Educators shared their experience of embedding virtual gaming into a nursing school curriculum (Verkuyl et al., 2021).

Purpose: Share the lessons learned from the development and incorporation of virtual gaming into a nursing course of study.

Design: How to decide the best virtual gaming simulation (VGS) that aligns with the course content and meets the course learning objectives; and the importance of having a prebrief before the virtual game, enactment, debriefing, and evaluation of the virtual simulation game.

Methods: Educators are continuously challenged to actively engage learners. The researchers in this study created virtual gaming simulations to augment their learners' education. The VGS presented learners with a realistic scene of a nurse–client encounter. After viewing the film clip, the learners were presented with options on how to proceed. If they chose incorrectly, they were directed to choose another answer and continue with the simulation. Learners were given a summary of their achievement during the simulation and the opportunity to repeat the VGS as often as they would like.

Results: The researchers believe having both the educators and the learners involved in the development of VGS will improve the acceptance and applicability of this type of simulation. They also stress the importance of a prebrief before and a debrief after the simulation. Evaluation of the experience is essential to learn from the experience and to make improvement on future VGS offerings.

**Conclusions:** There is an exponential increase in the use of VGS in education. Learning from and sharing best practice in virtual gaming will help establish best-practice guidelines in this emerging field of active education.

*(continued)*

**Evidence-Based Simulation Practice 13.2**

A pilot study was designed to teach airway insertion skills to nursing faculty and students using immersive virtual reality (I-VR; Samosorn et al., 2020).

**Purpose:** Teach students difficult airway management skills using virtual reality (VR) intervention.

**Design:** Survey sampling was combined with a quasi-experimental, one-group, pretest–posttest design to assess the fidelity, realism, potential adverse effects, and efficacy of a VR intervention for airway management among undergraduate nursing faculty and students.

**Methods:** The airway management VR laboratory is a computer-generated I-VR (CG-I-VR) delivered over a PC-VR setup (Oculus Rift) with dynamic haptic feedback delivered through the handheld controllers. This voiceover narration-guided intervention consists of six lessons orienting learners to basic skills and processes associated with airway management for an unresponsive and apneic patient. Detailed step-by-step instructions and dynamic positive reinforcement haptic feedback were added to keep the users engaged. Gamification in the form of level unlocks was also added as a reward mechanism. The total instruction time was 20 minutes. Web-based survey instruments included a presence questionnaire which assessed the realism of the experience, a VR sickness questionnaire which assessed cybersickness, and a validated knowledge test.

**Results:** 10 faculty members and 21 students participated in this study. The faculty and students rated the VR airway laboratory as having high presence, no cybersickness, and significantly improving knowledge of airway management ($p < .0001$). The faculty and students, overall, felt the airway management intervention oriented them very well.

**Conclusions:** The authors argue that immersion brings about psychological fidelity within VR, which actively promotes learner engagement. Immersive spatial representations coupled with vestibular and proprioceptive senses can have a positive effect on memory recall. The VR airway laboratory is an efficacious means of teaching difficult airway management skills to nursing students.

# ▶ SUMMARY

This chapter discussed VL modalities, including I-VR, VPs, VRS, MUVE, and serious games, and has looked at the design of these modalities and their effectiveness in the learning environment. There are concrete advantages to using VL environments, which include promoting interprofessional collaboration and providing experiences that mimic real-life situations and are easily transferred to the clinical practice setting. Disadvantages of VL include the cost and extensive faculty development required to design the scenario. There are also health and safety issues associated with the use of VR. The learner must also be oriented to the VL platform in order to be successful in maneuvering within the scenario to enhance their learning experience. VL and VRS can be used in the education of healthcare professionals when there is an increased demand for clinical placement and, at the same time, fewer resources of time and space available for learning. The uses of VL and their outcomes are expanding in academia and show much promise in enhancing the learning environment and improving learning outcomes.

# ● CASE STUDY 13.1

Students in their last semester of nursing at a local university are enrolled in the community health nursing course. The course has been designed within the context of public health nursing. Disaster preparedness is one of the topics taught in the course. The faculty member has collaborated with the faculty in other disciplines, including medical students, physician-assistant students, and emergency management services (EMS), as well as paramedic students, to plan a virtual reality (VR) learning experience in the management of disasters. The faculty members are developing the scenario but are not sure how to design the simulation using Second Life as the virtual learning (VL) platform. How should they begin the process of designing the simulation so that it is a meaningful learning experience?

# ● CASE STUDY DISCUSSION

A major factor to consider is the cost of designing the virtual simulation. Does the university support the learning platform and is it willing to provide funds for the project? An initial action to be considered when designing a virtual serious game is determining the purpose of the activity. The scenario should be designed based on the objectives and outcomes of the exercise. This is the key factor in developing a VL situation. It is advisable to base the virtual world (VW) on a sound learning theory, which then influences the activities that are constructed within the activity. The faculty should receive some professional development on how to design the simulation using the Second Life platform. What computer requirements are needed for the learner to interact in the VW? Instructional technology services at the university need to be available to support both the faculty and the students through the process. The faculty should conduct an assessment of the students' abilities and/or needs to interact with technology and plan orientation based on the data obtained. The value of professional collaboration across disciplines, especially in disaster preparedness, should be emphasized prior to the start of the VL simulation so that learners from all of the disciplines are actively involved in the game.

1. The simulation educator is considering adding immersive virtual reality (I-VR) to complement a simulation program. Which of the following is an example of an I-VR simulation designed to be used for clinical education?

   A. Having a remote conference interviewing a standardized patient
   B. Viewing a single-display, computer-generated patient avatar
   C. Playing a clinical skill-based video game on a computer monitor
   D. Interacting with the hospital environment in three dimensions using a headset

2. Which of the following simulations is better suited for in person learning over immersive virtual reality (I-VR)?

   A. Rail crash disaster simulation
   B. Fire in the operating room
   C. Three dimensional anatomy and physiology education
   D. Abdominal palpation

3. What is the purpose of a virtual patient (VP) within a virtual world?

   A. Provide feedback to the learner during the simulation
   B. Practice clinical decision-making with a patient
   C. Repetitively practice an essential clinical skill
   D. Allow the learner to create a realistic avatar

4. Virtual gaming is a method of learning delivery that is associated with which educational theory?

   A. Behaviorism
   B. Realism
   C. Emancipatory
   D. Constructivism

5. A novice simulation educator is designing a virtual world (VW) for their learners to practice clinical decision-making. Which concept should drive the creation of a virtual reality simulation?

   A. VWs should offer the learner immersion and presence
   B. The simulation educator should create a fantasy world populated with imaginative characters
   C. VWs are personalized and do not allow for collaboration
   D. Experimentation with a VW is discouraged

1. **D) Interacting with the hospital environment in three dimensions using a headset**

Using a three-dimensional environment integrates virtual reality (VR). Remote learning, single-display computers, and videos are not considered VR.

2. **D) Abdominal palpation**

Learning about abdominal palpation may be better done in person so there is visual and haptic learning. Disasters such as rail crashes and fires in the operating room can be done effectively in I-VR. Three-dimensional education is effective for viewing human systems and learning anatomy and physiology.

3. **B) Practice clinical decision-making with a patient**

Enhancing students' quality decision-making is always the goal of healthcare education. Inserting patients does not necessarily provide feedback to students, assist with clinical skills (they could be providing healthcare information), or produce an avatar.

4. **D) Constructivism**

Virtual gaming allows students to build on previous knowledge, which is a basic tenet of the constructivist theory. Behaviorism works on a reward basis, realism emphasizes evidence, and emancipatory focuses on social justice.

5. **A) VWs should offer the learner immersion and presence**

VWs should offer learners an engaged experience in order for them to have a sense of responsibility about decision-making. VWs should not be a fantasy work or lack collaboration. Virtual learning should not be discouraged because it is a good method for many students' learning styles and can meet some specific learning outcomes.

6. The use of immersive virtual reality (I-VR) in simulation education is grounded in which of the following principles?

   A. Social learning
   B. Suspended disbelief
   C. Situated cognition
   D. Cognitive dissonance

7. The professor wants to teach the importance of identifying hospital stressors for autistic adults by showing facial expressions and subtle behavioral changes during a nurse–patient interaction. Which of these immersive technologies would BEST facilitate learning?

   A. Six degrees of freedom (6DoF) hospital room with computer-generated characters
   B. 360° virtual reality (VR) video with live actors in first-person view
   C. Multiuser virtual environment with haptic feedback
   D. Augmented reality overlay of a patient's vitals on a smartphone

8. The design of a virtual reality simulation based on the constructivist theory would include:

   A. Social interaction between learners
   B. Peer support for decision-making
   C. Moving from simple to complex
   D. Creating a realistic avatar

9. When developing an immersive virtual reality (I-VR), the first action the simulation educator must perform is:

   A. Determine the platform to use to design the game
   B. Require students to have taken a computer course
   C. Conduct a prebriefing about the experience
   D. Develop learning objectives for the activity

10. Which of the following is an example of the application of Kolb's experiential learning theory as it applies to virtual reality simulation (VRS)?

    A. Learners make decisions based on their avatar's role in the simulation
    B. VRSs are for learners to observe and not interact
    C. Learners alter the environment within virtual reality (VR) to increase realism
    D. Learners can apply their experience of the simulation to the real world

## 6. C) Situated cognition

I-VR is grounded in situated cognition, which uses the sense of self-location, the sense of agency, and the sense of body ownership, and is critical to learning. Social learning refers the larger picture in the community. Suspending disbelief is done for many simulation modalities, while cognitive dissonance is engaging in a learning activity that may not be pleasant but reaches a goal.

## 7. B) 360° virtual reality (VR) video with live actors in first-person view

The 360° VR video with live actors in first-person view would be the best methodology because students can visualize a live capture of real environments and real people using 360° cameras, which gives much more visual fidelity and leads to a more realistic decision-making. 6DoF hospital room, multiuser virtual environment, and augmented reality overlay are effective in many learning activities but do not show subtle changes.

## 8. C) Moving from simple to complex

Students have to move from novice to competent and so learning should be from simple to complex to be congruent with the learner's level. Constructivist does not need social interaction, peer support, or an avatar for students to learn. Constructivism should build on past experiences and become more complex as learning scaffolds.

## 9. D) Develop learning objectives for the activity

The first activity for all learning experiences should be to establish the objectives or learning outcomes. After establishing the objectives, the simulation educator can decide on the platform and develop the scenario, which should include a prebriefing. There is no need for students to take a computer course.

## 10. D) Learners can apply their experience of the simulation to the real world

Kolb's theory links experiential learning to clinical practice for healthcare professionals. Students need to engage in VR and make decisions based on their role, not the avatar's role. Realism in VR is dictated by the educator and the platform.

# REFERENCES

Arguel, A., Lockyer, L., Lipp, O. V., Lodge, J. M., & Kennedy, G. (2017). Inside out. *Journal of Educational Computing Research, 55*(4), 526–551. https://doi.org/10.1177/0735633116674732

Billings, D. M., & Halstead, J. A. (2009). *Teaching in nursing: A guide for faculty.* Saunders Elsevier.

Biocca, F. (1992). Virtual reality technology: A tutorial. *Journal of Communication, 42*(4), 23–72. https://doi.org/10.1111/j.1460-2466.1992.tb00811.x

Bracq, M.-S., Michinov, E., Arnaldi, B., Caillaud, B., Gibaud, B., Gouranton, V., & Jannin, P. (2019a). Learning procedural skills with a virtual reality simulator: An acceptability study. *Nurse Education Today, 79*, 153–160. https://doi.org/10.1016/j.nedt.2019.05.026

Bracq, M.-S., Michinov, E., & Jannin, P. (2019b). Virtual reality simulation in nontechnical skills training for healthcare professionals. *Simulation in Healthcare: The Journal of the Society for Simulation in Healthcare, 14*(3), 188–194. https://doi.org/10.1097/sih.0000000000000347

Brydon, M., Kimber, J., Sponagle, M., MacLaine, J., Avery, J., Pyke, L., & Gilbert, R. (2021). Virtual reality as a tool for eliciting empathetic behaviour in carers: An integrative review. *Journal of Medical Imaging and Radiation Sciences, 52*(3), 466–477. https://doi.org/10.1016/j.jmir.2021.04.005

Butt, A. L., Kardong-Edgren, S., & Ellertson, A. (2018). Using game-based virtual reality with haptics for skill acquisition. *Clinical Simulation in Nursing, 16*, 25–32. https://doi.org/10.1016/j.ecns.2017.09.010

Chen, F.-Q., Leng, Y.-F., Ge, J.-F., Wang, D.-W., Li, C., Chen, B., & Sun, Z.-L. (2020). Effectiveness of virtual reality in nursing education: Meta-analysis. *Journal of Medical Internet Research, 22*(9), e18290. https://doi.org/10.2196/18290

Choi, W., Dyens, O., Chan, T., Schijven, M., Lajoie, S., Mancini, M. E., Dev, P., Fellander-Tsai, L., Ferland, M., Kato, P., Lau, J., Montonaro, M., Pineau, J., & Aggarwal, R. (2017). Engagement and learning in simulation: Recommendations of the Simnovate engaged learning domain group. *BMJ Simulation and Technology Enhanced Learning, 3*(Suppl. 1), S23–S32. https://doi.org/10.1136/bmjstel-2016-000177

Dhar, P., Rocks, T., Samarasinghe, R. M., Stephenson, G., & Smith, C. (2021). Augmented reality in medical education: Students' experiences and learning outcomes. *Medical Education Online, 26*(1), 1953953. https://doi.org/10.1080/10872981.2021.1953953

Epp, S., Reekie, M., Denison, J., De Bosch Kemper, N., Willson, M., & Marck, P. (2021). Radical transformation: Embracing constructivism and pedagogy for an innovative nursing curriculum. *Journal of Professional Nursing, 37*(5), 804–809. https://doi.org/10.1016/j.profnurs.2021.06.007

Farra, S. L., Gneuhs, M., Hodgson, E., Kawosa, B., Miller, E. T., Simon, A., Timm, N., & Hausfeld, J. (2019). Comparative cost of virtual reality training and live exercises for training hospital workers for evacuation. *CIN: Computers, Informatics, Nursing, 37*(9), 446–454. https://doi.org/10.1097/cin.0000000000000540

Farra, S. L., Miller, E. T., & Hodgson, E. (2015). Virtual reality disaster training: Translation to practice. *Nurse Education in Practice, 15*(1), 53–57. https://doi.org/10.1016/j.nepr.2013.08.017

Gaba, D. M. (2004). The future vision of simulation in health care. *Quality and Safety in Health Care, 13*(Suppl. 1), i2–i10. https://doi.org/10.1136/qshc.2004.009878

Green, J., Wyllie, A., & Jackson, D. (2014). Virtual worlds: A new frontier for nurse education? *Collegian, 21*(2), 135–141. https://doi.org/10.1016/j.colegn.2013.11.004

Guise, V., Chambers, M., & Välimäki, M. (2012). What can virtual patient simulation offer mental health nursing education? *Journal of Psychiatric and Mental Health Nursing, 19*(5), 410–418.

Hamilton, D., Mckechnie, J., Edgerton, E., & Wilson, C. (2021). Immersive virtual reality as a pedagogical tool in education: A systematic literature review of quantitative learning outcomes and experimental design. *Journal of Computers in Education, 8*(1), 1–32. https://doi.org/10.1007/s40692-020-00169-2

Hogan, M., Kapralos, B., Cristancho, S., Finney, K., & Dubrowski, A. (2011). Bringing community health nursing education to life with serious games. *International Journal of Nursing Education Scholarship, 8*(1). https://doi.org/10.2202/1548-923X.2072

Jeffries, P. R. (2012). *Simulation in nursing education: From conceptualization to evaluation* (2nd ed.). National League for Nursing.

Jensen, L., & Konradsen, F. (2018). A review of the use of virtual reality head-mounted displays in education and training. *Education and Information Technologies, 23*(4), 1515–1529. https://doi.org/10.1007/s10639-017-9676-0

Keating, S. B. (2010). *Curriculum development and evaluation in nursing* (2nd ed.). Springer Publishing Company.

Kittel, A., Larkin, P., Elsworthy, N., Lindsay, R., & Spittle, M. (2020). Effectiveness of 360° virtual reality and match broadcast video to improve decision-making skill. *Science and Medicine in Football, 4*(4), 255–262. https://doi.org/10.1080/24733938.2020.1754449

Kolb, D. A. (1984). *Experiential learning: Experience as the source of learning and development* (Vol. 1). Prentice-Hall.

Kye, B., Han, N., Kim, E., Park, Y., & Jo, S. (2021). Educational applications of metaverse: Possibilities and limitations. *Journal of Educational Evaluation for Health Professions, 18*, 32. https://doi.org/10.3352/jeehp.2021.18.32

Lee, M. J. W., Georgieva, M., Alexander, B., Craig, E., & Richter, J. (2021). *State of XR & immersive learning outlook report 2021.* Immersive Learning Research Network.

Lerner, D., Mohr, S., Schild, J., Göring, M., & Luiz, T. (2020). An immersive multi-user virtual reality for emergency simulation training: Usability study. *JMIR Serious Games, 8*(3), e18822. https://doi.org/10.2196/18822

Liaw, S. Y., Carpio, G. A. C., Lau, Y., Tan, S. C., Lim, W. S., & Goh, P. S. (2018). Multiuser virtual worlds in healthcare education: A systematic review. *Nurse Education Today, 65*, 136–149. https://doi.org/10.1016/j.nedt.2018.01.006

Luo, H., Yang, T., Kwon, S., Li, G., Zuo, M., & Choi, I. (2021). Performing versus observing: Investigating the effectiveness of group debriefing in a VR-based safety education program. *Computers & Education, 175*, 104316. https://doi.org/10.1016/j.compedu.2021.104316

Moro, C., Phelps, C., Redmond, P., & Stromberga, Z. (2021). HoloLens and mobile augmented reality in medical and health science education: A randomised controlled trial. *British Journal of Educational Technology, 52*(2), 680–694. https://doi.org/10.1111/bjet.13049

Patel, V., Aggarwal, R., Cohen, D., Taylor, D., & Darzi, A. (2013). Implementation of an interactive virtual-world simulation for structured surgeon assessment of clinical scenarios. *Journal of the American College of Surgeons, 217*(2), 270–279.

Petit dit Dariel, O. J., Raby, T., Ravaut, F., & Rothan-Tondeur, M. (2013). Developing the serious games potential in nursing education. *Nurse Education Today, 33*(12), 1569–1575. https://doi.org/10.1016/j.nedt.2012.12.014

Pottle, J. (2019). Virtual reality and the transformation of medical education. *Future Healthcare Journal, 6*(3), 181–185. https://doi.org/10.7861/fhj.2019-0036

Ramakrishnan, A., Lieva, A., & Okupniak, C. (2020, March 2–4). *Virtual reality in clinical simulation: A modality for undergraduate nursing education* [Paper presentation]. 14th International Technology, Education and Development Conference, Valencia, Spain.

Ricciardi, F., & De Paolis, L. T. (2014). A comprehensive review of serious games in health professions. *International Journal of Computer Games Technology, 2014*, 1–11. https://doi.org/10.1155/2014/787968

Rodríguez, F. C., Dal Peraro, M., & Abriata, L. A. (2021). Democratizing interactive, immersive experiences for science education with WebXR. *Nature Computational Science, 1*(10), 631–632. https://doi.org/10.1038/s43588-021-00142-8

Rogers, L. (2011). Developing simulations in multi-user virtual environments to enhance healthcare education. *British Journal of Educational Technology, 42*(4), 608–615. https://doi.org/10.1111/j.1467-8535.2010.01057.x

Sailer, M., Hense, J. U., Mayr, S. K., & Mandl, H. (2017). How gamification motivates: An experimental study of the effects of specific game design elements on psychological need satisfaction. *Computers in Human Behavior, 69*, 371–380. https://doi.org/10.1016/j.chb.2016.12.033

Samosorn, A. B., Gilbert, G. E., Bauman, E. B., Khine, J., & Mcgonigle, D. (2020). Teaching airway insertion skills to nursing faculty and students using virtual reality: A pilot study. *Clinical Simulation in Nursing, 39*, 18–26. https://doi.org/10.1016/j.ecns.2019.10.004

Sankaranarayanan, G., Wooley, L., Hogg, D., Dorozhkin, D., Olasky, J., Chauhan, S., Fleshman, J. W., De, S., Scott, D., & Jones, D. B. (2018). Immersive virtual reality-based training improves response in a simulated operating room fire scenario. *Surgical Endoscopy, 32*(8), 3439–3449. https://doi.org/10.1007/s00464-018-6063-x

Singh, A., Ferry, D., & Mills, S. (2018). Improving biomedical engineering education through continuity in adaptive, experiential, and interdisciplinary learning environments. *Journal of Biomechanical Engineering, 140*(8). https://doi.org/10.1115/1.4040359

Singh, A., Ferry, D., Ramakrishnan, A., & Balasubramanian, S. (2020). Using virtual reality in biomedical engineering education. *Journal of Biomechanical Engineering, 142*(11). https://doi.org/10.1115/1.4048005

Society for Simulation in Healthcare. (2021). *Certified healthcare simulation educator handbook.* https://www.ssih.org/Portals/48/Certification/CHSE_Docs/CHSE%20Handbook.pdf

Somrak, A., Pogačnik, M., & Guna, J. (2021). Suitability and comparison of questionnaires assessing virtual reality-induced symptoms and effects and user experience in virtual environments. *Sensors (Basel), 21*(4), 1185. https://doi.org/10.3390/s21041185

Sultan, L., Abuznadah, W., Al-Jifree, H., Khan, M. A., Alsaywid, B., & Ashour, F. (2019). An experimental study on usefulness of virtual reality 360° in undergraduate medical education. *Advances in Medical Education and Practice, 10*, 907–916. https://doi.org/10.2147/amep.s219344

Tiffany, J., & Hoglund, B. A. (2014). Teaching/learning in second life: Perspectives of future nurse-educators. *Clinical Simulation in Nursing, 10*(1), e19–e24. https://doi.org/10.1016/j.ecns.2013.06.006

Tran, C., Toth-Pal, E., Ekblad, S., Fors, U., & Salminen, H. (2020). A virtual patient model for students' interprofessional learning in primary healthcare. *PLoS One, 15*(9), e0238797. https://doi.org/10.1371/journal.pone.0238797

Verkuyl, M., Lapum, J. L., Hughes, M., Mcculloch, T., Liu, L., Mastrilli, P., Romaniuk, D., & Betts, L. (2018). Virtual gaming simulation: Exploring self-debriefing, virtual debriefing, and in-person debriefing. *Clinical Simulation in Nursing, 20*, 7–14. https://doi.org/10.1016/j.ecns.2018.04.006

Verkuyl, M., Lapum, J. L., St-Amant, O., Hughes, M., & Romaniuk, D. (2021). Curricular uptake of virtual gaming simulation in nursing education. *Nurse Education in Practice, 50*, 102967. https://doi.org/10.1016/j.nepr.2021.102967

Vygotsky, L. S. (1978). *Mind in society: The development of higher psychological processes.* Harvard University Press.

Waltemate, T., Gall, D., Roth, D., Botsch, M., & Latoschik, M. E. (2018). The impact of avatar personalization and immersion on virtual body ownership, presence, and emotional response. *IEEE Transactions on Visualization and Computer Graphics, 24*(4), 1643–1652. https://doi.org/10.1109/tvcg.2018.2794629

# PART IV
**Educational Principles Applied to Simulation**

# Educational Theories, Learning Theories, and Special Concepts

Mary Hanson-Zalot, Julia Ward, and Ruth A. Wittmann-Price

*The teacher who is indeed wise does not bid you to enter the house of his wisdom but rather leads you to the threshold of your mind.*

—*Khalil Gibran*

This chapter addresses Domain III: Educational Principles Applied to Simulation (Society for Simulation in Healthcare [SSH], 2021).

## ▶ LEARNING OUTCOMES

- Discuss educational philosophies and theories in relation to simulation education.
- Identify learning and motivational theories used for simulation experiences.
- Define concepts related to simulation education.

## ▶ INTRODUCTION

Understanding educational and learning theories increases awareness of what, why, and how educators teach and how learners assimilate knowledge in the simulation laboratory or virtual reality (VR) session. A simulation or VR environment is an excellent milieu in which to synthesize content from the cognitive, psychomotor, and affective learning domains. Development of competence in all three learning domains is necessary for healthcare providers. The goals of simulation learning experiences are to promote patient safety and provide healthcare learners with the best possible safe learning environment (Guerrero et al., 2022).

Educational theories are contextual and spurn learning theories or how students grasp, understand, and apply knowledge. This chapter provides an overview of educational theories, including those educational concepts applied specifically to simulation learning and evaluation.

## ▶ EDUCATIONAL PHILOSOPHIES AND THEORIES

To facilitate learning in a simulation environment, a simulation educator must build experiences on sound theoretical foundations that include understanding the essence of educational philosophies, which:

- date back to ancient times, are never stagnant, and change as the larger social system matures
- provide the foundations on which learning theories and educational pedagogies are built
- consider the branch of philosophy that addresses why we teach, how we teach, where we teach, and what the goals of education are for learners and society (Watts & Hodges, 2021)

Traditional educational theories were teacher-centered and based on what the educator could provide to the student. Postmodern theories more often take into account the social meaning of learning and the relationship of knowledge and power, and are more likely to consider multiple and innovative ways of learning (Turner, 2017).

Worldviews about education categorize how an educational philosophy relates to the social context. Learning theories have more defined concepts that are more applicable to teaching situations. Teaching is the act of facilitating learning through instruction, guidance, and coaching. In today's social context, teaching is student-centered (Horberg et al., 2019).

Learning is described as how people understand information. The manner in which individuals store, connect, discover, and retrieve skills and information has been well studied and formalized into many theoretical frameworks. These frameworks explain how knowledge is built and what paradigms are used to advance healthcare research. Figure 14.1 shows the frameworks used in developing research knowledge for healthcare professionals (Win, 2016).

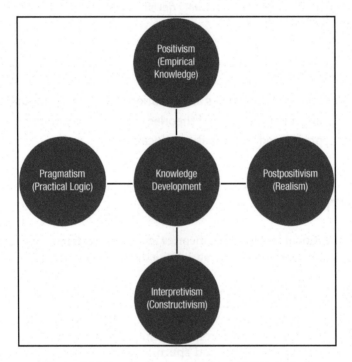

**Figure 14.1** Knowledge development philosophies.

The two main learning theories discussed and used currently in education are *behaviorism* and *constructivism*. Behaviorism is an ingrained theory in education and structures teaching plans. Constructivism is an ideal theory to encapsulate, ground, and expand what is done in the simulation laboratory because its major tenets promote active learning.

### Simulation Teaching Tip 14.1

Kim and Yoo (2022) remind faculty that high-fidelity simulation does not always ensure knowledge acquisition compared with using low-fidelity simulation.

## BEHAVIORISM

Behaviorism is a learning theory that was developed in the 1940s. The following are some of the major tenets of behaviorism:

- Learning is observable through behavior.
- Learning is reinforced by response.
- Behavior modification leads to control.
- Token economies may be used for classroom management.
- Instructional objectives guide learning (Tyler, 1949).
- Learning is shaped by others.
- Learning is teacher-centered.
- Behaviorists include Watson, Skinner, Pavlov, and Bandura.

Behaviorism posed a couple of difficult issues for education, including the following:

- Behaviorism does not explain the intrinsic motivation of the learner.
- All learning is not displayed in behavior.
- By predetermining objectives or outcomes, the depth and breadth of the learners' experiences may be squelched (Bevis & Watson, 1989; Diekelmann, 1997, 2005).

It is difficult, at best, to package the human intellect into a modifiable mold for convenience of grouping, evaluating, and justifying what is being taught or presented and what a learner carries forth from an experience. Behaviorism was made popular by Tyler's landmark book *Basic Principles of Curriculum and Instruction* (1949) in relation to writing instructional objectives or what the teacher expected the learner to learn by the end of a teaching session or course.

## CONSTRUCTIVISM

Currently, constructivism is the theoretical paradigm that best fits educational processes and the social context of today. Constructivists view learning as an active process that builds new knowledge on knowledge already obtained, thereby connecting what is unknown to what is known. Adaptive behaviors are produced when learners take received stimuli and convert or construct them into cognitive knowledge that makes sense to them. Constructivism is based in the reality of the learner and is therefore learner-focused. The role of faculty in constructivism includes coaching and facilitating (Le Coze, 2017). Learning using simulation fits well into the constructivist theoretical framework because it is problem-based and prompts individually constructed knowledge through experiential learning (Brown & Watts, 2016).

## ▶ LEARNING THEORIES

## EXPERIENTIAL LEARNING THEORY

A learning theory that fits within the constructivist framework is experiential learning. The experiential learning theory (ELT) is widely used in simulation experiences. It is defined as "the process whereby knowledge is created through the transformation of experience. Knowledge results from the combination of grasping and transforming an experience" (Kolb, 1984, p. 41).
There are four major concepts within Kolb's ELT:

- *Concrete experience* (*CE*), or experiences built from reality
- *Abstract conceptualization* (*AC*), or thinking about an experience

■ *Reflective observation* (*RO*), or taking in the experience
■ *Active experimentation* (*AE*), or using hands-on experiences to learn (Kolb et al., 1999)

ELT is student-centered because the learners are in control of the direction the simulation scenario takes. Although the student learning outcomes (SLOs) are formulated by the certified healthcare educator, the students are in control of their actions and the consequences. As students become more advanced in their healthcare studies, they are able to relinquish a more passive role in scenarios and increase their active roles and feelings of being prepared to participate in experiential learning (Bastin et al., 2017). The change from passive to active learning is depicted in Figure 14.2.

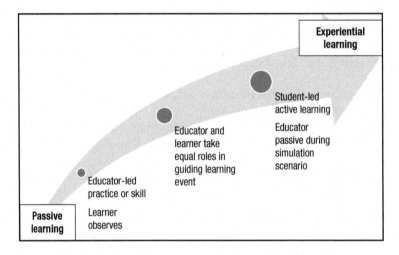

**Figure 14.2** Change in learning from passive to active.

Gibbs (1988) also has a model for planning experiential learning, which includes the following:

■ planning for action
■ carrying out the action
■ reflecting on the action
■ relating the action back to the theory

Grant and Marsden (1992) explain experiential learning as having the following components:

■ providing an experience
■ thinking about the experience
■ identifying improvements
■ planning the learning needed
■ putting the learning into practice

Simulation is well suited for experiential learning because it is a practiced experience in a controlled environment that allows for reflection (thinking) and ultimately changes in practice (doing) by adult professionals (Griffith et al., 2017). One of the main aims of simulation-based learning in undergraduate education is to impact future clinical practice to influence patient outcomes (Bruce et al., 2019).

## SCAFFOLDING LEARNING THEORY

Congruent with ELT is cognitive scaffolding. This theory was introduced by Vygotsky (1978) to explain how a novice learns to be an expert. Just as a scaffold supports a building under construction, the novice learner needs resources and support from experts or mentors to increase cognitive knowledge on a subject and build it progressively. The scaffolding sets the framework for learning and is intentionally established as a "stretch" for the learner. In order for the learner to reach higher levels of knowledge or understanding about a situation or process, support must be in place, such as:

- constructive feedback
- explanations
- reflection
- revision of knowledge building

Scaffolding learning has been noted to promote deeper learning and student confidence (Lauerer et al., 2017; Figure 14.3).

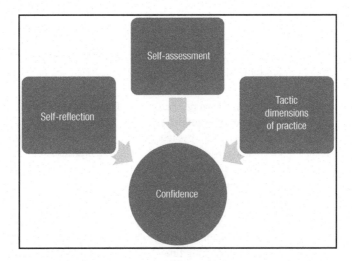

**Figure 14.3** Outcomes of scaffolding learning.

## SOCIAL LEARNING (COGNITIVE) THEORY

The social learning theory also incorporates reinforcement and modeling new behavior as learners observe it from certified healthcare educators. Behavior is determined by social determinants, such as demographics and economics, behavioral influences such as those characteristics innate to a person, and environmental elements such as resources (Sriramatr et al., 2016).

Another popular concept that was attributed to the social learning theory is self-efficacy coined by Bandura (1997). Self-efficacy is often measured in healthcare learners, and progressive or ongoing simulation experiences are an ideal environment for its measurement. Self-efficacy is the perception of confidence in one's self in a given situation. Self-efficacy is based on four principles:

- *Mastering experiences:* the learner's own history of success
- *Vicarious experiences:* the observed behaviors of a role model being successful at a task

- *Verbal persuasion:* telling individuals they will be successful
- *Physiologic states:* the person's "gut feeling" that success can be achieved

## ▶ PEDAGOGY VERSUS ANDRAGOGY AS EDUCATIONAL CONCEPTS

*Pedagogy* is generally defined as the art and science of teaching. It refers to the manner in which educators instruct. Its development was intended for children, but the development of all curricula incorporates pedagogy to some extent and developing effective pedagogy assists students in the learning process (Cadieux et al., 2017). *Andragogy* is the art and science of teaching adults and was coined by Malcolm Knowles in 1975 (Table 14.1).

**Table 14.1 Andragogy and Pedagogy**

| Educational Considerations | Andragogy | Pedagogy |
|---|---|---|
| Demands of learning | Learners have life demands besides school. | Learners can devote more time to the demands of learning because responsibilities are minimal. |
| Role of instructor | Learners are autonomous and self-directed. Educators facilitate the learning, but do not supply all the facts. | Learning is teacher-centered because the educator directs the learning. Surface learning is often used. |
| Life experiences | Learners have a tremendous amount of life experience. Learners connect the learning to their knowledge base. Learners must recognize the value of learning. | Learners do not have the knowledge base to make the connections of new knowledge to life experiences without facilitation. |
| Purpose of learning | Learners have a goal in sight for their learning. | Learners cannot always see the long-term necessity of information. |
| Permanence of learning | Learning is self-initiated and tends to last a long time. | Learning is compulsory and tends to disappear shortly after instruction. |

Adult learners display a variety of learning characteristics.

- The most common reason an adult enters any learning experience is to create change in the following:
  - skills
  - behavior
  - knowledge level
  - attitudes about things

Adult learners sometimes experience unique barriers to learning, which include the following:

- lack of time
- lack of confidence
- lack of information about opportunities to learn
- scheduling problems
- multiple role demands (Carpenter-Aeby & Aeby, 2013)

It is important to incorporate adult learning principles into simulated learning experiences to maximize learning potential for this population. The characteristics of an adult learner include the following:

- developed self-concept
- rich in experiences
- ready to learn
- prefers application of knowledge
- enjoys problem-based learning (PBL; Carpenter-Aeby & Aeby, 2013)

## ▶ SIMULATION LEARNING FRAMEWORKS

Several simulation learning frameworks describe how simulation specifically affects learning.

### KNEEBONE

Kneebone (2005) describes simulation learning using the following elements. Simulation should:

- allow for deliberate practice (DP) in a safe environment
- provide expert tutors to be available for the learners
- include experiences similar to real life
- be student-centered

### KIRKPATRICK

Kirkpatrick (1998) proposed four levels of learning which are applicable to simulation, as depicted in Figure 14.4. Each level follows in order of occurrence. The lowest level, level 1, is participant reactions. During the simulation experience, students can express their reactions to simulation during debriefing or reflection on the simulation. Level 2 is the learning that takes place by demonstrating the acquisition of knowledge and skills that occurred following the simulation experience. Level 3 relates to the degree to which learners changed their behavior outside the learning environment. At the top of the pyramid, level 4 is the results achieved through the previous levels as demonstrated by measuring outcomes such as improved clinical performance.

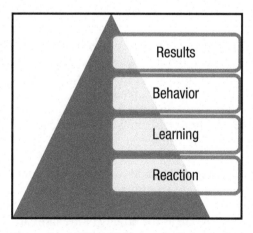

**Figure 14.4** Kirkpatrick's levels of simulation learning.

---

**Simulation Teaching Tip 14.2**

Thomas (2022) reminds educators that virtual reality should be cultivated in case another pandemic disrupts in person clinical learning experiences and simulation.

---

## DOERR AND MURRAY

Doerr and Murray (2008) describe the teaching–learning process of simulation by using the model of a four-step plan, which includes the following:

1. the plan
   - developing learning outcomes
   - description of the scenario and certified healthcare educator responses to the learners
   - scripts for standardized patients (SPs)
2. the situation
3. debriefing
4. transference

## MELLER

Meller (1997) describes the elements of activity in relation to simulation.

- *Passive elements:* things that try to stage the realism of the simulation experience, such as moulage (refer to Chapter 9, "Moulage in Simulation")
- *Active elements:* things that are programmed into the simulation experience that cause the learner to respond
- *Interactive elements:* changes that the certified healthcare educator makes in reaction to the actions of the learner

## ▶ REALISM IN SIMULATION

Although realism is a traditional worldview of education, it takes on a slightly different interpretation when applied to simulation. A certain amount of realism must be present during a scenario to meet SLOs. Some points about simulation scenario realism are as follows:

- The goal is to acquire experience in a safe environment.
- The scenario must be real enough to suspend disbelief.
- The scenario must mimic as closely as possible a real clinical scenario.
- SPs, along with manikins, increase the realism.
- The environmental setup is also important in producing a realistic scenario.
- SPs provide a transition from role-playing to real patients for healthcare professionals.
- SPs can provide learners with "authentic" assessment.

Patient-focused simulation (PFS) includes using a hybrid method of simulations either with a part-task trainer or a manikin along with an SP. PFS promotes realism because it combines the art of caring with learning clinical skills (Dunbar-Reid et al., 2015).

Realism is sometimes referred to as the fidelity of the simulation experience. Issenberg et al. (2010) describe fidelity as the exactness of duplication and remind us that simulation is never isomorphic with real life. The higher fidelity may be equated with increased realism. The goal of a simulated environment is to replicate a realistic situation. Fidelity in simulation includes the following:

- *Physical fidelity:* How real does the manikin appear?
- *Psychological fidelity:* How mentally prepared are the learners?
- *Equipment fidelity:* What can the manikin, task trainer, or VR platform do?
- *Environmental fidelity:* How do the surroundings look (Dieckmann et al., 2007)?
- *Conceptual fidelity:* Does the situation and its components make sense (Dieckmann et al., 2007; Rudolph et al., 2007)?

Dieckmann et al. (2007) warn that high fidelity does not necessarily equate to better learning outcomes. Laucken (2003) describes reality as three ways of thinking that are interactive with one another to create reality for the individual person in the experience. Figure 14.5 demonstrates the interconnectedness of Laucken's theory of how reality is conceptualized.

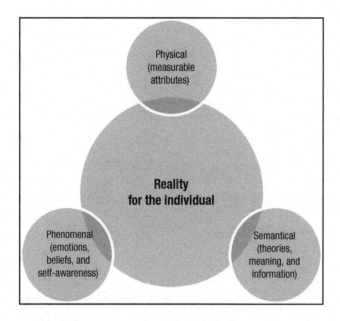

**Figure 14.5** Laucken's (2003) theory of conceptualizing reality.

## SUSPENDING DISBELIEF

Suspending disbelief or engaging in a fiction contract in a simulation experience encompasses the appropriate use of the "as-if" concept (Vaihinger, 1927). Certified healthcare educators running a scenario must integrate information that is believable and within the framework of the scenario, and learners must be open to changing information and understand that the scenario represents actual patient care. There have been elements that lead students to be able to suspend belief. Some elements, according to Muckler (2017), include "fidelity, psychological safety, emotional buy-in, the fiction contract, and how learners assign meaning" (p. 3).

Factors that prevent students from just pretending to actually suspending disbelief should be identified by research (Muckler, 2017).

## DELIBERATE PRACTICE

One of the founding teaching principles of simulation is DP. Ericsson et al. (1993) discussed DP as a method of teaching and reinforcing skills for healthcare providers; it is a forerunner to simulation. Ericsson et al. understood the implications of translating practice on nonhuman materials to the clinical area as a means to promote expertise and safety.

DP can help ensure competence, retention of skills, and mastery of learning (Gonzalez & Kardong-Edgren, 2017).

### Simulation Teaching Tip 14.3

In a study by Wells-Beede et al. (2022), students rated virtual reality (VR) positively and simulation in nursing was demonstrated to increase critical thinking skills. The authors recommend further development of VR for nursing education.

## TEAM-BASED LEARNING

Team-based learning (TBL) encourages cooperation in small groups and is appropriate for healthcare students. TBL has three main components:

- a preparation phase that the student completes individually prior to the group activity
- affirming the content is understood
- group activity

The first element requires students (Zachry et al., 2017). Simulation encourages TBL through open communication in a safe space that protects the discussion while leveling the playing field. The safe space concept of learning through simulation contains the following features.

Changuiti et al. (2022) have demonstrated that simulation increased the technical competencies of midwifery students.

## ▶ LEARNING DOMAINS

Learning is discussed as a process that takes place in three domains: cognitive, affective, and psychomotor, or as stated by the Quality and Safety Education for Nurses (QSEN) program (2005), knowledge, skills, and attitudes (KSAs; Case Western Reserve University, 2014). Learners in healthcare programs are evaluated for growth in all three domains due to the nature of the service work that they will provide to humanity. Bloom's taxonomy (1956; Table 14.2) identifies learning mainly in the cognitive (knowledge) domain. Psychomotor (skills) domains are evident in the application of knowledge, such as demonstrations, and are not difficult to evaluate because they produce observable behavior. Psychomotor learning is often related to procedures, skills, and interventions, all of which can be evaluated in the simulation laboratory. The affective (attitudes) domain of learning is more difficult to assess because it is related to judgment and values, such as changes in feelings, interests, and values (caring). Affective learning also includes metacognition or learning how to learn (Burwash & Snover, 2016).

**Table 14.2 Bloom's Taxonomy**

| Level | Concept | Verbs Used When Writing Learning Outcomes |
|---|---|---|
| **Evaluating** (formerly called *evaluation*) | Judgment, selection | Appraise, argue, assess, attach, choose, compare, defend, estimate, judge, predict, rate, select, support, value, evaluate |
| **Creating** (formerly called *synthesis*; this step formerly occurred before evaluating) | Productive thinking, novelty | Arrange, assemble, collect, compose, construct, create, design, develop, formulate, manage, organize, plan, prepare, propose, set up |
| **Analyzing** (formerly called *analysis*) | Induction, deduction, logical order | Analyze, appraise, calculate, categorize, compare, contrast, criticize, differentiate, discriminate, distinguish, examine, experiment, question, test |
| **Applying** (formerly called *application*) | Solution, application | Apply, choose, demonstrate, dramatize, employ, illustrate, interpret, operate, practice, schedule, sketch, solve, use, write |
| **Understanding** (formerly called *comprehension*) | Explanation, comparison, illustration | Classify, describe, discuss, explain, express, identify, indicate, locate, recognize, report, restate, review, select, translate |
| **Remembering** (formerly called *knowledge*) | Memory, repetition, description | Arrange, define, duplicate, label, list, memorize, name, order, recognize, relate, recall, repeat, reproduce, state |

*Source:* Adapted from Bloom, B., Englehart, M., Furst, E., Hill, W., & Drathwohl, D. (Eds.). (1956). *Taxonomy of educational objectives.* Longmans, Green.

Wong and Driscoll (2008) describe the learning development of the affective domain in five stages:

1. *Receiving:* Learners attend, listen, watch, and recognize.
2. *Responding:* Learners answer, discuss, respond, reply, and actively participate.
3. *Valuing:* Learners accept, adopt, initiate, or demonstrate a preference.
4. *Organizing:* Learners formulate, integrate, modify, and systematize.
5. *Internalizing:* Learners commit, exemplify, and incorporate professionalism into practice.

Simulation can evaluate students' knowledge acquisition in all three domains (Drasovean, 2017). Simulation learning can evaluate students in an environment that contains standard conditions. Evaluation of simulation experiences is thoroughly addressed in Chapter 19, "Evaluation of Simulation Activities."

# ▶ MODES OF THINKING

Laucken (2003) describes three modes of *realistic* learner thinking during a simulation experience.

- *Physical mode* of thinking includes the actual equipment and the fidelity of the equipment. Although manikins simulate humans, there are many unrealistic attributes, and the same is true for other laboratory equipment.
- *Semantical mode* of thinking includes the situation created in humans containing information that represents an event. For example, the situation of a patient having a

myocardial infarction would include EKG and vital sign changes that would indicate to a learner that this was the event taking place.

- *Phenomenal mode* of thinking includes learners' perceptions, emotions, and thinking process during the simulation experience, as well as participants' understanding of the relationship of the simulated experience to actual clinical practice.

Specifically in simulation experiences, the right fidelity in the experience needs to be used to emphasize the goal of the experience. The experience needs to be constructed with the goal in mind and framed within the learning outcomes. In addition, the fidelity being used should match the educational level of the student (Lubbers & Rossman, 2017).

## ▶ CRITICAL THINKING AND METACOGNITION

Critical thinking as an educational concept can be traced back to 1941, when Glaser defined the composites of knowledge (Glaser, 1941). Other historical developments in the concept of critical thinking are as follows:

- Miller and Malcolm (1990) adapted Glaser's definition into a model for critical thinking and advised educators to pay closer attention to learners' mental processes.
- In the early days of concept development, educators were concerned with finding an appropriate definition for critical thinking in order to evaluate learners.
- A multitude of definitions arose, and some of the more prominent ones are listed in Table 14.3.

**Table 14.3 Descriptions of Critical Thinking**

| Author | Description of Critical Thinking |
|---|---|
| Facione et al. (1994) | Critical thinking is the process of purposeful, self-regulating judgment. |
| Paul and Elder (2007) | Attitudes are central, rather than peripheral, to critical thinking, as is independence, confidence, and responsibility, which are needed to arrive at one's own judgment. |
| Bandman and Bandman (1995) | Critical thinking is the rational examination of ideas, inferences, assumptions, principles, arguments, conclusions, issues, statements, beliefs, and actions. It covers scientific reasoning, decision-making, and reasoning in controversial issues. It also includes deductive, inductive, informal, and practical reasoning. |

Educators can *role-model critical thinking* and *create opportunities for learners to develop their own critical thinking skills* by asking higher level questions and "thinking out loud," or dialoguing, about a simulation scenario from different perspectives in order to synthesize a solution. The authors of the *Indian State Nurses Foundation & Indian State Nurses Association* (2014) define attributes or characteristics that enhance and deter critical thinking; these are listed in Table 14.4.

**Table 14.4** Attributes or Characteristics That Enhance and Deter Critical Thinking

| Characteristics of Critical Thinking | Characteristics that Deter Critical Thinking |
|---|---|
| ■ Universal intellectual standards are upheld and include: <br>  ● Clarity <br>  ● Accuracy <br>  ● Precision <br>  ● Relevance <br>  ● Depth <br>  ● Breadth <br>  ● Logic <br>■ Intellectual humility as opposed to intellectual arrogance <br>■ Intellectual courage as opposed to intellectual cowardness <br>■ Intellectual empathy as opposed to intellectual narrow-mindedness <br>■ Intellectual autonomy as opposed to intellectual conformity <br>■ Intellectual integrity as opposed to intellectual hypocrisy <br>■ Intellectual perseverance as opposed to intellectual laziness <br>■ Confidence in reason as opposed to distrust of reason and evidence <br>■ Fair-mindedness as opposed to intellectual unfairness <br>■ Reasoning <br>■ Divergent thinking <br>■ Creativity <br>■ Clarification | ■ Egocentrism fallacy <br>  ● It is true because I believe it. <br>  ● It is true because we believe it. <br>  ● It is true because I want to believe it. <br>  ● It is true because I have always believed it. <br>  ● It is true because it is in my selfish interest to believe it. <br>■ Omnipotence fallacy <br>■ Invulnerability fallacy <br>■ The halo effect |

Source: Indian State Nurses Foundation & Indian State Nurses Association. (2014). Developing a nursing IQ—Part 1 Characteristics of critical thinking: What critical thinkers do, what critical thinkers do not do. *ISNA Bulletin, 41*(1), 6–14.

Ritchie and Smith (2015) propose that critical thinking is the seventh "C" needed in community health nursing, along with the following:

1. Care
2. Compassion
3. Competence
4. Communication
5. Courage
6. Commitment
7. Critical thinking

## Evidence-Based Simulation Practice 14.1

Roh et al. (2022) studied gender differences and psychological safety in simulation scenarios in 97 students who identified as female and 95 students who identified as male. A descriptive study demonstrated that lower academic safety was reported by those students who identified as female. Students who identified as male reported a higher germane load as opposed to a higher intrinsic load reported by those who identified as female. The researchers concluded that gender identity needs to be part of simulation learning design.

Assessment of learners' critical thinking skills has been completed by use of several different tools. The following are two of the most widely used tools:

- The California Critical Thinking Disposition Inventory is a tool that evaluates seven "habits of the mind," which are the following:
  - truth seeking
  - open-mindedness
  - analyticity
  - systematicity
  - self-confidence
  - inquisitiveness
  - cognitive maturity
- The Watson–Glaser Critical Thinking Appraisal (WGCTA; Watson & Glaser, 1964) is available in three different formats; the newest version has 16 scenarios and 40 items. There are five subcategories:
  - inference
  - recognition of assumptions
  - deduction
  - interpretation
  - evaluation

## MINDFULNESS

A related term to critical thinking is *mindfulness*. The *ISNA Bulletin* (2014) defines *mindfulness* as being "engaged with a certain activity, focused, and actively thinking about whatever it is you are undertaking at the moment" (p. 6).

## METACOGNITION

Metacognition is a different concept from critical thinking. "Metacognition is an active process of knowing, or being acutely aware of one's cognitive state with the ability to complete a given task" (Hsu & Hsieh, 2014, p. 234). Metacognition is the process of evaluating your own learning and ideas and being able to change them to understand and promote your own learning success.

### Evidence-Based Simulation Practice 14.2

Oxlad et al. (2022) studied psychology student (N = 84) experiences with simulation-based learning (SBL). In their descriptive study, students assessed SBL as a valid way to learn assessment and intervention skills. The students viewed SBL as a good way to learn clinical competencies.

## ▶ EVIDENCE-BASED SIMULATION PRACTICE

The foundations of evidence-based simulation practice (EBSP) are analogous to evidence-based practice (EBP). Healthcare educators use the same method of synthesizing and appraising evidence in the simulation environments in order to draw a conclusion or develop an opinion that is grounded and derived from logical, common ideas in the literature (Leibold, 2017).

Overall, more research needs to be completed in order to produce evidence to support specific learning activities. Pearson et al. (2007) opined that faculty members should use the acronym FAME when planning to make a change based on evidence:

F: feasibility
A: appropriateness
M: meaningfulness
E: effectiveness

---

### Evidence-Based Simulation Practice 14.3

Westphal et al. (2022) used high-fidelity simulation to teach nurse anesthesia students about the life-threatening complication of local anesthesia.

Local anesthetic systemic toxicity (LAST): The simulation-based learning experience was developed into a case scenario that demonstrated an improvement in student knowledge base about the appropriate interventions from 58.4% to 93.8%. There was also a significant increase in comfort level in dealing with patients with LAST from 4.8 to 8.4 (scale: 0–10).

---

## ▶ GOFFMAN'S THEORY OF FRAME ANALYSIS

In order to make sense out of a situation, such as a simulated experience, Goffman (1974), who developed a theory about experience interpretation, discusses human perception in frames.

- *Primary frames* describe how the learner's mind or cognition makes sense out of a situation.
- *Natural primary frames* are those that include natural law (physics, anatomy, and physiology).
- *Social primary frames* include human factors such as decision-making and communication.
- *Modulations* are learners' understanding that they are in a "what-if" situation that is predefined by the situation in the primary frame. Modulations should hold to learning rules, such as the following:
  - Be within the primary frame and not be a surprise or deception.
  - Have a time frame that is appropriate.
  - Know the rules and roles within the modulation (Muckler, 2017).

## ▶ THEORIES OF KNOWING

Healthcare education also draws on theories about how learners come to understand concepts. There are two classic models that have been significant in healthcare education for the past several decades and are widely used as the theoretical foundations for many studies and curricula, as well as learning activity development. They are Barbara Carper's (1978) ways of knowing and Patricia Benner's (1982) novice-to-expert theory.

---

### Simulation Teaching Tip 14.4

Simulation participants should introduce themselves during prebriefing and include their pronouns to promote inclusiveness.

Carper (1978) described four ways that healthcare professionals understand practice situations:

- *Empirical knowledge,* or scientific knowledge (this includes EBSP)
- *Personal knowledge,* or understanding how you would feel in the patient's position
- *Ethical knowledge,* or attitudes and understanding of moral decisions
- *Esthetic knowledge,* or understanding the situation of the patient at the moment

Munhall (1993) added a fifth way of knowing: *unknowing* or understanding that one cannot know everything about the patient and that one must place oneself in a position of willingness to learn from the patient's perspective.

## ▶ DEEP, SURFACE, AND STRATEGIC LEARNING

*Deep learning* is a term first described by Marton and Saljo (1976) to refer to a learning approach and type of knowledge acquisition. The approach a learner takes to the information presented in the classroom can be classified into three types of learning styles: deep, surface, and strategic.

- A deep learning approach is accomplished when a learner addresses a material with the intent to understand both the concepts and the meaning of the information.
  - The learner relates new ideas to existing experiences and formulates links in long-term memory.
  - The motivation for a deep learning approach is primarily intrinsic, created from the learner's interest and desire to understand the relevance of the information to applied practice.
- A surface learning, or atomistic, approach facilitates learning by:
  - Memorization of facts and details: Surface learning is similar to rote learning in that the learner assimilates information presented at face value.
  - Motivation for surface learning: This is primarily extrinsic and is driven by either the learner's fear of failing or the desire to complete the course successfully.
- When using a strategic learning approach, the learner does what is needed to complete a course. Strategic learning uses a mixture of both deep and surface learning techniques.
  - All three approaches to learning can be measured by the Approaches and Study Skills Inventory for Students (ASSIST; Entwistle, 1999; Ramsden & Entwistle, 1981).

### Evidence-Based Simulation Practice 14.4

Arslan et al. (2022) studied simulation programs to teach peripheral intravenous catheterization (PIVC) procedures. A systematic review and meta-analysis of randomized controlled trials (RCTs) and nonrandomized controlled trials (N-RCTs) found 12 studies. Analysis of the studies revealed that virtual IV training increased PIVC confidence compared with part-task trainer in both students and staff.

## ▶ MOTIVATIONAL THEORIES

Not only do simulation educators need to know how students acquire information, they also need to know why they learn. What are their motivating factors? Motivation has been linked to student retention and success. Many variables affect motivation; motivation can be influenced by the need for achievement or curiosity, or it can be a function of the situation at hand or a person's ability. A learner's *locus of control* can be *extrinsically or intrinsically motivated*. Motivation includes a student's goals, beliefs, perceptions, and expectations (Hanifi et al., 2013).

- Extrinsic motivations are those based on external variables, such as grades or earning money, and in today's environment there are many social pressures for students to become nurses.
- Intrinsic motivation has to do with the feeling of accomplishment, of learning for the sake of learning, or the feeling that being a nurse is something the learner always wanted to do. Hanifi et al. (2013) identified internal motivators as spirituality, selflessness, and serving people and that these assist students to remain in school (Nesje, 2015). Intrinsic motivation is correlated with the *self-determination theory* developed by Deci and Ryan (Deci et al., 1994). According to this theory, humans have three types of needs:
  - to feel competent
  - to feel related
  - to feel autonomous

The following are some traditional models to better explain student motivation:

## ARCS MODEL

In the ARCS model, Keller (1987) talks about the factors educators can implement to motivate learners.

- A: attention—Keep the learner's attention through stimulus changes in the environment.
- R: relevance—Make the information relevant to the learner's goals.
- C: confidence—Make expectations clear so the learner will engage in learning.
- S: satisfaction—Have appropriate consequences for the learner's new skills.

## BROPHY'S MODEL

Brophy (1986) listed the following methods by which motivation is formed:

- modeling
- communication of expectations
- direct instruction
- socialization by parents and educators

## VROOM'S EXPECTANCY MODEL

Vroom's expectancy model (VEM; Vroom, 1964) describes what people want and whether they are positioned to obtain it. The Vroom model describes three concepts:

- *Force (F):* the amount of effort a person will place into reaching a goal
- *Valence (V):* how attractive the goal is to the person
- *Expectancy (E):* the possibility of the goal being achieved

The equation for the VEM model is $F = V \times E$ (Vroom, 1964).

## DEYOUNG'S MOTIVATIONAL MODEL

DeYoung (2009) lists 10 principles to motivate learners; they are applicable to a laboratory and virtual learning environment as well as to a traditional setting.

- Use several senses.
- Actively involve the learner.
- Assess readiness.
- Determine whether the learner thinks the information is relevant.
- Repeat information.
- Generalize information.
- Make learning pleasant.
- Begin with what is known.
- Present information at an appropriate rate.
- Provide a learning-friendly environment.

## ▶ LEARNER SOCIALIZATION IN THE VIRTUAL, SIMULATION, AND SKILLS ENVIRONMENT

Simulation experiences are a social practice (Underman, 2015) because they encompass a goal-oriented situation that calls for participant interaction in a setting (module) that influences behavior. The simulation setting includes the following:

- introduction
- simulator briefing
- scenario
- debriefing, which can be done during the simulation or after the learning experience (Karkowsky et al., 2016)
- session ending (Dieckmann et al., 2007)

The social practice goal of simulation is to enhance positive learner socialization and extend it to healthcare practice. Socialization is the process of internalizing the norms, beliefs, and values of a professional culture to which one hopes to gain admission (Peddle et al., 2016).

- New healthcare students are instructed in the ways and attitudes of the organization and gradually adopt the attitudes, values, and unspoken messages within the organization (Rudd, 2014).
- It is important to note that a lack of socialization has been associated with negative job satisfaction, which results in high turnover rates (Yanchus et al., 2017).

The transition of a healthcare learner to the professional environment is challenging. Simulation environments are being used to decrease reality shock and familiarize learners using both social practice and social aspects within the clinical practice. Social aspects include interdisciplinary communication, teamwork, and role identification (Dieckmann et al., 2007).

Kramer (1974) describes *reality shock* as what takes place when a neophyte realizes that what was learned in school does not match that which is experienced in actual clinical practice.

Kramer's four phases of reality shock are:

1. honeymoon
2. shock or rejection
3. recovery
4. resolution

The need to evaluate the influence of simulation-based learning during undergraduate nursing education on the practice of a graduate nurse is a contemporary research opportunity for those seeking to better understand the longitudinal impact of simulation (El Hussein & Cuncannon, 2022).

## DESIGNED EXPERIENCES THROUGH "SERIOUS GAMING"

Another topic in simulation related to socialization is the use of serious gaming. Serious gaming uses a video game simulation platform to build educational programs that enhance learning by *being* or becoming the character in the game and by *doing* to create and organize for a functional epistemology. Using an epistemology in which one learns through doing and through performance is a new frontier in education, but this mode of simulation also lacks research. Some of the concepts associated with serious gaming include:

- *Interactivity:* Serious games can be played alone or as part of a community.
- *Agency:* The simulated world grants the player the right to create.
- *Parameters:* These are built-in barriers by the game designers (Squire, 2007).

Additional information about Second Life and gaming is provided in Chapter 13, "Virtual Reality."

## ▶ THE ART OF TEACHING SIMULATION

LeFlore and Anderson (2009) explain that most simulation scenarios begin with a "stem," or some information about the case, and then teaching during simulation experiences can take on one of the three levels of facilitation by certified healthcare educators:

- *Self-directed:* This approach allows experienced learners to proceed through scenarios without assistance from the certified healthcare educator.
- *Cueing students:* In this approach, the certified healthcare educator provides hints or cues to the learners to ensure they progress through the scenario.
- *Expert or instructor model:* This is an approach in which the certified healthcare educator instructs during the scenario as the learners are experiencing the situation.

## ▶ LEARNING OUTCOMES VERSUS LEARNING OBJECTIVES

Historically, healthcare education has used objectives for learning since Tyler's landmark book, *Basic Principles of Curriculum and Instruction* (1949), encouraged educators to develop behavioral objectives to organize their teaching. Therefore, objectives are part of the behavioral paradigm. To standardize the format of objectives, educators have incorporated the action verbs outlined in Bloom's taxonomy (1956), which were revised in 2001.

### BLOOM'S TAXONOMY

Bloom's *Taxonomy of Educational Objectives* (1956) describes an end behavior (see Table 14.2). The taxonomy uses "behavioral terms" to divide learning into leveled achievement, from knowledge acquisition to the synthesis of new ideas (Novotny & Griffin, 2006).

Most teaching sessions begin with objectives or learning outcomes to frame the content or experience. *Objectives* and *learning outcomes* are the two terms used often in healthcare education. Some professions will also use the term *goals*. All the terms are trying to depict what the student will have acquired by the end of the class, session, or scenario. The most common method of developing a measurable objective or learning outcome is depicted in Table 14.5.

**Table 14.5** Learning Outcomes

| Antecedent | Learner | Verb Describing Behavior | Content | Context | Criteria |
|---|---|---|---|---|---|
| "By the end of this session" | "The learner will" | "Demonstrate" | Sterile gloving | In clinical settings | 100% of the time |
| "By the end of this session" | "The learner will" | "Compare" | Different cultures | Related to childbearing experiences | By interviewing two culturally differed patients |

Depending on the length of the simulation scenario and the level of the practitioners, educators usually have several objectives in mind. The number of learning objectives/outcomes should be reasonable and related to the intent of the learning session and the time allotted to the scenario. Objectives and learning outcomes are reflected in the evaluation of the learning session. Most lists of objectives or learning outcomes are prefaced with the statement "By the end of this scenario the student will be able to . . ." Evaluating learning that takes place in simulation is addressed in Chapter 19, "Evaluation of Simulation Activities." Simulation as an evaluation tool has become widespread because it occurs in a controlled environment where all learners can be presented with testing in similar conditions. Traditional clinical experiences were not able to provide this because educational opportunities may differ from day to day (Drasovean, 2017).

## ▶ EVALUATING SIMULATION LEARNING EXPERIENCES

Simulation learning experiences are used for either formative and summative learner assessment or evaluation. Evaluation practices themselves need to be assessed so that healthcare professionals are more confident they are preparing competent practitioners for the future (Logue, 2017). Additionally, the frequency of simulation experiences may ultimately influence a student's ability to translate learning to the clinical environment as a practicing nurse (Bruce et al., 2019). Simulation-based evaluation is one method used to evaluate learning, and the goals of the students' learning can be short term, such as the following:

■ Has the student met the learning objectives/outcomes?
■ Did the scenario improve patient care and safety?

An important consideration when using simulation-based evaluation is validity. Is the simulation experience measuring what it is intended to measure? Kane (2006) discusses the evaluation process of testing by breaking it down into four key areas:

■ *Scoring:* Was the test provided to learners under fair and consistent conditions?
■ *Generalization:* Are the results reliable and consistent when the evaluation technique is used with different groups?
■ *Extrapolation:* Is the assessment measuring the construct it is supposed to measure and not extraneous variables?
■ *Decision/interpretation:* Are the scores being used for their intended purpose and without manipulation?

Current literature discusses developing instruments to evaluate students' learning through the use of simulation. Hung et al. (2016) developed a 37-item Simulation-Based Learning Evaluation Scale (SBLES) that is based on competencies and is valid and reliable. Some tools are specific, whereas others can be used in a variety of simulation learning experiences. The Team Performance Observation Tool was developed to assess interprofessional simulation experiences (Zhang et al., 2015). Chapter 21, "The Role of Research in Simulation," discusses in detail the current research being completed in relation to simulation learning and evaluation.

## ▶ GAGNE'S CONDITIONS OF LEARNING

Gagne's (1970) steps for instruction are a classic list of tasks that is still referenced today and suited for learning in a simulated environment. Gagne's (1970) nine events of instruction are shown in Table 14.6.

**Table 14.6 Gagne's Conditions of Learning**

| Instructional Event | Activities of Teaching–Learning |
|---|---|
| 1. Gains attention of the learner | Stimuli activate receptors |
| 2. Informs learners of the objectives | Sets expectations for the learner |
| 3. Stimulates recall of prior learning | Activates short-term memory and the retrieval of information by asking questions |
| 4. Presents the content | Presents content with features that can be remembered |
| 5. Provides "learning guidance" | Assists the learners in organizing the information for long-term memory |
| 6. Elicits performance (practice) | Asks the learners to perform to enhance encoding and verification |
| 7. Provides appropriate feedback (feedback about simulation experiences is covered in Chapter 18, "Standardized Patient Debriefing and Feedback") | Encourages performance |
| 8. Assesses performance | Evaluates performance |
| 9. Enhances retention and transfer | Reviews periodically to decrease memory loss of information |

## ▶ LEARNING ACTIVITIES USED IN SIMULATION ENVIRONMENTS

### INTERPROFESSIONAL LEARNING

Interprofessional learning is needed to prepare students for the future of healthcare (Labrugue et al., 2018). Team-based education is needed for quality patient care and is the focus of many healthcare education and simulation initiatives. The goal of interprofessional learning is to have all health professional learners "deliberately working together" as stated by the Interprofessional Education Collaborative (IPEC; 2016), which originally consisted of 6 professional organizations and now includes 15 national organizations. The IPEC outlined four core competencies needed for healthcare professionals to function effectively in interprofessional teams. The domains of the four major competencies and related criteria are fully explained in Chapter 6, "Interprofessional Simulation." In addition to the IPEC competencies, the simulation organization International Nursing Association for Clinical Simulation and Learning (INACSL) has developed standards for best practice for simulation-enhanced interprofessional education (sim-IPE; 2016). Sim-IPE enables learners from different healthcare professions to engage in a simulation-based experience to achieve linked or shared objectives and outcomes.

## PROBLEM-BASED LEARNING

PBL is a teaching strategy that was developed in the 1970s as a student-centered approach. It uses patient problems of increasing complexity to assist students in understanding clinical decision-making individually and in a group format (Jamshidi et al., 2021). Lee et al. (2017) studied PBL and simulation noting they have positive effects on team efficacy and on the learning attitudes of healthcare students.

## SELF-DIRECTED LEARNING

*Self-directed learning (SDL)* is another term often heard in healthcare education and refers to a collection of learning activities that are truly learner-focused. It originated with Knowles (1975) and is a process in which the learner decides their own learning needs. The learner formulates the goals, develops the networking and resources, does the learning, and evaluates the learning. Learners must be ready to take on the task of SDL and need to have the confidence, maturity, and tenacity to engage in SDL (Robinson & Persky, 2020). SDL activities can include virtual learning modules. To assess whether learners are ready for this type of knowledge acquisition, the Self-Directed Learning Readiness Scale (SDLRS) is used.

## REFLECTION

Reflection is a method used to develop critical thinking and is used extensively in simulation experiences through debriefing (see Chapter 17, "Debriefing") and feedback (see Chapter 18, "Standardized Patient Debriefing and Feedback"). Please refer to these chapters to better understand the essence of reflection, which is a critical component of simulation learning.

## ENVIRONMENTAL MANAGEMENT

The underpinning of positive learning environment management is respect for the learners. Once an atmosphere of trust and respect is established, there should be very few management issues. Chickering and Gamson's (1987) seven principles of good teaching practice are applicable to simulation learning environments and include:

- Encourage contact between learners and educators.
- Develop reciprocity and cooperation among learners.
- Encourage active learning.
- Give prompt feedback.
- Emphasize time on task.
- Communicate high expectations.
- Respect diverse talents and ways of learning.

According to Mulligan (2007), there are four pillars of classroom management and these are discussed here because they also fit the simulation learning environment very well.

- Pillar 1: Educators should use instructional strategies (active learning strategies) that motivate and keep learners interested and engaged.
- Pillar 2: Educators need to use instructional time wisely and take a proactive approach to teaching by charging the learners to be accountable for their learning.

- Pillar 3: Social behaviors that need attention and correcting should be dealt with immediately, face to face, and privately.
- Pillar 4: Educators need to create a flexible environment in order to adjust to the learners' needs.

## ▶ SUMMARY

Simulation as a learning tool has a history of success in healthcare education. The theoretical foundations of experiential learning and realism are well represented in simulation. Successful simulation in healthcare education contains the following best-practice attributes as identified in a mega-analysis completed by McGaghie et al. (2010).

- *Feedback:* formative or summative (discussed in Chapter 17, "Debriefing," and Chapter 18, "Standardized Patient Debriefing and Feedback")
- *DP:* encompasses nine educational goals:
  - occur with motivated learners
  - define the learning outcomes
  - keep the experience at the appropriate level for the learners
  - repeat the exercise or skill to gain proficiency
  - promote rigor in skill to ensure best practice
  - provide learners with feedback
  - promote self-regulation in learners
  - evaluate to reach a mastery standard
  - start the process again with another task (McGaghie et al., 2009)
- curriculum integration
- outcome measurement
- simulation fidelity
- skill acquisition and maintenance
- mastery learning
- transfer to practice
- team training
- high-stake testing
- instructor training
- educational and professional context

## ● CASE STUDY 14.1

A new faculty member is hired at a small baccalaureate school with premed, nursing, and prepharmaceutical programs. The faculty member is full time, tenure track, and working on their doctoral degree. The faculty member is assigned a mentor and a 12-credit/semester teaching load, which is normal for many institutions. They meet with their mentor, who goes over the syllabus. The mentor asks the new faculty member why they have so many assignments for the learners to do after they have completed their hybrid simulation experience. The new faculty member states that they believe that the learners' writing skills are lacking, and they need writing assignments. The assignment expands on the simulation day by describing the illness process of the simulated patient scenario in depth. If you were the mentor and saw a novice place 50% of the clinical course grade on writing assignments related to simulation, how would you handle it?

1. A healthcare simulation educator is developing a scenario for a student to learn newborn care and would like to use the constructivist theory as the foundation. The BEST method would be to:

   A. Have the student repeat a newborn assessment several times to get the procedures correct

   B. Decide after prebriefing the student's previous experiences with newborns

   C. Develop a scenario that changes the newborn's status if an assessment is performed wrong

   D. Change the newborn's status to mimic a healthy newborn if the assessment is done correctly

2. The student needs additional understanding when they state "A constructivist approach to this scenario includes . . .":

   A. Using the material we learned yesterday and applying it today

   B. Starting with what we know about this situation and then assessing the patient

   C. Approaching the patient as if we have no information

   D. Relating what is similar in this case to other cases we have worked through

3. During a team-based simulation scenario, one student takes the lead and approaches the patient first and takes the blood pressure when the manikin tells the group that they feel lightheaded. The student who assesses the blood pressure is displaying which learning style?

   A. Concrete experience (CE)

   B. Abstract conceptualization (AC)

   C. Reflective observation (RO)

   D. Active experimentation (AE)

4. The simulation healthcare educator has developed a simulation scenario based on the scaffolding learning theory and presents it to a group of students. The students are provided with an explanation of the case that becomes increasingly difficult. The group was unable to formulate a cohesive plan for the patient. One learning element that is most likely missing may have been:

   A. Instructor presence

   B. Realism

   C. Constructive feedback

   D. Knowledge

5. Guided by social learning theory, the healthcare simulation educator demonstrates to a student who has low self-efficacy how to insert chest tubes correctly. The principle that the healthcare simulation educator is using is:

   A. Mastering experience learning

   B. Vicarious experience learning

   C. Verbal persuasion

   D. Physiologic state

## 1. B) Decide after prebriefing the student's previous experiences with newborns

The constructivist theory should build on previous knowledge, and the teaching–learning modality should be established to fit the student's learning needs. Understanding what the student's previous experience is after the simulation educator prebriefs the student about the assessment is a good idea. Having the student repeat a newborn assessment several times to get the procedures correct reflects behaviorism through demonstration of repetition. Developing a scenario that changes the newborn's status if an assessment is performed wrong and changing the newborn's status to mimic a healthy newborn if the assessment is done correctly is a stimulus-response method or behaviorism.

## 2. C) Approaching the patient as if we have no information

"Approaching the patient as if we have no information" is not congruent with the constructivist theory, which builds on past experiences. The constructivist theory builds on what the student already knows or has experienced. Therefore, "Using the material we learned yesterday and applying it today," "Starting with what we know about this situation and then assessing the patient," and "Relating what is similar in this case to other cases we have worked through" all relate to past experiences.

## 3. D) Active experimentation (AE)

AE is using hands-on practice to learn the skill. CE: Taking the initiative to obtain blood pressure is not an example built from reality. AC: Taking the initiative to obtain blood pressure is not thinking about what to do. RO: Taking the initiative to obtain blood pressure is not a reflective activity.

## 4. C) Constructive feedback

Constructive feedback may be a missing element to the students' inability to construct a plan. The four components of Vygotsky's scaffolding learning theory are constructive feedback, explanations, reflection, and revision of knowledge. Instructor presence is not warranted to construct a plan. Realism is not part of formulating a plan. Knowledge is present but there is no indication that a revision of knowledge is necessary.

## 5. B) Vicarious experience learning

The healthcare simulation educator is using vicarious experience learning because the student is observing the healthcare simulation educator's demonstration of chest tube insertion. Mastering experience learning is incorrect because the student is not demonstrating their own history of success and is inactive during this simulation. Verbal persuasion is incorrect; there is no evidence that the healthcare simulation educator is providing verbal encouragement. Physiologic state is not correct because there is no evidence that either the healthcare simulation educator or the student expressed success in achieving chest tube insertion.

6. One of the healthcare students was previously an emergency medical technician (EMT) and during a simulation prebriefing they state that they would like to advance their splinting skills. The student is demonstrating which type of educational concept?

   A. Pedagogy
   B. Realism
   C. Behaviorism
   D. Andragogy

7. The new healthcare simulation educator needs additional information when they provide a list of Kneebone's (2005) simulation learning principles as:

   A. Occurring in a safe environment
   B. Tutors being available to learners
   C. Teacher-centered
   D. Mimicking real life

8. Kirkpatrick's (1998) simulation learning principles are orderly, and once learning is achieved the healthcare simulation educator should expect the students to:

   A. React to the debriefing questions
   B. Apply the learning to patient care with positive outcomes
   C. Learn through a premodule requirement
   D. Demonstrate a change in behavior

9. The last step of Doerr and Murray's (2008) simulation teaching–learning process is:

   A. Debriefing
   B. Transference
   C. Developing learning outcomes
   D. Creating the situation

10. A simulation educator is developing student objectives/learning outcomes and would like to assess students at the application level. Which objective/learning outcome would BEST fit the application level?

   A. Defining the hybrid simulation procedure
   B. Discussing the clinical decision for starting CPR
   C. Prioritizing the intervention
   D. Evaluating the intervention's effect

*(See answers next page.)*

### 6. D) Andragogy

Andragogy is correct because the student is advancing self by building on past experiences. Pedagogy is a method of learning used to teach passively, mostly to younger students without previous knowledge. Realism refers to the fidelity of the simulation and does not apply in this situation. Behaviorism is not correct because there is no evidence that the student is demonstrating learning through a behavior change.

### 7. C) Teacher-centered

Kneebone's simulation principles include a student-centered, not teacher-centered, principle. Additional principles include simulations occurring in a safe environment, having tutors available for the students, and ensuring the simulation mimics real life.

### 8. B) Apply the learning to patient care with positive outcomes

Apply the learning to patient care with positive outcomes is the highest level (level 4) in Kirkpatrick's pyramid. Reacting to the debriefing questions is an example of level 2. Learning through a premodule requirement is level 2. Demonstrating a change in behavior is level 3.

### 9. B) Transference

Transference is the last step in Doerr and Murray's simulation teaching–learning process, taking the knowledge learned in simulation and applying it to actual patients. Developing learning outcomes is the first step, creating the situation is the second step, and debriefing is the third step.

### 10. C) Prioritizing the intervention

Prioritizing the intervention is an application-level objective according to Bloom's taxonomy. Defining the hybrid simulation procedure would be a recall objective. Discussing the clinical decision for starting CPR would be an objective at the understanding level. Evaluating the intervention's effect would be an objective at the evaluating level, higher than application.

# REFERENCES

Arslan, S., Kuzu Kurban, N., Takmak, S., Sanlialp, Z., Arife, O. S., & Senol, H. (2022). Effectiveness of simulation-based peripheral intravenous catheterization training for nursing students and hospital nurses: A systematic review and meta-analysis. *Journal of Clinical Nursing, 31*(5/6), 483–496. https://doi.org/10.1111/jocn.15960

Bandman, E. L., & Bandman, B. (1995). *Critical thinking in nursing* (2nd ed.). Appleton & Lange.

Bandura, A. (1997). *Self-efficacy: The exercise of control.* W. H. Freeman.

Bastin, M. L., Cook, A. M., & Flannery, A. H. (2017). Use of simulation training to prepare pharmacy residents for medical emergencies. *American Journal of Health-System Pharmacy, 74*(6), 424–429. https://doi.org/10.2146/ajhp160129

Benner, P. (1982). From novice to expert. *American Journal of Nursing, 82*(3), 402–407.

Bevis, E., & Watson, J. (1989). *Toward a caring curriculum: A new pedagogy for nursing.* National League for Nursing.

Bloom, B., Englehart, M., Furst, E., Hill, W., & Drathwohl, D. (Eds.). (1956). *Taxonomy of educational objectives.* Longmans, Green.

Brophy, J. (1986). On motivating students. *Occasional Paper No. 101.* Institute for Research on Teaching, Michigan State University.

Brown, M. R., & Watts, P. (2016). Primer on interprofessional simulation for clinical laboratory science programs: A practical guide to structure and terminology. *Clinical Laboratory Science, 29*(4), 241–246. https://doi.org/10.29074/ascls.29.4.241

Bruce, R., Levett-Jones, T., & Courtney-Pratt, H. (2019). Transfer of learning from university-based simulation experiences to nursing students' future clinical practice: An exploratory study. *Clinical Simulation in Nursing, 35*, 17–24. https://doi.org/10.1016/j.ecns.2019.06.003

Burwash, S. C., & Snover, R. (2016). Up Bloom's pyramid with slices of Fink's pie: Mapping an occupational therapy curriculum. *Open Journal of Occupational Therapy, 4*(4), 1–8. https://doi.org/10.15453/2168-6408.1235

Cadieux, D. C., Lingard, L., Kwiatkowski, D., Van Deven, T., Bryant, M., & Tithecott, G. (2017). Challenges in translation: Lessons from using business pedagogy to teach leadership in undergraduate medicine. *Teaching & Learning in Medicine, 29*(2), 207–215. https://doi.org/10.1080/10401334.2016.1237361

Carpenter-Aeby, T., & Aeby, V. G. (2013). Application of andragogy to instruction in an MSW practice class. *Journal of Instructional Psychology, 40*(1–4), 3–13.

Carper, B. A. (1978). Fundamental patterns of knowing in nursing. *Advances in Nursing Science, 1*(1), 13–24. https://doi.org/10.1097/ANS.0b013e3181c9d5eb

Case Western Reserve University. (2014). *QSEN Institute.* http://qsen.org/about-qsen

Changuiti, O., Ouassim, A., Marfak, A., Saad, E., Hilali, A., & Youlyouz-Marfak, I. (2022). Simulation pedagogical program design for midwifery education using logic model. *Journal for Nurse Practitioners, 18*(6), 640–644. https://doi.org/10.1016/j.nurpra.2022.02.011

Chickering, A. W., & Gamson, Z. F. (1987). Seven principles for good practice in undergraduate education. *Wingspread Journal, 9*(2), 3–7. https://eric.ed.gov/?id=ED282491

Deci, E., Eghrari, H., Patrick, B. C., & Leone, D. R. (1994). Facilitating internalization: The self-determination theory perspective. *Journal of Personality, 62*(1), 119–142. https://doi.org/10.1111/j.1467-6494.1994.tb00797.x

Deyoung, C. G., & Gray, J. R. (2009). Personality neuroscience: Explaining individual differences in affect, behaviour and cognition. In P. J. Corr & G. Matthews (Eds.), *The Cambridge handbook of personality psychology* (pp. 323–346). Cambridge University Press. https://doi.org/10.1017/CBO9780511596544.023

Dieckmann, P., Gaba, D., & Rall, M. (2007). Deepening the theoretical foundations of patient simulation as social practice. *Simulation in Healthcare, 2*, 183–193. https://doi.org/10.1097/SIH.0b013e3180f637f5

Diekelmann, N. L. (1997). Creating a new pedagogy for nursing. *Journal of Nursing Education, 36*(4), 147–148. https://doi.org/10.3928/0148-4834-19970401-03

Diekelmann, N. L. (2005). Engaging the students and the teacher: Co-creating substantive form with narrative pedagogy. *Journal of Nursing Education, 44*(6), 249–252.

Doerr, H., & Murray, W. B. (2008). How to build a successful simulation scenario = obstacle course + treasure hunt. In R. R. Kyle & W. B. Murray (Eds.), *Clinical simulation: Operations, engineering and management* (pp. 745–749). Elsevier/Academic Press.

Drasovean, Y. (2017). Optimizing learner assessment in a respiratory therapy clinical simulation course. *Canadian Journal of Respiratory Therapy, 53*(1), 17–22.

Dunbar-Reid, K., Sinclair, P. M., & Hudson, D. (2015). Advancing renal education: Hybrid simulation, using simulated patients to enhance realism in haemodialysis education. *Journal of Renal Care, 41*(2), 134–139. https://doi.org10.1111/jorc.12112

El Hussein, M. T., & Cuncannon, A. (2022). Nursing students' transfer of learning from simulated clinical experiences into clinical practice: A scoping review. *Nurse Education Today, 116*, 105449. https://doi.org/10.1016/j.nedt.2022.105449

Entwistle, N. J. (1999). Approaches to studying and levels of understanding: The influences of teaching and assessment. In J. C. Smart (Ed.), *Higher education: Handbook of theory and research* (pp. 1–18). Agathon Press.

Ericsson, K. A., Krampe, R. T., & Tesch-Römer, C. (1993). The role of deliberate practice in the acquisition of expert performance. *Psychology Review, 100*(3), 363–406. https://doi.org/10.1037/0033-295X.100.3.363

Facione, N. C., Facione, P. A., & Sanchez, C. A. (1994). Critical thinking disposition as a measure of competent judgment: The development of the California Critical Disposition Inventory. *Journal of Nursing Education, 33*, 345–350. https://doi.org/10.3928/0148-4834-19941001-05

Gagne, R. (1970). *The conditions of learning* (2nd ed.). Holt, Rinehart and Winston.

Gibbs, G. (1988). *Learning by doing: A guide to teaching and learning methods*. Fell.

Glaser, E. M. (1941). *An experiment in the development of critical thinking*. Teacher's College, Columbia University.

Goffman, E. (1974). *Frame analysis. An essay on the organization of experience*. Northeastern University Press.

Gonzalez, L., & Kardong-Edgren, S. (2017). Deliberate practice for mastery learning in nursing. *Clinical Simulation in Nursing, 13*(1), 10–14. https://doi.org/10.1016/j.ecns.2016.10.005

Grant, J., & Marsden, P. (1992). *Training senior house officers by service based training*. Joint Conference for Education in Medicine.

Griffith, R. L., Steelman, L. A., Wildman, J. L., LeNoble, C. A., & Zhou, Z. E. (2017). Guided mindfulness: A self-regulatory approach to experiential learning of complex skills. *Theoretical Issues in Ergonomics Science, 18*(2), 147–166. https://doi.org/10.1080/1463922X.2016.1166404

Guerrero, J. G., Ali, S. A. A., & Attalah, D. M. (2022). The acquired critical thinking skills, satisfaction, and self confidence of nursing students and staff nurses through high-fidelity simulation experience. *Clinical Simulation in Nursing, 64*, 24–30. https://doi.org/10.1016/j.ecns.2021.11.008

Hanifi, N., Parvizy, S., & Joolaee, S. (2013). Motivational journey of Iranian bachelor of nursing students during clinical education: A grounded theory study. *Nursing & Health Sciences, 15*(3), 340–345. https://doi.org/10.1111/nhs.12041

Horberg, U., Galvin, K., Ekebergh, M., & Ozolins, L. L. (2019). Using lifeworld philosophy in education to intertwine caring and learning: An illustration of ways of learning how to care. *Reflective Practice, 20*(1), 55–69. https://doi.org/10.1080/14623943.2018.1539664

Hsu, L., & Hsieh, S. (2014). Factors affecting metacognition of undergraduate nursing students in a blended learning environment. *International Journal of Nursing Practice, 20*(3), 233–241. https://doi.org/10.1111/ijn.12131

Hung, C., Liu, H., Lin, C., & Lee, B. (2016). Development and validation of the simulation-based learning evaluation scale. *Nurse Education Today, 40*, 72–77. https://doi.org/10.1016/j.nedt.2016.02.016

Indian State Nurses Foundation & Indian State Nurses Association. (2014). Developing a nursing IQ part 1 characteristics of critical thinking: What critical thinkers do, what critical thinkers do not do. *ISNA Bulletin, 41*(1), 6–14.

International Nursing Association for Clinical Simulation and Learning Standards Committee. (2016, December). INACSL standards of best practice: Simulation^SM simulation-enhanced interprofessional education (sim-IPE). *Clinical Simulation in Nursing, 12*(S), S34–S38. http://doi.org/10.1016/j.ecns.2016.09.011

Interprofessional Education Collaborative. (2016). *Core competencies for interprofessional collaborative practice: 2016 update.* https://ipec.memberclicks.net/assets/2016-Update.pdf

Issenberg, S. B., McGaghie, W. C., Issenberg, E. R., Petrusa, D. L., & Scalese, R. J. (2010). Features and uses of high-fidelity medical simulations that lead to effective learning: A BEME systematic review. *Medical Teacher, 27*(1), 10–28. https://doi.org/10.1080/01421590500046924

Jamshidi, H., Parizad, N., & Maslakpak, M. H. (2021). Problem-based learning: A new pathway towards improving patient safety-based communication skills in nursing students. *Journal of Preventive Epidemiology, 6*(2), e25. https://doi.org/10.34172/jpe.2021.25

Kane, M. (2006). Validation. In R. L. Brennan (Ed.), *Educational measurement* (4th ed., pp. 17–64). American Council on Education/Praeger.

Karkowsky, C. E., Landsberger, E. J., Bernstein, P. S., Dayal, A., Goffman, D., Madden, R. C., & Chazotte, C. (2016). Breaking bad news in obstetrics: A randomized trial of simulation followed by debriefing or lecture. *Journal of Maternal–Fetal & Neonatal Medicine, 29*(22), 3717–3723. https://doi.org/10.3109/14767058.2016.1141888

Keller, J. M. (1987). Development and use of the ARCS model of motivational design. *Journal of Instructional Development, 10*(3), 2–10.

Kim, Y., & Yoo, J. (2022). Effects of manikin fidelity on simulation-based nursing education: A systematic review and meta-analysis. *Journal of Nursing Education, 61*(2), 67–72. https://doi.org/10.3928/01484834-20211213-03

Kirkpatrick, D. L. (1998). *Evaluating training programs: The four levels* (2nd ed.). Berrett-Koehler.

Kneebone, R. (2005). Evaluating clinical simulations for learning procedural skills: A theory-based approach. *Academic Medicine, 80*(6), 549–553.

Knowles, M. S. (1975). *Self-directed learning: A guide for learners and teachers.* Association Press.

Kolb, D. A. (1984). *Experiential learning: Experience as the source of learning and development.* Prentice Hall.

Kolb, D. A., Boyatzis, R. E., & Mainemelis, C. (1999). Experiential learning theory: Previous research and new directions. In R. J. Sternberg & L.-F. Zhang (Eds.), *Perspectives on thinking, learning, and cognitive styles* (pp. 227–247). Lawrence Erlbaum Associates Publishers.

Kramer, M. (1974). *Reality shock: Why nurses leave nursing.* Mosby.

Labrague, L. J., Hamdan, Z. A., & McEnroe-Petitte, D. M. (2018). An integrative review on conflict management styles among nursing professionals: Implications for nursing management. *Journal of Nursing Management, 26*(8), 902–917. https://doi.org/10.1111/jonm.12626

Laucken, U. (2003). *Theoretical psychology.* Biblioteks und Information system der Univeritat.

Lauerer, J., Edlund, B. J., Williams, A., Donato, A., & Smith, G. (2017). Scaffolding behavioral health concepts from more simple to complex builds NP students' competence. *Nurse Education Today, 51*, 124–126. https://doi.org/10.1016/j.nedt.2016.08.016

Le Coze, J. (2017). Reflecting on Jens Rasmussen's legacy (2) behind and beyond, a "constructivist turn." *Applied Ergonomics, 59*(Part B), 558–569. https://doi.org/10.1016/j.apergo.2015.07.013

Lee, M., Nam, K., & Kim, H. (2017). Effects of simulation with problem-based learning program on metacognition, team efficacy, and learning attitude in nursing students. *CIN: Computers, Informatics, Nursing, 35*(3), 145–151. https://doi.org/10.1097/CIN.0000000000000308

LeFlore, J. L., & Anderson, M. (2009). Alternative educational models for interdisciplinary student teams. *Simulation in Healthcare, 4*, 135–142. https://doi.org/10.1097/SIH.0b013e318196f839

Leibold, N. (2017). Virtual simulations: A creative, evidence-based approach to develop and educate nurses. *Creative Nursing, 23*(1), 29–34. https://doi.org/10.1891/1078-4535.23.1.29

Logue, N. C. (2017). Evaluating practice-based learning. *Journal of Nursing Education, 56*(3), 131–138. https://doi.org/10.3928/01484834-20170222-03

Lubbers, J., & Rossman, C. (2017). Satisfaction and self-confidence with nursing clinical simulation: Novice learners, medium-fidelity, and community settings. *Nurse Education Today, 48*, 140–144. https://doi.org/10.1016/j.nedt.2016.10.010

Marton, F., & Saljo, R. (1976). On qualitative differences in learning: I—Outcome and process. *British Journal of Educational Psychology, 46*(1), 4–11. https://doi.org/10.1111/j.2044-8279.1976.tb02980.x

McGaghie, W. C., Issenberg, S. B., Petrusa, E. R., & Scalese, R. J. (2010). A critical review of simulation-based medical education research: 2003–2009. *Medical Education, 44*, 50–63. https://doi.org/10.1111/j.1365-2923.2009.03547.x

McGaghie, W. C., Siddall, V. J., Mazmanian, P. E., & Myers, J. (2009). Lessons for continuing medical education from simulation research in undergraduate and graduate medical education: Effectiveness of continuing medical education: American College of Chest Physicians evidence-based educational guidelines. *Chest, 135*(Suppl. 3), 62–68. https://doi.org/10.1378/chest.08-2521

Meller, G. (1997). A typology of simulators for medical education. *Journal of Digital Imaging, 10*(3 Suppl. 1), 194–196. https://doi.org/10.1007/BF03168699

Miller, M. A., & Malcolm, N. S. (1990). Critical thinking in the nursing curriculum. *Nursing & Healthcare, 11*(2), 66–73.

Muckler, V. C. (2017). Exploring suspension of disbelief during simulation-based learning. *Clinical Simulation in Nursing, 13*(1), 3–9. https://doi.org/10.1016/j.ecns.2016.09.004

Mulligan, R. (2007). Management strategies in the educational setting. In B. Moyer & R. A. Wittmann-Price (Eds.), *Teaching nursing: Foundations of practice excellence* (pp. 109–125). F. A. Davis.

Munhall, P. L. (1993). Unknowing: Toward another pattern of knowing in nursing. *Nursing Outlook, 41*(3), 125–128.

Nesje, K. (2015). Nursing students' prosocial motivation: Does it predict professional commitment and involvement in the job? *Journal of Advanced Nursing, 71*(1), 115–125. https://doi.org/10.1111/jan.12456

Novotny, J., & Griffin, M. T. (2006). *A nuts-and-bolts approach to teaching nursing.* Springer Publishing Company.

Oxlad, M., D'Annunzio, J., Sawyer, A., & Paparo, J. (2022). Postgraduate students' perceptions of simulation-based learning in professional psychology training. *Australian Psychologist, 4*, 226–235. https://doi.org/10.1080/00050067.2022.2073807

Paul, R., & Elder, L. (2007). Critical thinking: The nature of critical and creative thought. *Journal of Developmental Education, 32*(2), 34–35.

Pearson, A., Wiechula, R., Court, A., & Lockwood, C. (2007). A reconsideration of what constitutes "evidence" in the healthcare professions. *Nursing Science Quarterly, 20*, 85–88. https://doi.org/10.1177/0894318406296306

Peddle, M., Bearman, M., & Nestel, D. (2016). Virtual patients and nontechnical skills in undergraduate health professional education: An integrative review. *Clinical Simulation in Nursing, 12*(9), 400–410. https://doi.org/10.1016/j.ecns.2016.04.004

Quality and Safety Education for Nurses. (2005). *Home page.* https://qsen.org/

Ramsden, P., & Entwistle, N. J. (1981). Effects of academic departments on students' approaches to studying. *British Journal of Educational Psychology, 51*, 368–383. https://doi.org/10.1111/j.2044-8279.1981.tb02493.x

Ritchie, G., & Smith, C. (2015). Critical thinking in community nursing: Is this the 7th C? *British Journal of Community Health, 20*(12), 578–579. https://doi.org/10.12968/bjcn.2015.20.12.578

Robinson, J. D., & Persky, A. (2020). Developing self-directed learners. *American Journal of Pharmaceutical Education, 84*, 3.

Roh, Y. S., Jang, K. I., & Issenberg, S. B. (2022). Gender differences in psychological safety, academic safety, cognitive load, and debriefing satisfaction in simulation-based learning. *Nurse Educator, 47*(5), E109–E113. https://doi.org/10.1097/NNE.0000000000001179

Rudd, A. (2014). *Examining professional stereotypes in an interprofessional education simulation experience* [Doctoral dissertation]. University of Alabama, Tuscaloosa.

Rudolph, J. W., Simon, R., & Raemer, D. B. (2007). Which reality matters? Questions on the path to high engagement in healthcare simulation. *Simul Healthcare, 2*(3), 161–163. https://doi.org/10.1097/SIH.0b013e31813d1035

Society for Simulation in Healthcare. (2021). *Certified healthcare simulation educator handbook.* https://www.ssih.org/Portals/48/Certification/CHSE_Docs/CHSE%20Handbook.pdf

Squire, K. D. (2007). Games learning, and society: Building a field. *Educational Technology*, 51–54. https://website.education.wisc.edu/~kdsquire/manuscripts/gls.pdf

Sriramatr, S., Silalertdetkul, S., & Wachirathanin, P. (2016). Social cognitive theory associated with physical activity in undergraduate students: A cross-sectional study. *Pacific Rim International Journal of Nursing Research*, 20(2), 95–105.

Thomas, S. (2022). Virtual reality: The next step in nursing education? *British Journal of Nursing*, 31(14), 756–757. https://doi.org/10.12968/bjon.2022.31.14.756

Turner, S. (2017). Using high-fidelity simulation scenarios in the classroom to engage learners. *Creative Nursing*, 23(1), 35–41. https://doi.org/10.1891/1078-4535.23.1.35

Tyler, R. W. (1949). *Basic principles of curriculum and instruction*. University of Chicago Press.

Underman, K. (2015). Playing doctor: Simulation in medical school as affective practice. *Social Science & Medicine*, 136, 180–188. https://doi.org/10.1016/j.socscimed.2015.05.028

Vaihinger, H. (1927). *The philosophy of the as-if system of the theoretical, pragmatic, and religious fictions of mankind based on an idealistic positivism*. Scientia.

Vroom, V. (1964). *Work and motivation*. Wiley.

Vygotsky, L. S. (1978). *Mind in society: The development of higher mental processes*. Wadsworth.

Watson, G., & Glaser, E. M. (1964). *Critical thinking appraisal*. Harcourt, Brace & Jovanovich.

Watts, S. O., & Hodges, H. F. (2021). Using invitational theory to examine nursing students' experiences of their learning environment. *Nursing Education Perspectives*, 42(6), 365–370. https://10.1097/01.NEP.0000000000000865

Wells-Beede, E., Garcia, B., Chunm, S., Kicklighter, C., & Seo, J. (2022). Creative solutions for complex circumstances: The utilization of virtual reality in a specialty course. *Clinical Simulation in Nursing*, 65, 82–85. https://doi.org/10.1016/j.ecns.2022.01.004

Westphal, C., Abdoue, A., Barsch, B., Cook, A., Golen, D., Greco, G., Murphy, J., & Olszowka, J. (2022). Simulating LAST to improve peri-anesthesia nursing knowledge. *Journal of PeriAnesthesia Nursing*, 37(4), e2–e2. NLM UID: 9610507

Win, W. (2016). Research philosophy in pharmacy practice: Necessity and relevance. *International Journal of Pharmacy Practice*, 24(6), 428–436. https://doi.org/10.1111/ijpp.12281

Wong, C. K., & Driscoll, M. (2008). A modified jigsaw method: An active learning strategy to develop the cognitive and affective domains through curricular review. *Journal of Physical Therapy Education*, 21(3), 15–23. https://doi.org/10.1097/00001416-200801000-00004

Yanchus, N. J., Periard, D., & Osatuke, K. (2017). Further examination of predictors of turnover intention among mental health professionals. *Journal of Psychiatric & Mental Health Nursing*, 24(1), 41–56. https://doi.org/10.1111/jpm.12354

Zachry, A. H., Nash, B. H., & Nolen, A. (2017). Traditional lectures and team-based learning in an occupational therapy program: A survey of student perceptions. *Open Journal of Occupational Therapy*, 5(2), 1–10. https://doi.org/10.15453/2168-6408.1313

Zhang, C., Miller, C., Volkman, K., Meza, J., & Jones, K. (2015). Evaluation of the team performance observation tool with targeted behavioral markers in simulation-based interprofessional eduction. *Journal of Interprofessional Care*, 29(3), 202–208. https://doi.org/10.3109/13561820.2014.982789

# Implementing Simulation in the Curriculum

**Nina Multak and Ruth A. Wittmann-Price**

*Learn from yesterday, live for today, hope for tomorrow. The important thing is not to stop questioning.*

—*Albert Einstein*

**This chapter addresses Domain III: Educational Principles Applied to Simulation (Society for Simulation in Healthcare [SSH], 2021).**

## ▶ LEARNING OUTCOMES

- ■ Describe the principles of integrating simulation into a curriculum.
- ■ Identify the learning domains to which simulation-based learning can be applied.
- ■ Discuss effective utilization of resources.

## ▶ INTRODUCTION

Simulation can be used to help learners acquire new knowledge and competencies and to better understand concepts needed for safe and effective patient care. By implementing simulation into healthcare curricula, educators will be able to more adeptly assess applied knowledge and competencies. Cantrell et al. (2022) and Heuer et al. (2022) describe the best practices of simulation in their critical review of simulation-based education.

### Evidence-Based Simulation Practice 15.1

Acosta et al. (2022) developed an in situ mixed-method simulation study to evaluate best practices for fall prevention. Researchers found that 80% of participants, who were frontline workers, would change current practice to best practice after a simulation-based education.

Curriculum integration of dozen practices is essential for the effective use of simulation (Price et al., 2022). It is widely accepted that simulation-based learning (SBL) is most effective when integrated with other learning events and focused on specific learning outcomes or entrustable professional activities (EPAs) or competencies. In addition, simulation-based healthcare education is complementary to clinical education (Olaussen et al., 2022).

Healthcare educators should understand the principles of integrating simulation into a curriculum and identify the curricular areas in which simulation can be effectively implemented. Resources should be used effectively and efficiently. Simulation-based education (SBE) and evaluation needs to be planned, scheduled, and carried out with consideration given to the entire curriculum (Rim & Shin, 2022). Simulation should involve all educational stakeholders and garner the necessary administrative support, including funding and materials (Huth et al., 2022).

# ▶ DEVELOPMENT OF A CURRICULUM

Healthcare educators seeking to implement simulation into the curriculum should consider the mission of the educational department or organization and the needs of the learners throughout their educational process. Educators should consider learners to be at the novice student level, progressing in the curriculum to competent graduate level and utilizing a vertical or threaded approach to curricular integration. Consideration should also be given to integrating simulation with inclusion of learners from other professions and disciplines (Altmiller et al., 2022).

It is important to keep measurable objectives in mind, as the design of the simulation activity is critical to its success. Effective simulation is designed using sound methods and principles with the goal that students gain competence in or observe and assess the outlined learning objectives within a safe, learning-conducive environment. Simulation activities are commonly developed in the areas of education (conceptual knowledge, competency), assessment, system integration, and for research purposes (Huth et al., 2022; Palaganas et al., 2015).

The initial steps of curriculum development, according to Kern et al. (2009), can be effectively applied to simulation.

The first step in the model of Kern et al. (2009) is problem identification with a subsequent needs assessment. Effective simulation activities begin with a needs assessment that identifies the learners, the knowledge of the learners, and the competencies or EPAs that are needed by the graduate. The needs assessment assists educators in developing measurable learning objectives or competency milestones or benchmarks throughout the curriculum. This should include an evaluation of the need or competency, identifying both the current educational approach and the ideal educational approach. Following a structured needs assessment will assist the simulation educator in developing more educationally sound and meaningful simulation programs.

The next step includes a focused assessment of the learners and the most ideal learning environment. For simulation-based healthcare education, the educator should decide in which of the following environments the information would best be learned: a simulation laboratory, a skills laboratory, a classroom, or in situ. It is important to identify the participants in the simulation curriculum. The knowledge and skills that novices need to learn are not the same as the knowledge needed by advanced students, and so it is important to develop learning objectives and competency milestones or benchmarks that provide the appropriate balance of guidance and autonomy for students' levels of sophistication and to identify whether students will be evaluated individually or as part of a team.

The Certified Healthcare Simulation Educator® (CHSE®) should analyze the current educational approach along with practitioners and the healthcare educational system to address the students' current educational needs. The difference between the ideal approach and the current approach represents a gap and identifies a general needs assessment. A targeted needs assessment should include an assessment of the following:

- the needs of a specific learner group or the competencies or EPAs needed as graduates
- the healthcare institution and the specific learning environment, which may differ from the needs of a specific student population (Kern et al., 2009; Wittmann-Price & Gittings, 2021)

Setting goals and objectives serves as a basis for assessment, and specific measurable learning objectives and EPAs should be considered. These include:

- cognitive (knowledge) domain
- affective (attitudinal) domain
- psychomotor domain (skill and behavioral; Kern et al., 2009; Wittmann-Price & Gittings, 2021)

The educational strategies considered should be specific to the learners and to the content of the curriculum.

The healthcare faculty are often challenged with identifying educational strategies that depart from structured learning and reactive thinking to reflective and proactive thinking. Experiential learning strategies using active learning approaches in which students become engaged with educational materials as active learners are replacing some of the classroom-based instruction (Jeffries & Clochesy, 2012). Simulation-based education bridges the classroom and the clinical arena and engages learners with broad perspectives to reflect and reframe their understanding of concepts important for clinical practice. Educators use simulation as a way to provide rich learning experiences that can imitate clinical experiences and integrate simulation into the curriculum with clear connections toward achievement of student learning outcomes.

Implementation of simulation in a curriculum requires consideration of many variables, including:

- obtaining political support
- reviewing the mission of the educational unit
- identifying and procuring resources
- raculty professional development and buy-in
- identifying and addressing barriers to implementation
- introducing the curriculum (piloting or phasing-in)
- administering the curriculum and refining the curriculum over successive cycles (process improvement and systematic evaluation)

The final step in the model of Kern et al. (2009) includes evaluation and feedback. This can be used to drive ongoing support, justify additional resources, and answer research questions about the effectiveness of specific curriculum elements. Table 15.1 outlines the model's steps and acknowledges the actual work needed to complete the steps.

**Table 15.1 Steps to Curriculum Development According to the Model of Kern et al. (2009)**

| Steps | Work Needed to Complete the Steps |
|---|---|
| Step 1: needs identification and general assessment<br>■ Identify the educational gap.<br>■ Identify the current approach (who is doing what, when, and how; resource limitations).<br>■ Identify the ideal approach.<br>■ Ideal approach − current approach = general assessment. | Work for steps 1 and 2<br>■ Systematic review of literature<br>■ Needs assessment report<br>■ Assessment tool |
| Step 2: needs analysis of targeted learners<br>■ Identify the learners, level of training, previous experience, current performance, learning styles, and preferences.<br>■ Identify barriers or enabling factors.<br>■ Identify the available resources for this group (simulation, faculty, and clinical experiences).<br>■ Identify multiple ways to obtain information/ needs assessment (Kern et al., 2009). | |

*(continued)*

**Table 15.1** Steps to Curriculum Development According to the Model of Kern et al. (2009) (*continued*)

| Steps | Work Needed to Complete the Steps |
|---|---|
| Step 3: goals and objectives<br>■ Review the types and levels of objectives.<br>■ Learning domains include cognitive, psychomotor, and affective.<br>■ Review Bloom's taxonomy of educational objectives.<br>■ Write specific, measurable, achievable, relevant, and timely objectives.<br>■ Identify EPAs and competencies needed by the graduate. | Work for steps 3 and 4<br>■ Identification of a new educational tool or method<br>■ Development of simulation scenarios<br>■ Research on the merits of educational processes or tools |
| Step 4: educational strategies<br>■ Use multiple educational methods and match methods to objectives.<br>■ Review/discuss the pros and cons of different methods.<br>■ Choose methods that are feasible in terms of resources.<br>■ Consider different simulation options.<br>  ● Computer-based virtual patients<br>  ● Role-playing<br>  ● Standardized (simulated) patients<br>  ● Task trainers or models<br>  ● Virtual reality simulators<br>  ● Manikin simulators<br>  ● Hybrid simulation<br>  ● Group learning projects<br>  ● Supplemental interactive activities | |
| Step 5: implementation<br>■ Consider resources: personnel, time, facilities, and funding/costs<br>■ Administration and operations<br>■ Piloting, phasing-in, and full Implementation | Work for steps 5 and 6<br>■ Descriptive study of curriculum implementation<br>■ Cost-effective analysis report<br>■ Assessment tool |
| Step 6: evaluation and feedback<br>■ Identify users and use (formative, summative), resources for evaluation, questions to ask, and evaluation design.<br>■ Select the measurement method.<br>■ Assess ethical issues.<br>■ Perform data collection and analysis.<br>■ Identify the results. | |

EPAs, entrustable professional activities.
*Source:* Adapted from Kern, D. E., Thomas, P. A., & Hughes, M. T. (2009). *Curriculum development for medical education: A six step approach* (2nd ed.). Johns Hopkins University Press.

A needs assessment for a curriculum can be accomplished by many methods, including the following:

■ informal discussions
■ questionnaires

- surveys
- interviews
- focus groups
- observations
- tests
- literature review
- available published documents

# ▶ DELIBERATE PRACTICE

Research on expert performance has transformed the way healthcare educators approach how clinicians acquire clinical competence and how expertise is defined (Ericsson, 2004, 2008; Price et al., 2022).

Deliberate practice is the path to acquiring expertise and the goal is to improve performance. Repeated behaviors become automatic habits. Students who master the art of deliberate practice are committed to being lifelong learners—always exploring and experimenting and refining. This requires sustained effort and concentration. The concept of deliberate practice, in which education is focused on improving particular tasks, has been essential to the development of the simulation-based experiential learning paradigm and has been implemented by healthcare educators across many disciplines (Price et al., 2022).

## Evidence-Based Simulation Practice 15.2

Price et al. (2022) implemented online practice and in person simulation as a quality improvement project for pediatric residents for 60 competencies using deliberate practice for skill attainment. Out of the 60 procedures, 12 were evaluated for residents' perceptions at 1-year intervals. There was a 12.7% increase in positive perceptions from the pediatric residents about using deliberate practice simulation to master competencies.

# ▶ LEARNING DOMAINS

Simulation can measure outcomes in the cognitive, affective, and psychomotor domains. Cognitive domain learning may include the acquisition and recall of facts and figures, concepts, and principles. Cognitive learning outcomes have been identified as a basic strategy for the assessment of student learning. A traditional lecture followed by a multiple-choice or short-answer exam is an example of cognitive evaluation. Healthcare simulation offers an opportunity for teaching and evaluation of higher level cognitive functions, such as the application, synthesis, and evaluation of healthcare knowledge (Kardong-Edgren et al., 2010; Lattner et al., 2022).

Learning in the affective domain includes the values, attitudes, and beliefs that are essential for a healthcare provider. Assessment of the affective domain requires educators to identify and verify that healthcare learners have absorbed the values, attitudes, and beliefs essential for a healthcare provider and that these are reflected in their professional practice. Manikin simulation allows opportunities for learners to reveal their competency in the affective domain through participation in simulation scenarios (Gillespie et al., 2021).

Technical skill performance is an example of assessment of psychomotor learning. Using task trainers, virtual reality simulators, and manikin simulators, the simulation educator can assess the acquisition of technical skills (Haidari et al., 2022; Jeffries & Norton, 2005). Using a case scenario to evaluate technical skills allows simulation educators to teach and evaluate psychomotor skills in a setting that is more realistic than a traditional skills station (such as suturing on a task trainer or starting an intravenous [IV] line using a simulated IV arm) and much safer than an actual patient care setting, such as a live patient in an ED. Evaluation instruments that measure preestablished outcomes may be used for a comprehensive evaluation of learning (Haidari et al., 2022; Kardong-Edgren et al., 2010).

## ▶ INTEGRATING SIMULATION

Simulation training can be implemented into various components of a curriculum.

- Basic science courses can effectively use simulation modalities. Pharmacologic effects can be simulated on a manikin for usual dosage ingestion or overdose. Medication effects can also be taught in code or advanced cardiac life support scenarios.
- Simulators can be used to teach healthcare learners about vital sign assessment as well as evaluation of cardiac and pulmonary conditions.
- Crisis management training can be implemented with consideration of complex details of realistic case scenarios.

Effectively directing simulation resources can result in an educator's ability to successfully implement simulation in the educational curriculum. These resources are shown in Figure 15.1. Organizational barriers can hinder the implementation of SBE in the curriculum. Scheduling

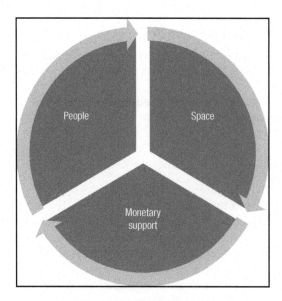

**Figure 15.1** Resources needed to include simulation in a curriculum.

trainees to attend simulation activities can be a challenge. It is suggested that leaders in the institution support simulation programming by encouraging the faculty to become involved and avoid learner scheduling and space issues (Exhibit 15.1). The faculty and financial resources can also be supported by administrative personnel (McGaghie et al., 2010; Sessions et al., 2020).

| **EXHIBIT 15.1 CONSIDERATIONS FOR SIMULATION IMPLEMENTATION** | | | |
|---|---|---|---|
| **Type of Knowledge, Skill, Attitudes, or Behavior Addressed in Simulation** | | | |
| Conceptual knowledge | Technical skills | Decision-making skills | Attitudes and behavior |
| **Purpose** | | | |
| Education | Assessment | Clinical training | Research |
| **Experience Level of Participants** | | | |
| Preprofessional education | Initial professional education | Clinical competency/ residency | Continuing education |

*Source:* Gaba, D. M. (2004). The future vision of simulation in health care. *Quality & Safety in Health Care, 13,* i2–i10. https://doi.org/10.1136/qshc.2004.009878

# ▶ SIMULATION CONCEPTS

It is important to embed simulation throughout a curriculum instead of implementing simulation exercises as independent curricular elements (Hill et al., 2022). It is also vital to consider a vertical as well as a horizontal approach to implementing simulation in the curriculum. Simulations should be developed for novice, experienced, and expert clinicians. An interprofessional or multidisciplinary approach to simulation programming should also be implemented in order to give learners experience developing their skills in a team-based setting. Establishing the best approach to integrating simulation in a curriculum can be determined by the institution as well as by the discipline and can address the potential effect of combining simulation-based healthcare education with other educational strategies (Hill et al., 2022; McGaghie et al., 2010).

Prior to curricular implementation, educators should consider the following simulation-based considerations:

- *Realism:* Educational goals should match simulation type. Task trainers should be used for procedural skills, whereas complex events should involve a high-fidelity manikin simulator (McGaghie et al., 2010; Monesi et al., 2022).
- *Reliability (e.g., assessment tools, implementation process):* The development of effective evaluation tools should follow an organized process with a clearly defined endpoint (Kardong-Edgren et al., 2010; Wilson et al., 2022).
- *Validity (e.g., content, construct):* Ideally, simulation evaluation instruments validly measure each of the three domains of student performance: cognitive, psychomotor, and affective. Several types of validity need to be considered when using tools for evaluation, including the following:
  - *Content validity:* refers to the appropriateness of each item and the comprehensiveness of the measurement
  - *Construct validity:* refers to the process of establishing that an action accurately represents the concept being evaluated (Kardong-Edgren et al., 2010; Wilson et al., 2022)
  - *Face validity:* refers to whether the evaluation tool appears to be measuring the concept it is supposed to measure
  - *Predictive ability:* refers to whether there is a correlation between the responses and the expectation (Gillies et al., 2020; Zheng & Agresti, 2000)
- *Feasibility (e.g., efficient, effective, achievable):* There should be possibilities for replication of some or nearly all of the essential aspects of a clinical situation so that the situation can be readily understood and managed when it occurs in actual clinical practice (Ansquer et al., 2021; Cant & Cooper, 2010).

- *Learner-centered education:* Students can use deliberate practice in a focused manner to master skills at their own pace (Ericsson, 2004; Wittmann-Price & Gittings, 2021).
- *Interprofessional education:* Interprofessional education (IPE) has been recognized by various international professional societies (e.g., World Health Organization, Institute of Medicine) and accreditation organizations as foundational to achieving safe, high-quality, accessible, patient-centered care (Acosta et al., 2022).
- *Teamwork:* Critical teamwork competencies should be identified and used as a focus for training content; teamwork simulations need to be designed to improve team processes (Monesi et al., 2022; Salas et al., 2008).
- *Human factors:* Engaging learners in repetitive practice is suggested as a primary factor in studies showing skill transference to real patients. With increased simulator availability, learning curves are shortened, leading to faster skill automaticity. Simulators must be made available at a location that is convenient to learners and accommodates their schedules (Issenberg et al., 2005; Phang et al., 2021).
- *Patient safety:* Simulation is an important educational technique to improve clinical training and patient safety (Groves et al., 2017; Phang et al., 2021).

## Simulation Teaching Tip 15.1

Simulation program development should occur in conjunction with other curriculum programming. Simulation can be used for both formative and summative assessments and is therefore most valuable when integrated throughout the training curriculum. Involving the faculty in the development of assessment tools enables more faculty involvement in simulation programming.

# ▶ SUMMARY

Simulation educators should continue to focus on evidence-based information which supports the best practices of simulation (Acosta et al., 2022; McGaghie et al., 2010). Implementing simulation in the curriculum is one of the top objectives in the best-practice list according to research. Other best practices noted in this research include feedback, deliberate practice, outcome measurement, appropriate fidelity, attention to competency acquisition and maintenance, mastery in learning, transference to practice, team training, high-stakes training, instructor training, and appropriate educational and professional context.

# ● CASE STUDY 15.1

Schools of health sciences are being developed in academic institutions all over the country to accommodate the market demand for healthcare practitioners. As the founding dean of a health sciences program that includes the disciplines of nursing, physician assistant studies, physical therapy, and occupational therapy, how could a founding dean develop an interprofessional simulation program in order to integrate simulation throughout all curricula?

1. The novice simulation educator needs more understanding about integrating simulation throughout the curriculum when they state:

    A. "Resources are needed for personnel and equipment."
    B. "A new building may be needed to accommodate the program."
    C. "High-fidelity equipment should be purchased."
    D. "Faculty buy-in is not necessary; it doesn't affect them."

2. The first step in integrating simulation throughout a curriculum should be to:

    A. Acquire equipment
    B. Develop student learning outcomes
    C. Review the mission and values
    D. Perform a needs assessment

3. The novice simulation educator needs better understanding when they state that simulation competencies should include which of the following domains?

    A. Psychomotor
    B. Cognitive
    C. Empathetic
    D. Affective

4. The final step of developing an integrative simulation curriculum is:

    A. Systematic program evaluation
    B. Deciding on teaching methods
    C. Developing student learning outcomes
    D. Discussing the mission

5. The simulation educator understands deliberate practice when they state:

    A. "It has an outcome of developing perfect skills."
    B. "It is a method to evaluate and grade students."
    C. "It is a method to ensure appropriate formative evaluation."
    D. "It is a method to use to become competent in skills."

6. A student who is practicing insertion of central lines in a hybrid simulation with a standardized patient is learning mainly in which domains?

    A. Affective and psychomotor
    B. Psychomotor and psychosocial
    C. Cognitive and affective
    D. Psychosocial and cognitive

## 1. D) "Faculty buy-in is not necessary; it doesn't affect them."

Faculty buy-in is always needed to make a successful simulation program. Resources are needed in both areas: personnel and equipment. A new building may be needed if space resources are scarce. High-fidelity equipment will be needed for a complete simulation laboratory learning experience.

## 2. D) Perform a needs assessment

Performing a needs assessment is always the first step to evaluate if a simulation program is needed. The next step would be to review the mission and then the student learning outcomes. Equipment can be purchased later.

## 3. C) Empathetic

Empathy is a needed attribute in healthcare but is not a learning domain. Psychomotor, cognitive, and affective are the traditional learning domains. Empathy falls within the affective learning domain.

## 4. A) Systematic program evaluation

A systematic program evaluation should be ongoing in order to make program improvements in real time. Teaching methods, student learning outcomes, and discussing the "fit" of the mission are all part of program development and all should be systematically evaluated.

## 5. D) "It is a method to use to become competent in skills."

Deliberate practice is used as a teaching method to assist learners in becoming competent in a skill. Deliberate practice is not used for formative or summative evaluation and the intent is not perfection. The intent is competence.

## 6. A) Affective and psychomotor

A standardized patient represents the human to human interaction needed in the affective domain, while a hybrid manikin or part-task trainer is used to promote skill development, which is mainly in the psychomotor domain. Cognitive domains address "why" something is being done, while psychosocial is not a labeled domain.

7. A scenario in which a student is telling family members "bad news" about a patient is developing skills in which domain?

   A. Affective
   B. Psychomotor
   C. Cognitive
   D. Psychosocial

8. A student who is calculating the correct morphine dosage in a simulation to complete a patient-controlled analgesic (PCA) pump setup is developing skills in which domain?

   A. Affective
   B. Psychomotor
   C. Cognitive
   D. Psychosocial

9. A fundamental simulation principle for educators to consider is:

   A. Student learning outcomes should match the simulation being designed
   B. Always use the lowest simulation type to accomplish an educational task
   C. The more real the environment, the better the learning outcome will be
   D. All students should be exposed to all simulation types for best practice

10. The novice simulation educator needs a better understanding when they include which of the following attributes when describing simulation feasibility?

    A. Efficient
    B. Effective
    C. Available
    D. Achievable

### 7. A) Affective

Affective domain development is needed to discuss critical information with patients and families. Cognitive is important for knowing why, psychomotor is not usually a major factor, and psychosocial is not a domain.

### 8. C) Cognitive

Cognition is needed to understand correct calculation and correct dosage. Psychomotor comes into play when setting up the pump, and affective is how the treatment is described to the patient and the family. Psychosocial is not a domain.

### 9. A) Student learning outcomes should match the simulation being designed

Student learning outcomes should drive the simulation methodology. Although using the lowest simulation type is good to conserve resources, it may not impact learning. Realism does not always ensure the objectives/student learning outcomes are met. Making sure all students are exposed to all simulation types is not necessary.

### 10. C) Available

Available is not one of the attributes of feasibility. Feasibility has to do with the transferability of simulation skills to the clinical environment. The skills are needed to be effective and efficient, and the competency or skill should be achievable.

# REFERENCES

Acosta, D. J., Rinfert, A., Plant, J., & Hsu, A. T. (2022). Using patient simulation to promote best practices in fall prevention and postfall assessment in nursing homes. *Journal of Nursing Care Quality, 37*(2), 117–122. https://doi.org/10.1097/NCQ.0000000000000599

Altmiller, G., Alexy, E., Dzubaty, D., Jakubowski, T., & Kartoz, C. (2022). Systematic curriculum mapping of virtual patient assignments to end-of-program outcomes. *Nurse Educator, 47*(2), 69–74. https://doi.org/10.1097/NNE.0000000000001107

Ansquer, R., Oriot, D., & Ghazali, D. A. (2021). Evaluation of learning effectiveness after a simulation-based training pediatric course for emergency physicians. *Pediatric Emergency Care, 37*(12), e1186–e1191. https://doi.org/10.1097/PEC.0000000000001961

Cant, R., & Cooper, S. (2010). Simulation-based learning in nurse education: Systematic review. *Journal of Advanced Nursing, 66*(1), 3–15. https://doi.org/10.1111/j.1365-2648.2009.05240.x

Cantrell, M. A., Mariani, B., & Lengetti, E. (2022). A quantitative research study protocol to advance simulation science in nursing education. *Nursing Education Perspectives, 43*(2), 103–108. https://doi.org/10.1097/01.NEP.0000000000000891

Ericsson, K. A. (2004). Deliberate practice and the acquisition and maintenance of expert performance in medicine and related domains. *Academic Medicine, 79*(10), S70–S81. https://doi.org/10.1097/00001888-200410001-00022

Ericsson, K. A. (2008). Deliberate practice and acquisition of expert performance: A general overview. *Academic Emergency Medicine, 15*(11), 988–994. https://doi.org/10.1111/j.1553-2712.2008.00227.x

Gaba, D. M. (2004). The future vision of simulation in health care. *Quality & Safety in Health Care, 13*, i2–i10. https://doi.org/10.1136/qshc.2004.009878

Gillespie, G. L., Farra, S. R., Saundra, L., & Brammer, S. V. (2021). Impact of immersive virtual reality simulations for changing knowledge, attitudes, and behaviors. *Nurse Education Today, 105*, 4–11. https://doi.org/10.1016/j.nedt.2021.105025

Gillies, C. E., Taylor, D. F., Cummings, B. C., Ansari, S., Islim, F., Kronick, S. L., Medlin, R. P., Ward, K. R., & Medlin, R. P. (2020). Demonstrating the consequences of learning missingness patterns in early warning systems for preventative health care: A novel simulation and solution. *Journal of Biomedical Informatics, 110*, 103528. https://doi.org/10.1016/j.jbi.2020.103528

Groves, P. S., Bunch, J. L., Cram, E., Farag, A., Manges, K., Perkhounkova, Y., & Scott-Cawiezell, J. (2017). Priming patient safety through nursing handoff communication: A simulation pilot study. *Western Journal of Nursing Research, 39*(11), 1394–1411. https://doi.org/10.1177/0193945916673358

Haidari, T. A., Bjerrum, F., Hansen, H. J., Konge, L., & Petersen, R. H. (2022). Simulation-based VATS resection of the five lung lobes: A technical skills test. *Surgical Endoscopy, 36*(2), 1234–1242. https://doi.org/10.1007/s00464-021-08392-3

Heuer, A., Bienstock, J., & Yingting, Z. (2022). Simulation-based training within selected allied health professions: An evidence-based systematic review. *Journal of Allied Health, 51*(1), 59–71.

Hill, P. P., Diaz, D. A., Anderson, M., Talbert, S., & Maraj, C. (2022). Live help using simulation-based education to teach interruption management skills: An integrative review. *Clinical Simulation in Nursing, 64*, 46–57. https://doi.org/10.1016/j.ecns.2021.12.002

Huth, K., Henry, D., Cribb, F. C., Coleman, C. L., Frank, B., Schumacher, D., & Shah, N. (2022). A multistakeholder approach to the development of entrustable professional activities in complex care. *Academic Pediatrics, 22*(2), 184–189. https://doi.org/10.1016/j.acap.2021.09.014

Issenberg, S. B., McGaghie, W. C., Petrusa, E. R., Gordon, D. L., & Scalese, R. J. (2005). Features and uses of high-fidelity medical simulations that lead to effective learning: A BEME systematic review. *Medical Teacher, 27*, 10–28. https://doi.org/10.1080/01421590500046924

Jeffries, P. R., & Clochesy, J. M. (2012). Clinical simulations: An experiential, student-centered pedagogical approach. In D. M. Billings & J. A. Halstead (Eds.), *Teaching in nursing: A guide for faculty* (4th ed., pp. 352–368). Elsevier Health Sciences.

Jeffries, P. R., & Norton, B. (2005). Selecting learning experiences to achieve curriculum outcomes. In D. M. Billings & J. A. Halstead (Eds.), *Teaching in nursing: A guide for faculty* (2nd ed., pp. 187–212). Elsevier.

Kardong-Edgren, S., Adamson, K. A., & Fitzgerald, C. (2010). A review of currently published evaluation instruments for human patient simulation. *Clinical Simulation in Nursing, 6*, e25–e35. https://doi.org/10.1016/j.ecns.2009.08.004

Kern, D. E., Thomas, P. A., & Hughes, M. T. (2009). *Curriculum development for medical education: A six step approach* (2nd ed.). Johns Hopkins University Press.

Lattner, C., Badowski, D., Otremba, D., Gieger, J., & Klass, J. (2022). Creating an asynchronous telehealth simulation for advance nursing practice students. *Clinical Simulation in Nursing, 63*, 5–9. https://doi.org/10.1016/j.ecns.2021.11.005

McGaghie, W., Issenberg, S. B., Petrusa, E. R., & Scalese, R. J. (2010). A critical review of simulation-based medical education research: 2003–2009. *Medical Education, 44*, 50–63. https://doi.org/10.1111/j.1365-2923.2009.03547.x

Monesi, A., Imbriaco, G., Mazzoli, C., Giugni, A., & Ferrari, P. (2022). Pandemic in Italy: Advantages and challenges. In-situ simulation for intensive care nurses during the COVID-19. *Clinical Simulation in Nursing, 62*, 52–56. https://doi.org/10.1016/j.ecns.2021.10.005

Olaussen, C., Steindal, S. A., Jelsness-Jorgensen, L., Aase, I., Stenseth, H., & Tvedt, C. R. (2022). Integrating simulation training during clinical practice in nursing homes: An experimental study of nursing students' knowledge acquisition, self-efficacy and learning needs. *BMC Nursing, 21*(1), 1–11. https://doi.org/10.1186/s12912-022-00824-2

Palaganas, J. C., Maxworthy, J. C., Epps, C. A., & Mancini, M. (2015). *Defining excellence in simulation*. Society for Simulation in Healthcare.

Phang, R., Beck, S., Dar, O., Robertson-Smith, J., Fyfe, C., Scanlan, M., Thoams, S., Wrigley, R., & Anakin, M. (2021). Using systems thinking to identify staff and patient safety issues in infectious disease simulation scenarios. *Clinical Simulation in Nursing, 61*, 23–32. https://doi.org/10.1016/j.ecns.2021.08.026

Price, A., Greene, H. M., Stem, C. T., Titus, M. O., Rutman, L. E., & Greene, H. M. (2022). Sticking it straight: Pediatric procedure curriculum initiative. *Pediatric Emergency Care, 38*(2), 79–82. https://doi.org/10.1097/PEC.0000000000002324

Rim, D., & Shin, H. (2022). Development and assessment of a multi-user virtual environment nursing simulation program: A mixed methods research study. *Clinical Simulation in Nursing, 62*, 31–41. https://doi.org/10.1016/j.ecns.2021.10.004

Salas, E., Diaz-Granados, D., Weaver, S. J., & King, H. (2008). Does team training work? Principles for health care. *Academic Emergency Medicine, 11*, 1002–1009. https://doi.org/10.1111/j.1553-2712.2008.00254.x

Sessions, L., Nemeth, L. S., Catchpole, K., & Kelechi, T. (2020). Use of simulation-based learning to teach high-alert medication safety: A feasibility study. *Clinical Simulation in Nursing, 47*, 60–64. https://doi.org/10.1016/j.ecns.2020.06.013

Society for Simulation in Healthcare. (2021). *Certified healthcare simulation educator handbook*. https://www.ssih.org/Portals/48/Certification/CHSE_Docs/CHSE%20Handbook.pdf

Wilson, M., Elki-Brown, N. S., James, L., James, S. M., Stevens, K., & Butterfield, P. (2022). Psychometric evaluation of the Creighton Competency Evaluation Instrument in a population of working nurses. *Journal of Nursing Measurement, 30*(1), 148–167. https://doi.org/10.1891/JNM-D-20-00083

Wittmann-Price, R. A., & Gittings, K. K. (2021). *Fast facts about competency-based education in nursing: How to teach competency mastery*. Springer Publishing Company.

Zheng, B., & Agresti, A. (2000). Summarizing the predictive power of a generalized linear model. *Statistics in Medicine, 19*, 1771–1781. https://doi.org/10.1002/1097-0258(20000715)19:13<1771::AID-SIM485>3.0.CO;2-P

# Planning Simulation Activities

**Karen K. Gittings**

*It takes as much energy to wish as it does to plan.*

—*Eleanor Roosevelt*

This chapter addresses Domain III: Educational Principles Applied to Simulation (Society for Simulation in Healthcare [SSH], 2021).

## ▶ LEARNING OUTCOMES

- ▪ Discuss the importance of developing goals and objectives/outcomes for simulation activities that are relevant to student learning outcomes.
- ▪ Describe formative and summative methods that can be used to evaluate learning outcomes for simulation activities.
- ▪ Design a simulation day or simulation activities to promote learning.

## ▶ INTRODUCTION

Simulation activities are a valuable adjunct for student learning and evaluation if linked appropriately to student learning outcomes. Planning ahead is vitally important for the overall success and effectiveness of simulation activities. The process begins with an assessment of learner needs, after which the goals of the simulation activities and measurable learning objectives/outcomes must be identified. The educator must then decide on whether the evaluation should be formative or summative and what methods of evaluation would be most appropriate. After these initial steps are completed, the simulation activities are designed with consideration of the resources needed and those that are available. A well-planned simulation activity will minimize problems in the implementation phase. The focus of this chapter is to discuss the planning process for simulation activities; a sample simulation day is reviewed to illustrate each step in the process.

## ▶ NEEDS ASSESSMENT

The first step in the planning process for simulation activities is to identify the needs of the learners. This can be accomplished through several methods. In some instances, it may be helpful to administer a formal needs assessment at the onset of the planning process; this allows learners to self-identify their educational needs. The needs assessment can also be done informally by the educator who is responsible for the simulation activities and has the most knowledge of the context in which the simulation is being used and how it links to student learning outcomes. Both methods will serve to provide a starting point for the planning process and further guide the development of goals and objectives/outcomes.

**Simulation Teaching Tip 16.1**

Educators should make a conscious effort to be aware of their body language during the debriefing process. An open posture in which the educator leans forward with arms at their sides invites learners to share, whereas an educator who is leaned back with their arms crossed sends a message of disagreement or disinterest (Grant et al., 2018).

## ▶ GOAL DEFINITION

Once learner needs have been assessed, it is important to set achievable goals for the day. The words *goals* and *objectives/outcomes* are often erroneously used interchangeably. Goals are usually statements that serve as a long-term target; they describe the expected outcome at the end of the teaching–learning process. Goals can be used to broadly identify the purpose and final outcomes of the day and lead to the development of more specific objectives/outcomes (Bastable, 2019).

## ▶ LEARNING OBJECTIVES/OUTCOMES

Learning objectives/outcomes are specific actions that are measurable, tangible, and designed to support attainment of the goals. Written to be short term, objectives/outcomes are statements about a single behavior that is to be accomplished after a teaching session or within a short period of time. Objectives/outcomes are often used to describe a behavior or performance that the learner must accomplish before being considered competent (Bastable, 2019).

The number of learning objectives/outcomes depends on the number of simulation activities and the time involved, but generally varies from one to four. In addition to being relevant, the learning objectives/outcomes should also be at the appropriate level for the learner; for example, the learning objectives of a simulation activity should be different if the learner is a student compared with an experienced practitioner. When running the simulation activities, it is important to always keep the learning objectives/outcomes in mind. Objectives/outcomes are the starting point for designing the simulation and will further guide the development of the scenario pertaining to content and complexity (Bailey, 2017).

## ▶ COMPETENCIES

Many health profession programs are moving away from objectives/outcomes to evaluate student learning and are using competencies. Competencies are embedded in the curriculum and extend to the simulation learning experiences. *Competency-based education* (CBE) is defined by Sargeant et al. (2018) as "[a]n outcomes-based approach to the design, implementation, assessment, and evaluation of education programs using an organizing framework of competencies" (p. 128). CBE has four essential components:

- CBE is responsive to society because graduates have the skills needed as practicing professional nurses.
- Curriculum design is based on abilities or competencies.
- CBE is focused on outcomes that can be assessed by multiple evaluation methods (Sargeant et al., 2018).
- CBE is learner-centered and congruent with constructivism, in which students understand the educational goals and independently construct knowledge themselves to reach the goals (Wittmann-Price et al., 2022).

CBE integrates milestones or benchmarks throughout the curriculum and provides the time and support for learners to reach the milestones/benchmarks. The competencies needed for a practicing health professional are evaluated at the end of the program to ensure graduates provide safe and quality patient care (Wittmann-Price & Gittings, 2021).

## ▶ TYPES OF EVALUATION

Evaluation of simulation activities can be formative or summative. Formative evaluation is done during the learning activity, allowing the educator to assess learners' progress toward achieving competencies or objectives/outcomes. As educators provide feedback throughout the process, learners are able to self-reflect on their performance. In this manner, the learning activity is used to facilitate learning and identify student learning deficits; the activity can also be evaluated and improved upon (Arrogante et al., 2021).

Summative evaluation is completed at the conclusion of a learning activity, course, or program. The focus is generally on evaluating the extent to which learning, outcomes, or competencies were met, leading to a grade assignment. These assessment results are often used to determine readiness for licensure, certification, and/or practice. Because summative evaluation occurs at the end, the biggest disadvantage is that nothing can be done to alter the results (Arrogante et al., 2021).

## ▶ EVALUATION METHODS

After determining the type of evaluation to be used, different methods of evaluation must be considered. Debriefing is considered an integral part of the teaching–learning process that occurs with high-fidelity simulation. This follow-up discussion provides learners the opportunity to process what they have learned. Learners are able to assess their own performance and, through feedback from faculty and peers, confirm their knowledge and identify areas that need improvement. It is the debriefing process that leads to the long-term acquisition of knowledge (Abelsson & Bisholt, 2017).

When other low-fidelity simulations are used, observation and feedback may be a more appropriate means of evaluation. *Observation* is the direct visualization of a learner's performance of a task or behavior. This is a useful method for evaluating skills competence. Faculty members observing learner performance are able to provide immediate feedback; in addition, learners have the opportunity to remediate and improve on skills. Using an objective tool with observation is important to avoid bias and accurately record information (Billings & Halstead, 2020).

Feedback is an important evaluative mechanism, but in order for it to be effective there must be a clear understanding of what constitutes good performance of the expected standards (Allen & Molloy, 2017). In order to provide appropriate feedback, observation must have occurred. The person providing feedback must also know the standard against which the learner is being compared; for this reason, it is important that the person providing feedback has expertise in the content area.

To evaluate the effectiveness of the simulation day, a survey with a rating scale can be used to elicit learners' and faculty's feedback on the extent to which the day's objectives/outcomes were met. Objectivity of the evaluation process is increased by using a rating scale (Billings & Halstead, 2020). Information from the survey can identify issues with the learning activities and lead to improvement for future simulation day activities.

**Evidence-Based Simulation Practice 16.1**

In a systematic review conducted by Wooding et al. (2020), the authors appraised 19 studies to explore the validity of teamwork tools utilized to assess interprofessional simulation teamwork training for healthcare professionals and students. The authors concluded that the Team Emergency Assessment Measure (TEAM), Team Performance Observation Tool (TPOT), and Assessment of Obstetric Team Performance (AOTP) and Global AOTP showed the strongest psychometrics.

## ▶ EVALUATION TOOLS

Measurements of learners' performance can range from self-reporting surveys to external reviewers using validated assessment tools. Many educators use subjective evaluation, such as self-reports of satisfaction and confidence, to evaluate learning objectives and outcomes. Surveys may include questions such as "what did you learn today" or "rate yourself on your ability to perform an assessment." For educators unskilled in tool development, self-reporting provides a means of evaluation that is easily obtained, although not necessarily a valid measure of simulation effectiveness. In order to evaluate the effectiveness of the simulation and attainment of outcomes, some form of objective evaluation should be included (Bjerrum et al., 2018). With the widening knowledge to practice gap in nursing, it becomes increasingly important to evaluate for outcomes relevant to clinical practice. The objective structured clinical examinations (OSCEs) are well-known as valid assessment tools used in medical schools for evaluation, but can also be used to objectively evaluate clinical nursing skills (Tseng et al., 2021). Several evaluation tools that use checklists or evaluation scales are documented in the literature, but many have not been evaluated for reliability or validity. In comparison with other methods of evaluation, OSCEs have been found to have better reliability, validity, and objectivity. New instruments are being developed that demonstrate appropriate psychometric properties for evaluation of OSCEs (Tseng et al., 2021).

## ▶ DESIGNING THE SIMULATION ACTIVITY

Planning and organizing the simulation activities are vital to a successful simulation day. Decisions must be made about the time frame allotted for the learning activities. For example, will the simulations be run during class or clinical time? If simulation activities occur on a clinical day, what will the learners do if simulation activities are completed in less time than their designated clinical hours?

Simulation activities that are consistent with the course's student learning outcomes must be planned. What simulation activities would reinforce student learning and promote achievement of student learning outcomes? How many simulation activities would be appropriate?

Consideration must also be given to the number of learners enrolled in the course. Simulation activities are most effective when learners are placed in small groups. Even when using low-fidelity simulations, fewer learners allow for more time for interaction with faculty members and hands-on practice. This leads to questions about how to schedule the learners in smaller numbers and still fit into the simulation laboratory schedule.

## ▶ SELECTING THE SIMULATION MODALITY

After designing the simulation day and activities, careful consideration must be given to the selection of modalities that will best support the learning objectives/outcomes. Simulation modalities are referred to as *high fidelity* and *low fidelity*, with *fidelity* often defined based on technology or complexity. *High fidelity* generally refers to the use of computer-driven technology and full-body manikins, which are utilized to perform procedural, high-risk skills in dynamic, authentic situations. *Low fidelity* refers to the traditional task trainers or standardized patients that are used for the practice and acquisition of nontechnical skills in an informal environment. *Mixed-fidelity* scenarios, which integrate the use of manikins and standardized patients, have been found effective in assessing skill competency and needs for further development (Melling et al., 2018).

## ▶ RESOURCE IDENTIFICATION

Once the simulation day has been planned, it is important to identify the resources that will be needed, as well as those that are available. First to consider is the location. Although many nursing/medical schools have simulation laboratories, size and room availability may be limited. Scheduling and reserving space are an early priority.

Equipment needs should also be identified. This should include a detailed list of everything that is needed at each simulation station. In addition to equipment needs, when planning for the simulation, it is also important to consider whether props or moulage are needed to achieve the desired look for the manikin. A medical record may also be necessary for the scenario to proceed. It is important to carefully plan the details in advance so that the necessary resources are available (Billings & Halstead, 2020).

It is also important to identify the content experts/educators and their availability for the simulation activities. Although some low-fidelity simulation activities can be designated as self-directed, generally a monitor is needed at each station to orient learners to the activity and keep them on target. For simulations done in nursing/medical schools, learners who are at a higher class level could be used to monitor some of the low-fidelity stations. For activities that involve high-fidelity or more complex learning activities, an adjunct clinical instructor or a graduate-level learner would be able to function as the content expert in instructing and assisting learners in meeting the learning objectives/outcomes. Some schools have dedicated laboratory personnel or technicians whose responsibilities include simulation and management of laboratory activities.

Simulation activities that are carried out in healthcare organizations are usually developed and organized by the staff of the education department. The educators have the primary responsibility of providing and managing the simulation activities, but other resources are often available. Healthcare personnel within the organization have unique knowledge and skills that make them valuable resources in assisting with simulation activities. In addition, healthcare organizations that have collaborative relationships with nursing/medical schools can invite faculty to participate in simulation activities.

## ▶ SIMULATION TEAM

Once the resources have been identified, it is important to organize the simulation team. Educators/content experts must be recruited to participate in simulation day activities. In the academic setting, if other faculty are to be used, consideration must be given to their workload and responsibilities. If the simulation activities are to be conducted on the learners' clinical days, the adjunct clinical instructors can be requested to assist with leading the simulation activities on the day their learners are in the laboratory setting. Adjunct clinical instructors may be recruited to assist with other days, but it must be clear whether additional pay is expected and whether departmental or laboratory budgets can support this. Graduate learners can also be recruited, as an example, from the nurse educator students; simulation hours may be used to fulfill hour requirements in a practicum course.

In the healthcare organizational setting, educators who are recruiting assistance from other agency personnel must often request release of the employees from their primary department. Arrangements need to be made as early as possible to prevent scheduling conflicts. This is also true when collaborating with faculty from nursing/medical schools.

If standardized (simulated) patients are used, actors must also be recruited. In collaboration with the drama department in academic settings, drama students may portray patients as part of an assignment. Other educators or faculty may also be used. Volunteers may be recruited as well. Professional actors skilled in playing standardized (simulated) patients are also available for hire, although their cost can be prohibitive.

Once the members of the simulation team have been recruited and confirmed, arrangements must be made to orient and train them for their roles. It can be challenging to schedule extra time for team members to train, especially when they have other jobs and responsibilities. This becomes less of an issue when the same content experts, whether clinical professionals, educators, or adjunct clinical instructors, are used frequently and simulation activities are done repetitively. Standardized (simulated) patients may require a more in-depth orientation and training depending on the role to be played.

## Evidence-Based Simulation Practice 16.2

In a study by Solli et al. (2020), nursing students' perspectives on the facilitator's role in briefing prior to a simulation were explored. Briefing is crucial in providing students with information necessary for a successful simulation; the facilitator's role in this is extremely complex. Facilitators must have expertise in simulation in addition to the ability to gauge the needs of diverse students and provide the necessary amount and degree of information.

# ▶ PREPARATIONS

Prior to the simulation day, multiple tasks must be accomplished to prepare the learners and the simulation team. A week in advance, the learners and team members should be sent an agenda with a schedule of the day's activities. The learners should additionally be provided information about the following:

- dress requirements
- equipment required (e.g., stethoscope)
- any preplanning work/assignment (Exhibit 16.1)

## EXHIBIT 16.1 LEARNER INSTRUCTIONS FOR SIMULATION DAY

**Please bring the following items on your simulation day:**

- Clinical uniform
- Stethoscope
- Simulation day agenda
- Class notes on nasogastric tubes
- Medical-surgical nursing textbook
- Nursing skills book
- Medications reference

The laboratory must also be prepared with all the equipment set up and ready for use. If the laboratory is heavily used, it may not be possible to set up until late in the preceding week. The laboratory setting should be fully prepared and functional so that simulation can be started and kept on schedule. When learners are required to stand around and wait due to lack of planning on the part of the coordinator, it reflects poorly on the simulation day overall. Learners appreciate well-run, organized learning activities.

It may be advisable to pilot a new simulation before conducting it with learners. This can be done in the form of a run-through or a field test and can be as simple as the course coordinator and simulation coordinator running the simulation scenario through with various unfolding events or endings. This process assists in identifying potential issues and problems that may occur during the simulation; in addition, this is an opportunity to ensure nothing has been forgotten, all necessary resources are available, and every simulation activity is running seamlessly. Prebriefing may also be used prior to the simulation in order to orient participants to the simulation and learning activities. During this time period, learners can review any relevant materials and familiarize themselves with the laboratory environment (Andrews, 2021). This also provides an opportunity for the faculty to ensure that any required preparatory work has been completed by the students.

## ▶ SUMMARY

Simulation days are very valuable to learners and can provide clinical skill practice that will be needed in the clinical area. Being true to the goals and objectives/outcomes of the experience is of utmost importance. Deciding on the logistics of how stations will be set up and what type of evaluation of skills will be accomplished is needed. It is also important to organize the day beforehand by setting up the laboratory, notifying people, and providing learners with expectations.

 ## CASE STUDY 16.1

A nurse educator is planning a simulation day for learners. To begin the process, they review the student learning outcomes of the Adult Health II course. The learners are first-semester seniors (third-semester nursing students) in a baccalaureate nursing program. The nurse educator identifies areas of new content and skills that will be introduced to the learners this semester, and from these determines the knowledge and skills that would be best taught through simulation activities. It is decided that the learners will be taught IV insertion and the principles of IV therapy during the simulation day.

In further assessing the learners' needs, the nurse educator recognizes that they gain little clinical experience in working with:

- Nasogastric (NG) tubes
- Small-bore feeding tubes
- Tube feedings
- Administration of medications through enteral feeding tubes

Even though learners are introduced to these skills in the fundamentals of nursing course, they may not have the opportunity to use them again due to clinical placement. It was therefore decided to include these skills as part of the simulation day for review and reeducation.

With an understanding of the learners' needs, the nurse educator is able to develop goals for the simulation day. It is important to keep in mind the course's student learning outcomes to ensure that the goals are relevant and support learning within the course.

*(continued)*

The goals include the following:
- The simulation day will enable learners to develop an understanding of IV insertion and the principles of IV therapy.
- The simulation day will enable learners to review knowledge and skills related to feeding tube insertion, tube feedings, and enteral medication administration.

After setting the goals for the simulation day, the nurse educator develops measurable objectives/outcomes that will be used to evaluate the effectiveness of the simulation activities. The objectives/outcomes include the following:

At the completion of the simulation day, learners will:
- Demonstrate correct technique in IV insertion using the IV simulator.
- Demonstrate the correct steps for hanging a secondary IV and programming the smart pump.
- Assess and perform nursing interventions for a simulated patient having abdominal pain.
- Demonstrate the correct technique for NG insertion and enteral administration of medications.

In deciding whether to use formative or summative evaluation, the nurse educator considers the goals for the day. Because the simulation day is designed to introduce new skills related to IV therapy and reinforce knowledge related to NG tubes and enteral medication administration, the nurse educator decides to use this day as a teaching opportunity with formative evaluation to assess learners' progress. At each learning station, students will be required to return and demonstrate their new skills. Faculty members are responsible for facilitating the learning of new skills and the correction of identified learning deficits.

As learners will only attend one simulation day associated with the Adult Health II course, a summative evaluation will be completed by learners and the faculty. This evaluation will be used to determine whether the learning activities were effective in meeting the planned goals and objectives/outcomes.

For the purposes of formative evaluation, the nurse educator elects to use debriefing, observation, and feedback. Debriefing will follow the high-fidelity simulation of the patient with abdominal pain. Each simulation will run 15 to 20 minutes, followed by a 30-minute debriefing. The simulation coordinator will lead the debriefing due to their expertise and advanced training in this skill. Faculty members will use observation and feedback at the three other low-fidelity simulation stations. Skills' checklists or other tools will be used to objectively document learner performance. Learners will be provided feedback during their performance to assist with process improvement.

Learners and the faculty will be asked to complete a brief survey at the conclusion of the simulation day. This tool will be developed with assistance from the simulation coordinator. Information will be collected anonymously and used to determine whether learning objectives/outcomes were met. Suggestions for further improvement will also be solicited.

Because the simulation day is designed to provide opportunities for learners to acquire new knowledge and skills, the nurse educator elects to use skills' checklists at the IV therapy and NG tube stations to evaluate learner performance. At the conclusion of the day, learners will be asked to complete a survey, which is a self-report of their satisfaction with the simulation day activities and their confidence in meeting the learning objectives/outcomes. In the future, when simulation activities are used to document competency, a more valid and reliable evaluation tool will need to be used.

In the nursing department where the nurse educator teaches, course coordinators are given the opportunity to schedule a week for simulation activities in their courses. The nurse educator elects to schedule the simulation week early in the semester so learners will have the opportunity to learn new skills (IV therapy) and review old skills (NG tubes) prior to starting back to clinical practice in the hospital setting. The nurse educator further decides to have four simulation stations that will support the identified learning objectives/outcomes. The first station will be an IV station, where learners will learn proper techniques for IV insertion. The second station will be an IV station, where learners will learn the principles of IV therapy, including hanging a secondary medication and programming the smart pump. At the third station, learners will be required to assess and intervene in a simulated patient having abdominal pain. Last, learners will review the procedures for inserting NG tubes and administering enteral medications. These simulation activities will be scheduled

*(continued)*

over a period of 7.5 hours. In order to keep the number of learners low, only two clinical groups (16 learners) will be scheduled per day. Learners will be divided into four groups of four. For a class of 50 learners, 3 to 4 days will be necessary to rotate all learners in the Adult Health II course through the simulation activities. A sample schedule for the simulation day is noted in Table 16.1.

### Table 16.1 Sample Schedule of a Simulation Day

| Times | Station 1 IV SIM | Station 2 IV Pump | Station 3 Simulator | Station 4 NG/ MEDS |
|---|---|---|---|---|
| 8:30–9:45 a.m. | Orientation | Orientation | Orientation | Orientation |
| 9:50–10:40 a.m. | Blue Team | Green Team | Purple Team | Red Team |
| 10:45–11:35 a.m. | Red Team | Blue Team | Green Team | Purple Team |
| 11:35–12:35 p.m. | Lunch | Lunch | Lunch | Lunch |
| 12:40–1:30 p.m. | Purple Team | Red Team | Blue Team | Green Team |
| 1:45–2:35 p.m. | Green Team | Purple Team | Red Team | Blue Team |
| 2:40–3:00 p.m. | Evaluations | Evaluations | Evaluations | Evaluations |
| 3:00–4:00 p.m. | Math Work | Math Work | Math Work | Math Work |

MEDS, medications; NG, nasogastric; SIM, simulator.

The nurse educator continues planning for the simulation day by identifying the simulation modalities that will be used at each station. At the first station, learners will work with the screen-based IV computer simulator to learn correct technique for IV insertion; because this program provides feedback at the conclusion of each scenario, learners will be provided with an objective evaluation of their technique.

At the second station, learners will have the opportunity to work with IV equipment and practice priming IV lines, hanging secondary IVs, and programming the smart pump. This simulation activity involves the use of a task trainer (smart pump) in which learners have the opportunity to practice IV therapy skills.

Learners will work with a high-fidelity manikin at the third station, where they will be required to assess and intervene with a patient having abdominal pain. Learners will be observed during the simulation activity and feedback will be provided as part of the debriefing process.

The fourth and final station will use low-fidelity simulation to allow learners to practice the technique of NG tube insertion and administration of enteral medications. A task trainer, which is a model of a human's head and upper torso, will be used to practice NG tube insertion. Enteral medication administration can be practiced with a very simple setup of an NG tube inserted into an empty jug. Evaluation will be through observation and feedback.

In order to plan for simulation and schedule laboratory space each semester, the simulation coordinator requests that course coordinators sign up for their simulation week at the end of the preceding semester. A master schedule is then generated so that all faculty are aware of their simulation week, as well as other courses using the laboratory. Prior to their assigned week, the nurse educator notifies the simulation coordinator of the planned learning activities and space needs so that rooms/space in the laboratory can be designated in advance.

After carefully considering each simulation activity, the nurse educator identifies potential personnel for each station. At the IV simulator station, a full-time faculty or trained adjunct faculty will need to run and demonstrate the IV simulator. The second station with IV therapy can be led by an adjunct clinical faculty member. As the third station involves a high-fidelity manikin, the simulation coordinator will lead the simulation and debriefing due to their advanced knowledge and skill in this area. The NG tube and enteral medication administration station has previously been designated as a self-directed station, but feedback from previous learners has led to this station also being directed by a content expert. This is a simulation activity that could be led by an adjunct clinical faculty or graduate learner.

*(continued)*

In order to have enough content experts to lead each simulation station, the nurse educator needs to recruit at least four additional members to the simulation team. The simulation coordinator is the first person recruited to run the high-fidelity simulation. Three clinical faculty will also be used.

- The first is an adjunct clinical faculty member who has worked in this adult health course for several years and has participated in multiple simulation exercises; as their expertise is IV therapy, they have been asked to lead this station.
- The second clinical faculty is actually a full-time faculty member with experience on the IV simulator, so they were asked to lead this particular station.
- The final clinical faculty member is new to this adult health course and simulation. Because their clinical experience is in acute care surgical nursing, they are very comfortable with NG tubes and have agreed to lead this station.

As the course coordinator, the nurse educator is also in the simulation laboratory with the learners to troubleshoot any problems that may occur.

In order to orient the team members to the simulation activities, the nurse educator sends out, in advance, an agenda with the day's schedule of activities. The learning objectives/outcomes are shared, and the simulation activities at each station are listed in detail. The goal of the simulation experience and the course coordinator's expectations for the day are made clear to all members. To accommodate everyone's schedule, training is held 1 hour prior to the learners' arrival. As three of the team members have participated in this simulation day previously, only a brief review is necessary. More time is spent with the new adjunct clinical faculty to familiarize them with the equipment and the learning objectives/outcomes for the station they are assigned. Because the new adjunct clinical faculty is an experienced nurse, they have no difficulty grasping the activities of this station.

Using the university's online learning platform, the nurse educator created a folder within the course's site with information pertaining to simulation day activities. Learners were also encouraged to visit the simulation site to meet their simulated patient and review their medical-surgical history. This provides learners with additional information about the high-fidelity simulation activity in an attempt to reduce anxiety and fear of the unknown.

As the simulation laboratory is in use at least 3 days a week, the nurse educator and the simulation coordinator prepare the simulation rooms the Friday before simulation activities are scheduled to begin for the adult health course. Handouts are prepared and copied for use at some stations. All equipment and supplies are laid out and organized; computerized simulators are calibrated as necessary. A final walk-through of the stations is conducted early Monday morning before the learners arrive. Because these four simulation activities have been used previously with success, no prior run-through was needed.

1. A novice educator is developing goals and objectives/outcomes for a planned simulation. Identify which statement is an example of a well-written objective.

   A. At the completion of the simulation, learners will understand the importance of good technique

   B. Following the simulation, learners will identify important concepts related to IV therapy

   C. Upon completion of the simulation, learners will appreciate the skill required to insert IV catheters

   D. After the simulation, learners will demonstrate the correct steps for IV insertion

2. A simulation educator is planning to use formative evaluation during a simulation exercise. Which statement indicates that additional knowledge of the types of evaluation is needed?

   A. "I plan to use a form to provide learners with feedback about their performance."

   B. "I will develop a rubric for faculty use in grading the learners' performance."

   C. "I will meet with learners individually to discuss any areas needing improvement."

   D. "I want to provide adequate time and opportunity for the learners to self-reflect."

3. A course coordinator is discussing debriefing with the clinical adjunct faculty. Which statement demonstrates that the educator has a clear understanding of debriefing?

   A. "Debriefing is a great method to use when teaching students using task trainers."

   B. "Incorporating debriefing is the best way for students to acquire short-term learning."

   C. "During the debriefing process, students have the opportunity to assess their performance."

   D. "Debriefing can be used as a graded evaluation of student learning."

4. Feedback is an important part of the evaluative process. Identify which one statement is MOST important in providing learners with effective, useful feedback.

   A. Standards or criteria should be developed so that the faculty are consistent in their grading

   B. Feedback should only be provided by the course or simulation coordinator

   C. Only positive feedback should be shared if the observer misses part of the simulation

   D. An observer can provide feedback even if they lack knowledge of good performance

5. A simulation educator is planning to use an objective structured clinical examination (OSCE) to evaluate learners at the conclusion of their Adult Health II course. Which statement is the MOST accurate description of an OSCE?

   A. OSCEs have only been found to be a reliable evaluation tool in medical education

   B. An OSCE is a valid assessment tool for evaluating competencies and judgment

   C. A self-assessment would provide a more valid method of evaluation than an OSCE

   D. A newly created checklist would have higher validity than an often-repeated OSCE

## 1. D) After the simulation, learners will demonstrate the correct steps for IV insertion

This objective precisely states a concrete, short-term behavior that the learner is expected to accomplish following the simulation. The verb that is used is specific, with little room for variance in interpretation. This objective is also written using the ABCD rule, which includes the audience, behavior, condition, and degree. The objective is measurable. *Understanding* is difficult to measure, *identify* is a low-level verb on Bloom's taxonomy, and *appreciate* is also difficult to measure.

## 2. B) "I will develop a rubric for faculty use in grading the learners' performance."

During formative evaluation, simulation educators provide feedback in order to facilitate learning and identify areas that need further reinforcement and/or improvement. Although formative evaluation can be graded, this is more often associated with summative evaluation. A form can be used, learners should be provided time to reflect, and students should be provided individual feedback for formative evaluations.

## 3. C) "During the debriefing process, students have the opportunity to assess their performance."

During debriefing, students have the opportunity to process what they have learned and to use feedback provided by the faculty and peers to reinforce their learning and identify areas for improvement and growth. Debriefing should be used for all simulation modalities used for learning and should add to students' long-term memory. Debriefing is not a grading process.

## 4. A) Standards or criteria should be developed so that the faculty are consistent in their grading

It is important that the person observing and providing feedback has expertise in the content and knowledge of what constitutes a good performance. Standards or criteria help ensure that all observers are consistent with their feedback; rubrics are often helpful in this regard. Feedback can be given by others such as simulated participants and feedback does not always have to be positive. Observers need to understand what competency standard is expected.

## 5. B) An OSCE is a valid assessment tool for evaluating competencies and judgment

OSCEs have been used for years as an evaluation tool in medical education, but they have also been found valid in the evaluation of skills and competencies of other health professional students. In choosing a tool for evaluation, it is important to consider the validity and reliability of the assessment. OSCEs can be used in many healthcare disciplines, self-assessment is a different type of evaluation, and a newly created checklist would need to be tested for validity and reliability.

6. A first-year faculty member is going to incorporate simulation into their adult health course for the first time. Which statement indicates that they have a clear understanding of the planning and organization of the simulation experience?

   A. "The simulation should last as long as the learners would have been in the clinical setting."
   B. "To minimize faculty time involvement, each simulation can include up to 12 learners."
   C. "Learners will have the opportunity for hands-on practice with skills during the simulation."
   D. "A scenario including a pediatric patient with asthma would be a great learning opportunity."

7. The simulation coordinator and the course faculty for the psychiatric mental health course are discussing the best way for learners to practice communication skills. Which modality would BEST assist learners in attaining this skill set?

   A. Low fidelity with a standardized patient
   B. High fidelity with a manikin
   C. Mixed fidelity with a manikin
   D. Low fidelity with a task trainer

8. A simulation educator is planning to use high-fidelity simulation for learners to utilize clinical judgment in a scenario in which the patient is rapidly deteriorating. Identify the one action that will BEST ensure that the simulation runs smoothly and effectively.

   A. List the equipment that will be needed for the simulation
   B. Identify additional content experts that can be used for future simulations
   C. Book simulation space at least 6 months in advance
   D. Schedule a trial run with key personnel in advance of the simulation

9. A team of faculty are planning a large simulation involving multiple standardized patients. Which statement indicates that the faculty need further guidance in their plans?

   A. "We need to consider budget funds available for paying professional actors."
   B. "We could work with faculty from theater to involve their students as standardized patients."
   C. "If our standardized patients don't show up, we can use any students or faculty available."
   D. "Alumni could be asked to volunteer as standardized patients."

10. While discussing prebriefing with their mentor, which statement by the new faculty member indicates that further information is needed?

   A. "During prebriefing, I plan to review information relevant to the simulation scenario."
   B. "Learners will have the opportunity to familiarize themselves with the laboratory during prebriefing."
   C. "I will orient the learners to the capabilities of the manikin during the prebriefing."
   D. "The learners will be able to complete all their prep work during prebriefing."

**6. C) "Learners will have the opportunity for hands-on practice with skills during the simulation."**
Students are able to practice skills/competencies and interact with the faculty to achieve the learning outcomes of the simulation and course. Simulation learning is not necessarily the same time commitment as direct clinical experiences because it is more intense. The number of learners depends on the scenario and the course objectives and can fluctuate. It is an adult health course, so a pediatric experience would not fulfill the student learning outcomes.

**7. A) Low fidelity with a standardized patient**
Standardized patients are effective in the practice and acquisition of nontechnical skills, such as communication, therapeutic use of self, and patient advocacy. High-fidelity manikins, mixed or hybrid simulation, and low-fidelity part-task trainers do not afford the interpersonal communication needed.

**8. D) Schedule a trial run with key personnel in advance of the simulation**
Scheduling a trial run is most important so that any barriers can be corrected before it is a learning situation. A trial run is necessary to ensure that key personnel have a shared understanding of the simulation, while providing an opportunity to identify potential problems. Planning in advance, including the resources, location, equipment, and availability of a content expert, is important to ensure the success of any simulation.

**9. C) "If our standardized patients don't show up, we can use any students or faculty available."**
Standardized patients are oriented to the simulation scenario. Putting others in the role may not yield the same results and may not be as effective. Paying professional actors to perform as standardized patients can be costly, so other alternatives such as alumni, drama students, and other healthcare students should be considered.

**10. D) "The learners will be able to complete all their prep work during prebriefing."**
Preparatory work should occur before students arrive for the simulation exercise. Prebriefing is a time to orient students to the simulation environment and equipment, discuss information relevant to the scenario, and answer any questions.

# ● REFERENCES

Abelsson, A., & Bisholt, B. (2017). Nurse students learn acute care by simulation—focus on observation and debriefing. *Nurse Education in Practice, 24*, 6–13. https://doi.org/10.1016/j.nepr.2017.03.001

Allen, L., & Molloy, E. (2017). The influence of a preceptor-student "daily feedback tool" on clinical feedback practices in nursing education: A qualitative study. *Nurse Education Today, 49*, 57–62. https://doi.org/10.1016/j.nedt.2016.11.009

Andrews, I. (2021). Prebriefing as a tool to building cultural competence during a study away program. *Journal of Cultural Diversity, 28*(1), 20–29.

Arrogante, O., Gonzalez-Romero, G. M., Lopez-Torre, E. M., Carrion-Garcia, L., & Polo, A. (2021). Comparing formative and summative simulation-based assessment in undergraduate nursing students: Nursing competency acquisition and clinical simulation satisfaction. *BioMed Central Nursing, 20*(1), 92. https://doi.org/10.1186/s12912-021-00614-2

Bailey, C. (2017). Human patient simulation. In M. J. Bradshaw & B. L. Hultquist (Eds.), *Innovative teaching strategies in nursing and related health professions* (pp. 245–267). Jones & Bartlett Learning.

Bastable, S. B. (2019). *Nurse as educator: Principles of teaching and learning for nursing practice* (5th ed.). Jones & Bartlett Learning.

Billings, D. M., & Halstead, J. A. (2020). *Teaching in nursing: A guide for faculty* (6th ed.). Elsevier.

Bjerrum, F., Thomsen, A. S. S., Nayahangan, L. J., & Konge, L. (2018). Surgical simulation: Current practices and future perspectives for technical skills training. *Medical Teacher, 40*(7), 668–675. https://doi.org/10.1080/0142159X.2018.1472754

Grant, V. J., Robinson, T., Catena, H., Eppich, W., & Cheng, A. (2018). Difficult debriefing situations: A toolbox for simulation educators. *Medical Teacher, 40*(7), 703–712. https://doi.org/10.1080/0142159X.2018.1468558

Melling, M., Duranai, M., Pellow, B., Lam, B., Kim, Y., Beavers, L., Miller, E., & Switzer-McIntyre, S. (2018). Simulation experiences in Canadian physiotherapy programmes: A description of current practices. *Physiotherapy Canada, 70*(3), 262–271. https://doi.org/10.3138/ptc.2017-11.e

Sargeant, J., Wong, B. M., & Campbell, C. M. (2018). CPD of the future: A partnership between quality improvement and competency-based education. *Medical Education, 52*, 125–135. http://doi.org/10.1111/medu.13407

Society for Simulation in Healthcare. (2021). *Certified healthcare simulation educator handbook.* https://www.ssih.org/Portals/48/Certification/CHSE_Docs/CHSE%20Handbook.pdf

Solli, H., Haukedal, T. A., Husebo, S. E., & Reierson, I. A. (2020). The art of balancing: The facilitator's role in briefing in simulation-based learning from the perspective of nursing students—a qualitative study. *BioMed Central Nursing, 19*(1), 99. https://doi.org/10.1186/s12912-020-00493-z

Tseng, L. P., Hou, T. H., Huang, L. P., & Ou, Y. K. (2021). Effectiveness of applying clinical simulation scenarios and integrating information technology in medical-surgical nursing and critical nursing courses. *BioMed Central Nursing, 20*(1), 229. https://doi.org/10.1186/s12912-021-00744-7

Wittmann-Price, R. A., & Gittings, K. K. (2021). *Fast facts about competency-based education in nursing.* Springer Publishing Company.

Wittmann-Price, R. A., Godshall, M., & Wilson, L. (Eds.). (2022). *Certified nurse educator (CNE) review manual* (4th ed.). Springer Publishing Company.

Wooding, E. L., Gale, T. C., & Maynard, V. (2020). Evaluation of teamwork assessment tools for interprofessional simulation: A systematic literature review. *Journal of Interprofessional Care, 34*(2), 162–172. https://doi.org/10.1080/13561820.2019.1650730

# Debriefing

Linda Wilson, John T. Cornele, and Kate Morse

*I think the big thing is don't be afraid to fail. It's a part of building character and growing.*
*—Nick Foles*

This chapter addresses Domain III: Educational Principles Applied to Simulation (Society for Simulation in Healthcare [SSH], 2021).

## ▶ LEARNING OUTCOMES

- Discuss the importance of simulation debriefing in the learning process.
- Discuss the principles of simulation debriefing.
- Describe a variety of simulation debriefing methodologies.

## ▶ INTRODUCTION

When using simulation as a learning tool, debriefing is an essential component of the learning process (Cantrell, 2008). Most simulation experts concur that the debriefing process of learners, which takes place after the simulation experience, is in effect the most important element of the learners' experience. Cant and Cooper (2009) describe debriefing as one of the "core components" of simulation learning. Alinier (2011) describes debriefing by stating that "[e]xperiential learning experience must then be reinforced and analyzed with the participants through a debriefing process that is as, if not more, important than the experience itself as it helps them to reflect about what happened and understand and assimilate the learning objectives" (p. 14). The ultimate goal of the learning process that takes place during debriefing is to foster clinical decision-making (Dreifuerst, 2009).

Dewey (1933, p. 9) suggests that reflection is a process and requires a process; he describes reflection as "active, persistent, and careful consideration." Furthermore, Dewey believed that reflection could be caused by "a state of doubt, hesitation, [or] perplexity" (p. 12). This active approach to reflection requires that the learner recognizes actions or events and enters a state of questioning of held beliefs and learned behaviors to identify issues and begin to problem solve.

## ▶ BACKGROUND

Debriefing was originally used in the military in order for personnel to describe what happened during a mission. Debriefing accomplished two objectives for the military. First, it assisted with operational understanding and strategic planning, and second it helped reduce the psychological impact of a traumatic event on the participant. Reconstructing the event through narrative was therapeutic for the participant. By conducting debriefing in groups, participants received several different perspectives (Fanning & Gaba, 2007).

# ▶ THE DEBRIEFING PROCESS

Learning in the simulation environment often requires learners to take risks, make mistakes, and admit lack of or faulty knowledge. To support this vulnerability, simulation educators must consider psychological safety in case design, prebriefing, and debriefing. *Psychological safety* can be defined as a learning space where the learners feel comfortable taking interpersonal risks, admitting error, discussing mistakes, sharing their thinking, and valuing diverse points of view (Edmonson et al., 2016; Rudolph et al., 2014). The idea of creating a safe and trusted learning space—psychological safety in learning—has been described in a concept analysis (Turner & Harder, 2018). The authors describe the three defining attributes of psychological safety as the ability of the learners to make mistakes without consequences, the qualities of the educator influencing the creation and maintenance of psychological safety, and the inclusion of activities such as orientation, preparation, objectives, and expectations. Daniels et al. (2021), in a narrative literature, highlighted critical faculty behaviors that positively influenced undergraduate nursing learners' perceptions of psychological safety to include role clarification, explaining the learning objectives, outlining the fiction contract, orienting learners to the environment, and offering opportunities to ask questions. The positive impacts on learners included less anxiety, increased student motivation and engagement, and trust in the teacher–learner relationship.

The simulation educator who is facilitating the learning process has a pivotal role in creating (prebriefing) and maintaining (debriefing) psychological safety throughout the learning process. As we aspire for transformative learning in simulation-based education (SBE), psychological safety is a critical element for learners who are engaging in critical self-reflection. The learner, along with facilitation from the simulation educator, creates new ways of thinking leading to perspective transformation (Meizrow, 2003).

Learning is facilitated during the debriefing process of simulation (Dieckmann et al., 2010). Debriefing is a process that commonly involves face-to-face discussion between a group of learners and an educator after a simulation scenario has taken place (International Nursing Association for Clinical Simulation and Learning [INACSL] Standards Committee et al., 2021). Debriefing is often distinguished as a separate process from feedback, which can occur using different modalities (face-to-face, written, or electronic) and normally occurs between one learner and an educator after a simulation experience (Archer, 2010). When standardized patients (SPs) are used in simulation experiences, they are often included in the feedback process to provide insights to the learner, but they are not usually participants in the debriefing process (Barrows, 1993).

The debriefing process is normally facilitated retrospectively with the simulation participants as soon as possible after the experience is completed (Cantrell, 2008) and includes all the learners actively involved in the entire experience (Alinier, 2011). Timing of the debriefing process is important, and it is beneficial to provide debriefing as close to the simulation experience as possible (Cantrell, 2008).

Some simulation experts refer to the process of debriefing as *team debriefing*, which highlights the aspect that it is a group activity (Alinier, 2011). Debriefing should be facilitated by a certified educator who has observed the entire simulation learning experience and has taken physical or mental notes about the details of the experience (Alinier, 2011). Recording of the simulation experience is important to the debriefing process and can also effectively include videotaping of the experience. Videotaping may assist learners in analyzing their performance and provide structure to the debriefing process. At times, depending on the complexity of the scenario, learning is facilitated by having a second certified educator observing the simulation scenario and participating in the debriefing process in order to note all the details of the simulation experience (Alinier, 2011).

Debriefing sessions are often approximately 20 to 30 minutes in length, and researchers have noted that 10-minute debriefing sessions are inadequate to facilitate the learning process (Cantrell, 2008). Therefore, as a critical component of simulation learning, adequate time must be assigned to the debriefing process.

Another type of debriefing is called *in-simulation* debriefing. This debriefing technique is done by suspending the scenario to discuss a specific incident or aspect of learning (Van Heukelom et al., 2010). The learners should be informed that this method is being used prior to the start of the scenario so that they are ready and accepting of the interruptions caused by the process.

### Evidence-Based Simulation Practice 17.1

Matthews and Viens (1988) found that videotaping a simulation experience and having learners critically critique the experience during debriefing decreased learner anxiety.

Lederman (1984) describes the following seven components as the essential, structural elements of debriefing:

- debriefer, or simulation educator
- participants, or learners to debrief
- the simulation experience
- the impact of the simulation experience
- recollection of the simulation experience
- report about the simulation experience
- time required for debriefing (Lederman, 1984)

## ▶ DEBRIEFING AND THE LEARNING PROCESS

Using simulation experiences provides learners an opportunity to practice and acquire knowledge and clinical skills in a safe environment (McGaghie et al., 2010). Much of the knowledge acquisition is facilitated during the debriefing process because it is a teaching strategy (Cantrell, 2008).

Debriefing as a teaching strategy supports a constructivist theory of education, which is fully explained in Chapter 13, "Virtual Reality," and Chapter 14, "Educational Theories, Learning Theories, and Special Concepts." Some of the learning processes that take place during debriefing include the following:

- promoting communication skills
- appropriately integrating emotions into the learning process
- reinforcing skill acquisition (Cantrell, 2008)

Debriefing is a learning process that ties in all three domains of learning:

- *Psychomotor*: During debriefing, skills are analyzed.
- *Affective*: Feelings and emotions are discussed.
- *Cognitive*: Learning takes place by having the events deconstructed (Cantrell, 2008).

Warrick et al. (1979) defined the objectives of debriefing as:

- identification of the different perceptions and attitudes that have occurred
- linking the exercise to specific theory or content and skill-building techniques
- development of a common set of experiences for further thought
- opportunity to receive feedback on the nature of one's involvement, behavior, and decision-making
- reestablishment of the desired classroom climate, such as regaining trust, comfort, and purposefulness

## ▶ DEFINING ATTRIBUTES OF DEBRIEFING

Dreifuerst (2009) described the following defining attributes of debriefing in a concept analysis:

- reflection
- emotions
- reception
- integration
- assimilation

Each attribute is described in the following text.

### REFLECTION

An important aspect of the debriefing process as pointed out by Dieckmann et al. (2007) is that no one has the "correct view." Debriefing comprises perceptions of the educators and the learners of what took place in the simulation experience. Different views assist learners with understanding different elements of the scenario, and in this way it mimics clinical situations. Debriefing discussions should begin with asking participants about their view of the situation just experienced and initiate the reflective learning process (Dieckmann et al., 2007).

Fanning and Gaba (2007) call reflection "the cornerstone" of both experiential learning and lifelong learning. The following text lists the different ways to conceptualize reflection and some important points about using reflection as a learning activity.

- In 1983, Schön published his landmark book, *The Reflective Practitioner: How Professionals Think in Action*, and called on educators to develop themselves as reflective practitioners in order to gain competence in their individual practices.
- Boud et al. (1985) defined *reflection* as "an important human activity in which people recapture their experience, think about it, mull it over, and evaluate it" (p. 19).
- Reflection is a technique that encourages critical thought, either with oneself (self-dialogue) or another individual or group (dialogue; Shor, 1992).
- Reflection is a thoughtful and self-regulating process (Kaakinen & Arwood, 2009).

Reflection can be facilitated in different ways.

- Many certified healthcare educators use the technique after an experience in a free-flow attempt to assist learners in uncovering what affective behaviors they can identify as assets and highlight those behaviors that may be deficits.

## Simulation Teaching Tip 17.1

Several issues must be considered when asking learners to reflect.

■ Reflection is a self-disclosing process that can elicit sensitive information.
■ What one does with information revealed during reflective sessions may become an ethical issue.

■ Others pose reflective questions to learners, such as "What was the one thing (incident or patient) that affected you most?" or "What was the best thing that happened to you during the experience?"
■ Usually, questions like these are followed up with questions such as "What one thing would you do differently if you were in that situation again?"

Having learners reflect facilitates finding deeper meanings and thinking critically about experiences, especially critical incidents (Montagna et al., 2010).

Scanlon and Chernomas (1997) identified three stages of reflection:
1. awareness
2. critical analysis
3. new perspective

Riley-Doucet and Wilson (1997) describe a three-step process for reflection:
1. *Critical appraisal* is done by a learner in free form to drill down to the meaning of the experience.
2. *Peer group discussions* share questions that the learners might have become aware of during the experience.
3. *Self-awareness* or *self-evaluation* is the last step and relates the learning outcomes for evaluative purposes.

Montagna et al. (2010) also recommend that the educator's feedback to learners be done with care and that certain resources are available if needed.

## EMOTIONS

Debriefing provides the learner the opportunity to reexamine the experience and deal with emotions, thereby providing an emotional release as well as a thinking process (Dreifuerst, 2009).

## RECEPTION

Reception has to do with how "open" the learner is to accepting the information provided or revealed during debriefing. The simulation educator needs to establish an environment that facilitates positive reception by:

■ presenting learners' strengths and challenges in a nonthreatening manner
■ maintaining learner–facilitator respect at all times
■ providing confidentiality as appropriate (Dreifuerst, 2009)

## INTEGRATION

Using a conceptual framework that is familiar to the learners in their discipline and integrating the context of the simulation scenario fosters learning. Integration links knowledge gained from the simulation experience to knowledge already familiar from the learning. By facilitating integration, the simulation educator is promoting deep learning (Dreifuerst, 2009). Refer to Chapter 14, "Educational Theories, Learning Theories, and Special Concepts," for an explanation of deep, surface, and strategic learning.

## ASSIMILATION

Assimilation has to do with the ultimate goal of simulation, which is the transfer of knowledge from the experience to actual clinical practice. Further assimilation studies are needed, but assimilation may be encouraged by techniques used by the facilitator, such as the Socratic dialogue. Dreifuerst (2009) reminds simulation educators that all attributes defined as elements of debriefing work together to promote learning, as shown in Figure 17.1.

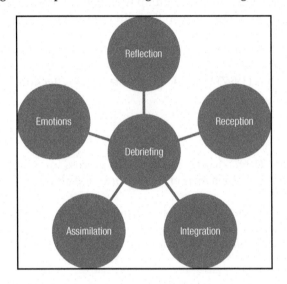

**Figure 17.1** Attributes of learning in debriefing as defined by Dreifuerst (2009).

*Source:* Data from Dreifuerst, K. T. (2009). The essentials of debriefing in simulated learning: A concept analysis. *Nursing Education Perspectives, 30*(2), 109–114.

## ▶ ORAL (SOCRATIC) QUESTIONING

Oral questioning, or Socratic dialogue, can promote learners' critical thinking and prompt them to reflect. Questions that involve synthesizing concepts rather than questions that can be answered with a "yes" or "no" or regurgitating facts are the most beneficial (Exhibit 17.1). Promoting thinking through questioning can be accomplished by using "what-if" questions and changing the situation to encourage learners to think beyond the experience (Dreifuerst, 2009).

---

**EXHIBIT 17.1 BENEFITS OF QUESTIONING**

- Increases motivation and participation
- Helps monitor learners' acquisition of knowledge and understanding
- Promotes higher cognition
- Assesses learners' progress
- Facilitates environmental management
- Encourages learners to ask and to answer questions
- Promotes dialogue/interaction/debate between and among educators and learners (Ralph, 2000)

## ▶ DEBRIEFING AS AN ASSESSMENT PROCESS

Debriefing, which usually involves a group of learners, is most often used as a formative evaluative mechanism. Summative evaluations of learners' performance are most commonly done on an individual basis using feedback (McGaghie et al., 2010). A method of using debriefing as an evaluation has been outlined by Rudolph et al. (2008), which is a four-step process and is shown diagrammatically in Figure 17.2.

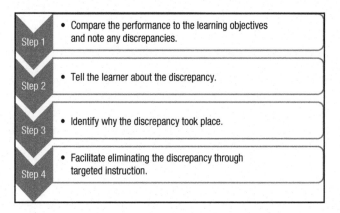

**Figure 17.2** The four-step evaluation process by Rudolph et al.

*Source:* Adapted from Rudolph, J. W., Simon, R., Raemer, D. B., & Eppich, W. J. (2008). Debriefing as formative assessment: Closing performance gaps in medical education. *Academic Emergency Medicine, 15*, 1010–1016. https://doi.org/10.1111/j.1553-2712.2008.00248.x

## ▶ FACILITATOR ROLE IN THE DEBRIEFING PROCESS

Fanning and Gaba (2007) described facilitator involvement in debriefing as high to low. Table 17.1 demonstrates the differences in involvement.

**Table 17.1** Involvement of Facilitators in Debriefing

| High-level facilitation | ■ The facilitator outlines the debriefing process.<br>■ The facilitator guides the discussion when necessary.<br>■ The facilitator has low-level involvement.<br>■ Learners are highly involved. |
|---|---|
| Low-level facilitation | ■ Facilitators take on an involved role.<br>■ Learners are less involved and have less initiative.<br>■ Facilitators use a direct debriefing process.<br>■ Simulation educators may overinstruct. |

*Source:* Fanning, R. M., & Gaba, D. M. (2007). The role of debriefing in simulation-based learning. *Simulation in Healthcare, 2*(2), 115–125. https://doi.org/10.1097/SIH.0b013e3180315539

# ▶ TYPES OF DEBRIEFING METHODS

## STRUCTURED DEBRIEFING

Debriefing sessions often begin with establishing group rules in order to focus the learners on the meaning of the scenario rather than have them focus on the fidelity of the scenario (Dieckmann et al., 2007). Cantrell (2008) used a structured debriefing process in her study with nursing learners and used guiding questions that were developed by Ham and O'Rouke (2004):

- What were the patient's goals for this episode of care?
- Were these goals met by your nursing behaviors?
- How did you prioritize the patient's needs?
- What would you do differently if actually caring for the patient and the family in an acute care setting?

Structured debriefing provides guidance in the learning process, facilitates the collection of data, and provides insight into the learners' thinking processes.

### Evidence-Based Simulation Practice 17.2

Birch et al. (2007) used debriefing in the simulation education of learners using a scenario about postpartum hemorrhage. The study found that learners who participated in the simulation experience and were debriefed had increased knowledge immediately after the scenario and at 3 months after the scenario.

## CASE STUDY ANALYSIS DEBRIEFING

One of the most common methods of debriefing is review of a case study. One method to accomplish this has been outlined in 12 steps by Salas et al. (2008):

1. Use debriefing to diagnose the case.
2. Provide a supportive environment.
3. Always note teamwork, which is critical to patient safety.
4. Team leaders should be educated in debriefing.
5. Members should not be threatened during a debriefing session.
6. Focus on critical incidents during the scenario.
7. Describe the interactions of the team.
8. Use objective data when possible.
9. Provide process feedback before outcome feedback.
10. Provide both individual and team feedback appropriately.
11. Provide feedback as soon as possible.
12. Record outcomes of the debriefing to use in the future.

## DEBRIEFING WITH GOOD JUDGMENT

A nonjudgmental approach to debriefing uses the simulation educator as a patient advocate by asking questions using "I" and referring to the patient (advocacy). The simulation educator then requests the learner to describe the thought process used, and this is the inquiry process (Rudolph et al., 2007). There are three phases in this method of debriefing: (a) reaction phase, (b) understanding phase, and (c) summary phase (Rudolph et al., 2007; Sawyer et al., 2016). An example is provided in Exhibit 17.2.

> ## EXHIBIT 17.2 AN EXAMPLE OF AN ADVOCACY-INQUIRY QUESTION
>
> **Dirty Question** (a question that—when asked—puts the learner on the defense): Why did you not verify the patient identification (ID) prior to giving that med?
>
> **Advocacy-Inquiry Question:** I noticed that you did not check the patient identification prior to giving the medication. That concerns me because verifying the correct patient is an important part of medication administration. Can you tell me what you were thinking at that time?
>
> By using the advocacy-inquiry technique for questions, there is no "guess what I am thinking." We need to understand the thinking behind actions in order to change them.
>
> *Source:* Adapted from Rudolph, J. W., Simon, R., Rivard, P., Dufresne, R. L., & Raemer, D. B. (2007). Debriefing with good judgment: Combining rigorous feedback with genuine inquiry. *Anesthesiology Clinics, 25,* 361–376. https://doi.org/10.1016/j.anclin.2007.03.007

## DEBRIEFING FOR MEANINGFUL LEARNING

This method of debriefing focuses on the following: (a) fostering students' reflective thinking and learning; (b) Socratic questioning; (c) the principles of active learning; and (d) the E5 model: engage, explore, explain, evaluate, and extend (or elaborate; Dreifuerst, 2015).

## PROMOTING EXCELLENCE AND REFLECTIVE LEARNING IN SIMULATION

Promoting Excellence and Reflective Learning in Simulation (PEARLS) is a blended approach to debriefing that includes (a) learners' self-assessment, (b) facilitating focused discussion, and (c) providing information via directive feedback and/or teaching. This method of debriefing has four phases: (a) reaction phase, (b) description phase, (c) analysis phase, and (d) summary phase (Eppich & Cheng, 2015; Sawyer et al., 2019). In 2019, Dube et al. published a modified PEARLS for systems integration (PSI; Dube et al., 2019).

## 3D MODEL OF DEBRIEFING

This method of debriefing begins with a prebrief. The debriefing then focuses on the aspects of defusing, discovering, and deepening where the learners will (a) reflect on the experience, (b) identify mental models that led to the specific behavior or cognitive process, and (c) build or enhance new mental models (Sawyer et al., 2019; Zigmont et al., 2011). The debriefing will end with a summary (Zigmont et al., 2011).

## PLUS DELTA DEBRIEFING

This method of debriefing focuses on what was accomplished or done well. To facilitate this debriefing, the simulation educator will use a two-column tool to have the group identify (a) what went well and (b) what can be changed next time (Gardner, 2013). This method of debriefing fosters a method of continuous improvement (Gardner, 2013).

## HOW DO YOU CHOOSE THE BEST METHOD OF DEBRIEFING FOR YOU?

To decide which method of debriefing is best for you, review all of the debriefing methods and compare them with your educational philosophy. You can also test various debriefing methods over time and evaluate them. Or possibly, your institution has selected a debriefing method that everyone is supposed to use so debriefing is done in a consistent manner.

There are many techniques used during the debriefing process. Table 17.2 describes some of these techniques.

**Table 17.2 Debriefing Techniques**

| Technique | Description of the Technique |
|---|---|
| Funneling | Learners are guided during debriefing, but the debriefer does not comment (Fanning & Gaba, 2007). |
| Framing | This is a technique used during debriefing to present the simulation experience to the participants in a relevant way (Fanning & Gaba, 2007). |
| Front-loading | This refers to providing specific questions before the debriefing to guide the direction of the debriefing (Fanning & Gaba, 2007). |
| Good cop–bad cop | This technique is used if there is more than one debriefer. This technique provides opposing sides to an issue (Fanning & Gaba, 2007). |
| Case review | This is an organized review of the patient's condition, starting with the diagnosis and then a review of systems. |

*Source:* Adapted from Fanning, R. M., & Gaba, D. M. (2007). The role of debriefing in simulation-based learning. *Simulation in Healthcare, 2*(2), 115–125. https://doi.org/10.1097/SIH.0b013e3180315539

## ▶ THE DEBRIEFING ENVIRONMENT

The environment where debriefing is conducted is also important. Besides having an appropriate amount of time set aside for debriefing, there should be enough room for the members being debriefed. Rooms for debriefing should be large, private, and comfortable. Large groups of learners pose special challenges to debriefing. The following are two methods used to overcome group learning that may exclude individuals:

### Simulation Teaching Tip 17.2

Dieckmann et al. (2007) discussed the importance of simulation educators paying attention to the semantical sense that learners develop during the analysis of a scenario during debriefing. The use of words and language in descriptions of the scenario can provide insight into how learners phenomenally experienced the scenario.

- *Separate groups:* Have more than one debriefer and separate the large group into smaller groups.
- *Use the fishbowl method:* Have an inner circle of learners and an outer circle. Debrief the learners in the inner circle and then have the learners switch to the outer circle and the outer circle learners move in for debriefing (Fanning & Gaba, 2007).

### Simulation Teaching Tip 17.3

Steinwachs (1992) described using a process of seating that avoids "energy gaps." In order to facilitate this concept, learners must sit next to each other and there should be no empty spaces. Decker (2007) suggested a circular design for seating that allows spherical movement while questioning the learners as discussion is promoted.

An additional consideration for establishing an environment that feels safe for debriefing is a space away from where the simulation was conducted, a comfortable and private area (Decker, 2007).

## ▶ DEBRIEFING DIFFICULTIES

Debriefing sessions are goal-oriented, but at times difficulties can occur when learners interpret debriefings differently than what was intended in the learning outcomes. In this case, extra time is often needed to explain what was supposed to occur as opposed to what did occur. Many simulation educators then reenact the scenario to accomplish the intended learning outcomes (Dieckmann et al., 2010).

 ## CASE STUDY 17.1

An undergraduate student wrote an email to their advisor stating the following:

During simulation laboratory learning today I was assigned a very complex patient and I was not prepared for the complexity. I did the best that I could, but the simulation faculty stopped the learning experience and brought my entire group into the debriefing session. We discussed all the things that went wrong, and I felt belittled and unsupported.

The simulation faculty's perspective was the following:

Students were provided a prebrief and a case study outlining the patient's condition 2 days before the simulation learning experience. It was obvious that the students did not prepare for the experience and the experience had to be stopped because basic competencies were not being met.

As the simulation director, how would you handle this situation?

1. The novice simulation educator needs further instruction when they are facilitating a debriefing by:

   A. Observing the entire simulation
   B. Taking notes on observations during the simulation
   C. Using an experienced debriefer as a consult
   D. Starting debriefing students one at a time

2. A simulation educator is very new to the debriefing process. Which method of debriefing might be easier for the educator to start with?

   A. Debriefing with good judgment
   B. Case study debriefing
   C. Debriefing for meaningful learning
   D. Advocacy inquiry

3. Ideally, the debriefing time should be:

   A. 5 to 20 minutes long
   B. Half the time needed to complete the simulation
   C. Equal to the time needed to complete the simulation
   D. Double the time needed to complete the simulation

4. The debriefing method in which the simulation educator facilitates the identification of what went well compared with what can be changed next time is called:

   A. Debriefing with good judgment
   B. Case study debriefing
   C. Debriefing for meaningful learning
   D. Plus delta

5. The debriefing method in which the simulation educator focuses on defusing, discovering, and deepening is called:

   A. Plus delta
   B. Debriefing with good judgment
   C. 3D model of debriefing
   D. Debriefing for meaningful learning

6. The simulation educator wants to learn how to be an effective debriefer. The BEST method to use to learn debriefing is to:

   A. Read a book about debriefing
   B. Practice with an experienced debriefer
   C. Watch a video of a debriefing session
   D. Attend a lecture on debriefing

## 1. D) Starting debriefing students one at a time

Debriefing should be completed in a group format and not one student at a time. Simulationists should watch the entire scenario, take notes, or use a consult if needed.

## 2. B) Case study debriefing

Case study debriefing may be less intimidating because healthcare educators are used to using case studies in didactic and clinical education. Debriefing with good judgment, debriefing for meaningful learning, and advocacy inquiry are techniques that are very effective but take professional development and practice.

## 3. D) Double the time needed to complete the simulation

Debriefing is where much of the learning takes place and should not be rushed; it usually takes approximately double the time of the simulation scenario. Trying to debrief in a short amount of time may not allow learners to reflect and synthesize what happened and what could be learned from the situation.

## 4. D) Plus delta

Plus delta is the technique that starts with the things that went well and then moves to process improvement. Case study debriefing discusses aspects of a case in chronological order. Debriefing for meaning learning and debriefing for good judgment are more issue-focused, reflective discussions.

## 5. C) 3D model of debriefing

The 3D model of debriefing uses the techniques of defusing any immediate issues, learners discovering a learning opportunity, and the debriefing coaching learners to understand the meaning of the issue on a deeper level; the other techniques do not provide these elements. Plus delta debriefing approaches learning from starting what was done correctly and then moving to process improvement. Debriefing with good judgment shares critical information without producing defensiveness. Debriefing for meaningful learning focuses on clinical judgment by reflecting on the student's care and the patient's response.

## 6. B) Practice with an experienced debriefer

Practicing with an experienced debriefer is very valuable and provides hands-on experience and valuable feedback. Practicing with an expert may be more effective than a video, book, or lecture.

7. A novice simulationist needs further understanding when they state that the best way to choose a debriefing method is to:

   A. "Review all available methods of debriefing."
   B. "Compare each debriefing method with your personal educational philosophy."
   C. "Test out each type of debriefing method."
   D. "Choose a method that works when time is limited."

8. Which debriefing method includes a technique called *advocacy inquiry*?

   A. Plus delta
   B. Debriefing with good judgment
   C. 3D model of debriefing
   D. Debriefing for meaningful learning

9. The simulation-based educator is beginning the debriefing and the opening statement is "I want to encourage you to share your thinking, this is a time to puzzle through your decisions and actions together." This is an example of which of the following positive educator behaviors?

   A. Orienting learners and building trust
   B. Establishing learner and educator roles
   C. Placing the responsibility of learning on the learners
   D. Placing the responsibility of learning on the simulation educator

10. A new simulation educator is learning the process of case design, prebriefing, and debriefing and is struggling with the concept of psychological safety. The mentor defines psychological safety as which of the following?

   A. A nice learning environment where difficult topics do not get discussed and the educator sidesteps all challenging questions
   B. A learning environment where the instructor sets the stage as being instructor-focused and learners can only ask questions when invited
   C. A learning environment where learners can take interpersonal risks, speak up, ask questions, and discuss mistakes without fear of retribution
   D. A learning environment where learners respect the educator, only speak when spoken to, and with hierarchy maintained

### 7.  D) "Choose a method that works when time is limited."

Debriefing time should not be rushed or limited. Reviewing methods, understanding one's own philosophy, and testing techniques are all important steps to finding a comfortable and effective debriefing method.

### 8.  B) Debriefing with good judgment

Debriefing with good judgment contains the advocacy-inquiry technique. Plus delta, 3D model of debriefing, and debriefing for meaningful learning do not contain the advocacy-inquiry technique.

### 9.  A) Orienting learners and building trust

The simulation-based educator is using an opening statement that orients the learners to how the discussion will be focused and their role (to share their thinking), so it builds trust by laying out the objective. It does not establish educator roles; it does not place the responsibility of learning on the learner or on the educator. Learning is a shared responsibility

### 10.  C) A learning environment where learners can take interpersonal risks, speak up, ask questions, and discuss mistakes without fear of retribution

A team or learning environment where participants can take interpersonal risks, speak up, ask questions, and discuss mistakes is the definition of psychological safety. A psychologically safe learning environment is not instructor-centered, nor is it "nice" where participants cannot tackle hard topics. Behaviors that do not promote psychological safety include demanding respect, not inviting speaking up, and maintaining hierarchy.

# REFERENCES

Alinier, G. (2011). Developing high-fidelity health care simulation scenarios: A guide for educators and professionals. *Simulation and Gaming, 42*(1), 9–26. https://doi.org/10.1177/1046878109355683

Archer, J. C. (2010). State of the science in health professional education: Effective feedback. *Medical Education, 44*, 101–108. https://doi.org/10.1111/j.1365-2923.2009.03546.x

Barrows, H. S. (1993). An overview of the uses of standardized (simulated) patients for teaching and evaluating clinical skills. *Academic Medicine, 68*(6), 443–451. https://doi.org/10.1097/00001888-199306000-00002

Birch, L., Jones, N., Doyle, P. M., Green, P., McLaughlin, A., Champney, C. T., Williams, D., Gibbon, K., & Taylor, K. (2007). Obstetric skills drills: Evaluation of teaching methods. *Nurse Education Today, 27*(8), 915–922. https://doi.org/10.1016/j.nedt.2007.01.006

Boud, D., Keogh, R., & Walker, D. (Eds.). (1985). *Reflection: Turning experience into learning* (pp. 7–8). Routlage.

Cant, R. P., & Cooper, S. J. (2009). Simulation-based learning in nursing education: Systematic review. *Journal of Advanced Nursing, 66*(1), 3–15. https://doi.org/10.1111/j.1365-2648.2009.05240.x

Cantrell, M. A. (2008). The importance of debriefing in clinical simulation. *Clinical Simulation in Nursing, 4*, e19–e23. https://doi.org/10.1016/j.ecns.2008.06.006

Daniels, A., Morse, C., & Breman, R. (2021). Psychological safety in simulation-based prelicensure nursing education: A narrative review. *Nurse Educator, 46*(5), E99–E102. https://doi.org/10.1097/NNE.0000000000001057

Decker, S. (2007). Integrating guided reflection into simulated learning experiences. In P. R. Jeffries (Ed.), *Simulation in nursing education: From conceptualization to evaluation* (pp. 73–85). National League for Nursing.

Dewey, J. (1933). *How we think: A restatement of the relation of reflective thinking to the educative process.* D. C. Health.

Dieckmann, P., Gaba, D., & Marcus, R. (2007). Deepening the theoretical foundations of patient simulation as social practice. *Simulation in Healthcare, 2*(3), 183–193. https://doi.org/10.1097/SIH.0b013e3180f637f5

Dieckmann, P., Lippert, A., Glavin, R., & Rall, M. (2010). When things do not go as expected: Scenario life savers. *Simulation in Healthcare, 5*, 219–225. https://doi.org/10.1097/SIH.0b013e3181e77f74

Dreifuerst, K. T. (2009). The essentials of debriefing in simulated learning: A concept analysis. *Nursing Education Perspectives, 30*(2), 109–114.

Dreifuerst, K. T. (2015). Getting started with debriefing for meaningful learning. *Clinical Simulation in Nursing, 11*(5), 268–275. https://doi.org/10.1016/j.ecns.2015.01.005

Dube, M., Reid, J., Kaba, A., Cheng, A., Eppich, W., Grant, V., & Stone, K. (2019). PEARLS for system integration. *Simulation in Healthcare, 14*, 333–342. https://doi.org/10.1097/SIH.0000000000000381

Edmonson, A. C., Higgins, M., Singer, S., & Weiner, J. (2016). Understanding psychological safety in health care and educational organizations: A comparative perspective. *Research in Human Development, 13*(1), 65–83. https://doi.org/10.1080/15427609.2016.1141280

Eppich, W., & Cheng, A. (2015). Promoting excellence and reflective learning in simulation (PEARLS). *Simulation in Healthcare, 10*(2), 106–115. https://doi.org/10.1097/SIH.0000000000000072

Fanning, R. M., & Gaba, D. M. (2007). The role of debriefing in simulation-based learning. *Simulation in Healthcare, 2*(2), 115–125. https://doi.org/10.1097/SIH.0b013e3180315539

Gardner, R. (2013). Introduction to debriefing. *Seminars in Perinatology, 37*(3), 166–174. https://doi.org/10.1053/j.semperi.2013.02.008

Ham, K., & O'Rourke, E. (2004). Clinical strategies. Clinical preparation for beginning nursing students: An experiential learning activity. *Nurse Educator, 29*(4), 139–141. https://doi.org/10.1097/00006223-200407000-00006

International Nursing Association for Clinical Simulation and Learning Standards Committee, Watts, P., McDermott, D., Alinier, G., Charnetski, M., Ludlow, J., Horsley, E., Meakim, C., & Nawathe, P. (2021). Healthcare simulation standards of best practice simulation design. *Clinical Simulation in Nursing, 58*, 14–21. https://doi.org/10.1016/j.ecns.2021.08.009

Kaakinen, J., & Arwood, E. (2009). Systematic review of nursing simulation literature for use of learning theory. *International Journal of Nursing Education Scholarship*, 6(1), 1–20. https://doi.org/10.2202/1548-923X.1688

Lederman, L. (1984). Debriefing: A critical reexamination of the post experience analytic process with implications for its effective use. *Simulation Games*, 15, 415–431. https://doi.org/10.1177/0037550084154002

Matthews, R., & Viens, D. C. (1988). Evaluating basic nursing skills through group video testing. *Journal of Nursing Education*, 27(1), 44–46. https://doi.org/10.3928/0148-4834-19880101-11

McGaghie, W. C., Issenberg, S. B., Petrusa, E. R., & Scalese, R. J. (2010). A critical review of simulation-based medical education research: 2003–2009. *Medical Education*, 44, 50–63. https://doi.org/10.1111/j.1365-2923.2009.03547.x

Meizrow, J. (2003). Transformative learning as discourse. *Journal of Transformative Education*, 1(1), 58–63. https://doi.org/10.1177/1541344603252172

Montagna, L., Benaglio, C., & Zannini, L. (2010). Reflective writing in nursing education: Background, experiences and methods. *Assistenza Infermieristica e Ricerca*, 29(3), 140–152.

Ralph, E. (2000). Oral-questioning skills of novice teachers: Any questions? *Journal of Instructional Psychology*, 26(4), 286–296.

Riley-Doucet, C., & Wilson, S. (1997). A three-step method of self-reflection using reflective journal writing. *Journal of Advanced Nursing*, 25, 964–968. https://doi.org/10.1046/j.1365-2648.1997.1997025964.x

Rudolph, J. W., Raemer, D. B., & Simon, R. (2014). Establishing a safe container for learning in simulation: The role of the presimulation briefing. *Simulation in Healthcare*, 9, 339–349. https://doi.org/10.1097/SIH.0000000000000047

Rudolph, J. W., Simon, R., Raemer, D. B., & Eppich, W. J. (2008). Debriefing as formative assessment: Closing performance gaps in medical education. *Academic Emergency Medicine*, 15, 1010–1016. https://doi.org/10.1111/j.1553-2712.2008.00248.x

Rudolph, J. W., Simon, R., Rivard, P., Dufresne, R. L., & Raemer, D. B. (2007). Debriefing with good judgment: Combining rigorous feedback with genuine inquiry. *Anesthesiology Clinics*, 25, 361–376. https://doi.org/10.1016/j.anclin.2007.03.007

Salas, E., Klein, C., King, H., Salisbury, M., Augenstein, J. S., Birnbach, D. J., Robinson, D. W., & Upshaw, C. (2008). Debriefing medical teams: 12 evidence-based best practices and tips. *Joint Commission Journal on Quality and Patient Safety*, 34, 518–527. https://doi.org/10.1016/S1553-7250(08)34066-5

Sawyer, T., Eppich, E., Brett-Fleegler, M., Grant, V., & Cheng, A. (2019). More than one way to debrief. *Simulation in Healthcare*, 11, 209–217. https://doi.org/10.1097/SIH.0000000000000148

Sawyer, T., Loren, D., & Halamek, L. P. (2016). Post-event debriefings during neonatal care: Why are we not doing them, and how can we start? *Journal of Perinatology*, 36(6), 415–419. https://doi.org/10.1038/jp.2016.42

Scanlon, J. M., & Chernomas, W. M. (1997). Developing the reflective teacher. *Journal of Advanced Nursing*, 25(6), 1138–1143. https://doi.org/10.1046/j.1365-2648.1997.19970251138.x

Schön, D. A. (1983). *The reflective practitioner: How professionals think in action.* Basic Books.

Shor, I. (1992). *Empowering education: Critical teaching for social change.* University of Chicago Press.

Society for Simulation in Healthcare. (2021). *SSH certified healthcare simulation educator handbook.* https://www.ssih.org/Portals/48/Certification/CHSE_Docs/CHSE%20Handbook.pdf

Steinwachs, B. (1992). How to facilitate a debrief. *Simulation Gaming*, 23, 186–195. https://doi.org/10.1177/1046878192232006

Turner, S., & Harder, N. (2018). Psychological safe environment: A concept analysis. *Clinical Simulation in Nursing*, 18, 47–55. https://doi.org/10.1016/j.ecns.2018.02.004

Van Heukelom, J. N., Begaz, T., & Treat, R. (2010). Comparison of postsimulation debriefing versus in-simulation debriefing in medical simulation. *Simulation in Healthcare*, 5, 91–97. https://doi.org/10.1097/SIH.0b013e3181be0d17

Warrick, D. D., Hunsaker, P. L., Cook, C. W., & Altman, S. (1979). Debriefing experiential learning exercises. *Journal of Experiential Learning and Simulation*, 1, 91–96.

Zigmont, J. J., Kappus, L. J., & Sudikoff, S. N. (2011). The 3D model of debriefing: Defusing, discovering, and deepening. *Seminars in Perinatology*, 35(2), 52–58. https://doi.org/10.1053/j.semperi.2011.01.003

# Standardized Patient Debriefing and Feedback

Anthony Errichetti and Denise Antonelle

*Thinking is easy, acting is difficult, and to put one's thoughts into action is the most difficult thing in the world.*

—*Johann Wolfgang von Goethe*

This chapter addresses Domain III: Educational Principles Applied to Simulation (Society for Simulation in Healthcare [SSH], 2021).

## ▶ LEARNING OUTCOMES

- Discuss debriefing as a self-reflective learning process.
- Describe how debriefing and feedback are necessary components in the patient simulation learning process, requiring learners to reflect on their work.
- Compare the different roles the clinical educators and standardized patients (SPs) have in the debriefing process.
- Discuss SP selection and training for the debriefing–feedback process.

## ▶ INTRODUCTION

The terms *standardized patient* and *simulated patient* (SP) are often used interchangeably. They refer to a person trained to portray a patient in realistic and repeatable ways (Lewis et al., 2017). SPs have been used for more than 50 years to teach and assess clinical skills (Barrows, 1993). Originally used to facilitate medical learner training through SP encounters, SPs are now used in high-stakes licensure examinations (Dillon et al., 2004). Their full potential, however, is realized when used in formative assessment exercises where skills assessment and debriefing are part of an educational plan. Selection of appropriate SPs and preparation for the debriefing and feedback process are required. This chapter presents an overview of how SPs can be selected and prepared for debriefing, with suggestions for basic to advanced debriefing approaches.

## ▶ DEBRIEFING FOUNDATIONS

Debriefing, as we know it today, has roots in the military and in adult and experiential learning theories and practices. The military "after-action review" (AAR) is a professional discussion of an event that enables soldiers and units to discover for themselves what happened and develop a strategy for improvement (Bartone & Adler, 1995).

An AAR is not a critique. No one, regardless of rank, position, or strength of personality, has all of the information or answers. After-action reviews maximize training benefits by allowing soldiers, regardless of rank, to learn from each other. (Department of the Army, 1993, p. 1)

Simulation learning is experiential learning, that is, learning through direct experience (Itin, 1999). American educator John Dewey noted, however, that experience alone does not guarantee learning, but that learning occurs when experience is reflected on or "reconstructed" (Dewey, 1933). Experiential learning therefore requires the learners to reflect on their actions (Kolb, 1984) and, in the context of simulation learning, actions taken during SP and other simulation exercises. It integrates personal experience with academic learning, structures opportunities for reflection, is inquiry-based, and facilitates face-to-face communication (Hatcher, 1997).

Debriefing is a process that facilitates learner self-reflection. It is a "rigorous reflection process" (p. 361) that focuses on clinical (e.g., critical thinking and actions) and behavioral (e.g., interpersonal communication) issues raised by a simulation exercise (Rudolph et al., 2007). Feedback, a tool of debriefing, is information given to the learners about their performance intended to be used to promote positive and desirable development (Archer, 2010). For feedback to be effective, the debriefer must be aware of the needs of the learner and be able to judge whether the learner is ready to accept it.

Adult learners, the focus of simulation education, have life experience, opinions, emotions, and assumptions ("frames"); well-developed personalities; and relationship patterns that drive their behaviors (Rudolph et al., 2007). They expect learning to be goal-directed, relevant, and applicable. Simulation learning, the antithesis of teacher-led classroom learning, is learning through experience and interaction with experts who understand adult learners' mind-set. Vygotsky's (1978) "zone of proximal development" (p. 86) describes the stage at which we find many adult learners who are, for example, students of healthcare science, that is, between unsupervised and supervised practice. This transition occurs with expert guidance (Vygotsky, 1978), the type of guidance that could come from a debriefing encounter.

## ▶ STANDARDIZED PATIENTS CORE COMPETENCIES

SPs are professionals trained to accurately simulate medical problems and conditions, document and assess skills, and provide feedback (Boulet & Errichetti, 2008; Knopp et al., 2022). They must continually demonstrate a number of "core competencies" to remain effective. The following is a list of those competencies, from the basic/foundational to the advanced, all of which are directly or indirectly related to mastering the debriefing process (Exhibit 18.1).

---

**EXHIBIT 18.1 STANDARDIZED PATIENT CORE COMPETENCIES**

**Foundational Skills**

- Professional conduct
- Acting/simulating

**Advanced Skills**

- Documenting skills (checklists)
- Assessing communication
- Debriefing–feedback

# FOUNDATIONAL COMPETENCIES

## Professional Conduct

SPs are required to demonstrate professional behaviors that guide their actions. These include the following:

- *Reliability:* being on time and carrying out scheduled activities as planned
- *Emotional intelligence:* the ability to be aware of and monitor one's own emotions as well as others' (Mayer & Salovey, 1997)
- *Social intelligence:* the awareness of how one interacts in social situations (Goleman, 2006; Thorndike, 1920)
- *Lifelong learning:* the willingness and ability to learn new things (e.g., medical problems and conditions) in new ways (e.g., through experiential and web-based learning)

## Acting/Simulating

SPs have the ability to learn patient roles and credibly simulate or imitate a patient's condition, including physical symptoms, believably enough to convince learners that they are in an authentic clinical encounter. It requires SPs to play a role while simultaneously observing the learner for postencounter assessment and debriefing. Overidentifying with a role (e.g., when portraying an illness one actually has) or getting too deeply into it (e.g., through "method acting") undermines the learner's assessment and debriefing. SPs must come out of the character immediately and prepare for postencounter activities.

Professionalism and credible acting may be all that are needed for clinical simulations that do not require the following advanced competencies.

## Evidence-Based Simulation Practice 18.1

Foley and Robinson (2021) used acting students from the university's theater school using improvisational techniques of "yes . . . and" to enhance nursing students' assessments of psychiatric mental health patients.

# ADVANCED COMPETENCIES

## Documentation

When history taking and physical examination skills are used, SPs must be able to memorize the checklist items, observe the learner during the encounter, and then document on the checklists what the learner accomplished.

## Communication Assessment

SPs are in the best position to assess the interaction and communication skills of the learner. They are in close proximity to the learner in the exam room during the encounter and are observing such skills as rapport building, empathic responses, nonverbal communication, eliciting information, active listening, information exchange, and physical examination quality.

## Debriefing and Feedback

The *Healthcare Simulation Dictionary* distinguishes between feedback and debriefing. In providing feedback, critical information is relayed back to the learner. Debriefing, however, involves the process of providing feedback and asking the learner to respond with their thoughts about actions taken (Lopreiato, 2016). In this regard, feedback and debriefing are often used synonymously.

Debriefing and feedback are arguably the most difficult skills for SPs to master, requiring SPs to come out of their characters immediately, assess the learner, and quickly formulate a debriefing agenda. The Association of Standardized Patient Educators acknowledges in its *Standards of Best Practice* document that feedback is an essential skill in simulation learning, and that SPs, when properly trained, can provide a unique perspective to learners (Lewis et al., 2017). SPs, using their social and emotional intelligence, engage the learner for a short, productive review of the encounter. They must be prepared to work with learners whose responses to the SP exercise can range from apathy to engagement. Most importantly, SPs must create a climate of psychological safety in which learners disclose and discuss needed areas of improvement (Schön, 1983). Indeed, empathy and compassion for the learner are key debriefing requirements.

## ▶ SELECTING STANDARDIZED PATIENTS FOR DEBRIEFING: SCREENING PROCESS

Not every SP is appropriate for debriefing and feedback activities. These are tasks requiring maturity, psychological awareness, discernment, and the ability to communicate with and coach learners. Before SPs can be used for this purpose, they must be rigorously screened to determine whether they have the potential to demonstrate the communication assessment and debriefing core competencies. They must be literate, have the ability and willingness to learn, and demonstrate the goodwill toward learners that is critically important to debriefing (Adamo, 2003). A robust screening process will determine whether SP candidates can be trained to engage learners in debriefing. The following are suggested steps to SP selection.

### PRESCREENING STANDARDIZED PATIENT CANDIDATES

The following suggested activities can evaluate an SP's capabilities:

- Candidates should submit a curriculum vitae (CV) to evaluate their experience and assess their writing skills.
- Candidates should complete an electronic application to determine their comfort level with technology.
- Provide candidates with an "SP Program Information Sheet," listing job skills, activities, and requirements to review before the first interview.
- A phone or video (e.g., Skype) interview with the SP recruiter should be conducted to evaluate the candidate's motivation, for example, their attitude toward the medical healthcare field, why they want to do this work, and whether they have read and comprehended the SP Program Information Sheet. The candidate's work history, understanding of SP work, and comfort level with educational technology can also be assessed during this online interview.

### Evidence-Based Simulation Practice 18.2

Barton et al. (2022) used standardized patients (SPs) as vaccine-hesitant patients and studied residents' communication skills. This randomized study ($N = 53$) used the Announce, Inquire, Mirror, Secure (AIMS) Method for Healthy Conversations. The study demonstrated that SPs increased residents' confidence and communication skills. SPs were useful in studying the effectiveness of structured communication training.

## STANDARDIZED PATIENT INFORMATION MEETING

If candidates are appropriate, they are invited to an unpaid "information meeting," an extended group interview and exercise that provides a didactic and experiential overview of the work. The goal of the meeting is to get an impression of the candidates' abilities to demonstrate and master the SP core competencies.

### Group Interview and Introduction
- Candidates introduce themselves.
- Group question: "What draws you to this work?"
- The SP trainer provides an overview of SP work through, for example, presentation of SP–learner encounter videos.
- Candidates are asked to give their opinion about the quality of the work demonstrated by the learners on the videos.
- "Veteran" SPs discuss their experience.

This process allows candidates to present themselves as they might be when functioning as SPs and reveals their potential to provide debriefing. For example, some candidates will demonstrate respect and consideration for other candidates, will listen and respond appropriately, and will ask questions. The process may also reveal candidates who lack emotional and social intelligence, for example, by "grandstanding" or making themselves the center of attention. Or candidates may appear to be overly reticent to speak, ask questions, or render an opinion. By reviewing and discussing videos, one can assess whether candidates view learners' behaviors in a positive light. A "red flag" would be raised if candidates are overly judgmental in their opinion of a learner (Exhibit 18.2).

---

**EXHIBIT 18.2 STANDARDIZED PATIENT SELECTION PROCESS: STEPS**

1. Prescreening
   - Submission of CV and application
   - Phone/video interview
2. SP information meeting
   - Group interview
   - SP exercise
   - Candidate debriefing

CV, curriculum vitae; SP, standardized patient.

---

### Experiential Standardized Patient Exercise
Candidates learn a short sample SP case in order to assess their reading ability and memory. They are then asked to voluntarily play the case as an SP several times and provide feedback to a simulated "learner" played by an SP. The feedback given could include how the learner communicated and interacted with the SP. This exercise provides candidates the opportunity to "try out" different components of SP work and for the trainer to determine candidates' capabilities.

### Standardized Patient Candidate Debriefing
Following this exercise, the candidates are debriefed about the SP information meeting. "What was the meeting like for you?" "What did you learn about SP work?" "What did you learn about yourselves?" "Any suggestions about how to improve this process?" It is important

that the SP trainer conducting the meeting understands and demonstrates an empathic debriefing approach as a prelude to preparing new SPs for debriefing training, that is, they try to understand how SPs think about the experience and whether they are able to provide the trainer with useful feedback.

## ▶ PREPARING STANDARDIZED PATIENTS FOR DEBRIEFING AND FEEDBACK

After determining whether SPs have the potential ability to provide debriefing and feedback, they are then trained for the process. Although there is considerable variability among SP programs regarding how debriefing and feedback are conducted, the following learning points are general guidelines for all programs.

### DEBRIEFING CONCEPTS FOR STANDARDIZED PATIENTS

- *Understand the difference between debriefing and feedback.* If debriefing is a process used to reflect on work, feedback is a tool of debriefing that clearly articulates "positive feedback" (what was done well) and "constructive feedback" (what could be improved upon with continued practice).
- *Coaching follows debriefing.* The debriefer engages the learner to assist them in reflecting on their work.
- *Debriefing is conducted in an empathic but straightforward way* that models the ideal healthcare encounter SPs expect from learners. It creates a climate of "psychological safety" in which learners can disclose without shame or humiliation.
- *Feedback and inquiry are linked.* The debriefer seeks to understand the learner through *empathic inquiry* (Rudolph et al., 2007).
- *SP debriefing is focused on interpersonal and communication skills.* Because debriefing potentially has a medical/healthcare component (e.g., reviewing how a differential diagnosis was determined, critical thinking and problem-solving, and patient management) and an interpersonal and communication component, an experienced clinician would address the healthcare issues and the SP would address the interpersonal and communication element.
- *Understand the goals and objectives of the exercise.* SPs are briefed on what the learners are expected to accomplish during a given exercise.
- *Understand the learner's level of training and expertise.* SPs are instructed, for example, to not expect expertise in novice learners and to avoid comparing student learners with the ideal healthcare provider.

### SMALL GROUP DEBRIEFING AND FEEDBACK EXERCISES

Moving from concepts to practice, the following small group training methods help SPs understand how they will follow a debriefing plan:

- *Review and discuss* the debriefing–feedback model used.
- *View videos depicting "gold standard" debriefing examples.* These can come from actual encounters or simulated encounters that illustrate appropriate debriefing and feedback approaches.
- *View SP–learner encounter videos and rate communication* as a group, compare ratings, and discuss: "What positive and constructive feedback would you give this learner?"
- *Role-play and discuss.* SPs greatly benefit from small group practice and receiving immediate feedback. *Role-play option:* Pair SPs, one playing the learner, the other playing

the SP who will give feedback. The SP as the learner can be coached to portray a common learner issue, for example, a nervous learner who has difficulty making eye contact.

■ *Use side coaching.* The trainer sits close to the SP and quietly gives instructions or redirects actions during role-play training.
■ *Use earbud coaching.* A variation of side coaching, the SP in training wears an earbud during debriefing and receives instructions or redirections from the trainer.

---

**Simulation Teaching Tip 18.1**

Watch a prerecorded actual learner–standardized patient (SP) encounter, make notes on learner communication issues to be addressed, and then have one SP portray the learner and the other assume the role of the SP who gives feedback.

---

## ▶ DEBRIEFING AND FEEDBACK MODELS

Models of debriefing range from the basic (giving positive and constructive feedback) to the reflective/exploratory (encouraging learner self-reflection and exploring learner "frames of reference"). All models require giving specific feedback on observable behavior. Also, the SP debriefer must prepare by reviewing learner communication ratings and/or exercise objectives and identifying areas to review.

The following are several examples of feedback and debriefing for SP encounters.

### BASIC FEEDBACK APPROACH

The *feedback sandwich* (Chowdhury & Kalu, 2004) softens constructive feedback by *sandwiching* it between two examples of positive performance (Exhibit 18.3).

■ *Advantages:* It is easy to teach to SPs and is satisfactory to learners who want specific feedback: "Tell me what I did well and what I could have done better."
■ *Disadvantages:* It is prescriptive and formulaic, it reinforces passivity on the part of the learner, and is more a report than a reflection on the work done.

---

**EXHIBIT 18.3 FEEDBACK SANDWICH**

**Positive Feedback:** "This is what I thought you did well."
**Constructive Feedback:** "When you did *x*, I would have preferred *y*."
**Positive Feedback:** "This is another example of what I thought you did well."

---

### PENDLETON'S RULES

*Pendleton's Rules* (Exhibit 18.4) structures feedback so that positive feedback is highlighted first, followed by a discussion of "what could have been done differently" (Pendleton et al., 1984, p. 247).

---

**EXHIBIT 18.4 PENDLETON'S RULES: STEPS**

**Learners**

- Self-assess performance.
- List two things done well and two things the learner could improve on with more practice.

**SPs**

- Assess the learner.
- List two things done well and two things the learner could improve on with more practice.

**SP and Learner**

- Compare notes, discussing areas of agreement and disagreement, and actions that could improve performance.

SP, standardized patient.

---

- *Advantages:* Learners actively prepare themselves for debriefing by identifying strengths and areas to improve. SPs can address and focus on areas to improve identified by the learners.
- *Disadvantages:* By rigidly focusing on the positives first, valuable debriefing time that could have been spent discussing more relevant issues may be lost.

## REFLECTIVE DEBRIEFING MODEL

Based on the work of Rudolph et al. (2006, 2007), this approach promotes reflection on the work between the learner and the SP, in which the SP encourages self-reflection, provides concrete and specific feedback, and most importantly attempts to understand the learner's "frame of reference" or assumptions about why they did what they did (Exhibit 18.5). In this approach, the SP debriefer raises issues of concern (e.g., why the learner did not demonstrate empathy during a "giving bad news" exercise) but tries to understand the learner's point of view. The SP models empathy and the desire to understand the other, a fundamental stance of patient-centered treatment. This, like other feedback and debriefing models, requires the debriefing facilitator to create a climate of psychological safety in which the learner will feel comfortable discussing and critiquing their work. The SP is a learner in this process as well because the learner's frame of reference is inferred and not always evident through their actions. Therefore, the learner's rationale for their actions may be either accepted ("Now I understand, that makes sense") or challenged ("Now I understand what you were doing, but let's explore another option").

- *Advantages:* It promotes mutual understanding of the learner's frame of reference, models empathy, and promotes true experiential learning.
- *Disadvantages:* It requires a high level of training, maturity, and psychological sophistication on the part of the SP learner.

---

**EXHIBIT 18.5 STANDARDIZED PATIENT REFLECTIVE DEBRIEFING STEPS**

**Standardized Patient**
- Encourage learner self-reflection by first taking the *emotional pulse* of the learner.
  - "How are you? How did you feel during the encounter?" (Focus on the learner's affect.)
- Encourage the learner to self-reflect on *positive actions*.
  - "What do you think went well?"
- Encourage the learner to self-reflect on *future actions*.
  - "With enough practice, what do you think could be improved?"
- When done well, the learner's concerns and questions are the primary focus of attention.

**When Feedback Is Given**
- Positive, specific feedback is given when appropriate.
- Constructive feedback (areas of questions or concerns) is given, but the learner's frame of reference is explored.
  - "Here is some feedback . . . help me to understand why you did x."
- Empathically explore the learner's thinking and be prepared to change your mind about your own assumptions or make rational challenges.

## DEBRIEFING THE PHYSICAL EXAMINATION

If the physical examination was technically correct but of poor quality, or if done with thoroughness and care but technically incorrect, SPs are encouraged to have the learners retry the exam in question and correct the technique.

## ▶ STARTING DEBRIEFING

The following are suggested openings appropriate for all types of debriefing and feedback.

### SET THE STAGE

- *Debriefing dress:* Wear a robe, gym pants, and so on over the exam gown if wearing one.
- *Welcome the learner:* Open the door, invite the learner in, and make the individual feel comfortable: "Please come in and have a seat."

### SET THE COLLABORATIVE AGENDA

"We have x minutes to discuss your work. We're going to focus on your communication and our patient–clinician relationship. I will not be reviewing your clinical reasoning, the questions you asked, and so forth. This is a dialogue so please ask me any questions. How does this sound?"

## ▶ ADDITIONAL APPROACHES TO ENSURE DEBRIEFING QUALITY

- To ensure debriefing and feedback quality, SP encounters should be video-recorded and those videos reviewed on a regular basis. A debriefing quality assurance checklist can be used to note SP behaviors. Such a checklist would note, for example, whether the SP

began the debriefing appropriately, maintained a positive attitude toward the learner, modeled empathy by attempting to understand the learners' frame of reference, and ended the debriefing encounter on a respectful note.
■ Prepare learners for debriefing. If learners are to get the most from the debriefing–feedback process, they can be instructed on how the process works, what they should expect from the SP, how they can participate in the process, and how they should prepare themselves for the debriefing.

### Evidence-Based Simulation Teaching 18.3

Berger-Estilita et al. (2021) developed a tool to frame the communication content of debriefings. The qualitative content analysis was linked to the student learning outcomes. The tool was used ($N = 20$) with 9 main categories and 81 subcategories. The types of debriefing used were advocacy, inquiry, illustration, and confirmation, and researchers found that debriefer questions and participant inputs were positively related to student learning outcomes, in contrast to other communications that included guess-what-I-am-thinking, apologies, observations, use of materials, participant descriptions, and simple repetition of statements, which were not positively related to student learning outcomes.

## ▶ SUMMARY

Debriefing and feedback are sophisticated skills, arguably among the most difficult to master. SPs must be screened for appropriateness. Although there are no formal screening exams to determine skill and psychological readiness, the experienced SP trainer can determine, through experiential exercises and communication assessment training, the most appropriate candidates. SPs must have a high degree of emotional and social intelligence and have the ability to distinguish between low- and high-quality performances appropriate for the level of the learner. They must practice, receive feedback, and be debriefed in a way that closely approximates the model of debriefing used. Indeed, debriefing trainers must model debriefing and feedback's best practices.

 ## CASE STUDY 18.1

You are interviewing three standardized patients (SPs) and ask them to role-play a patient with active appendicitis. The first one doubles over and moans continuously while you are trying to examine them. The second SP states a pain level of 3 on a scale of 0 to 10 and is sitting on the table smiling. The third one asks several questions about the condition and asks whether they can "read up" on it first on their electronic device. Assess all three SPs for their appropriateness to provide SP service and feedback to learners.

1. The novice simulation educator understands feedback when they state, "Feedback is . . .":

   A. Just another term for *debriefing*
   B. One tool of debriefing
   C. Best delivered by peers
   D. A process of self-reflection

2. The simulation educator prepares the learners for debriefing:

   A. To teach them debriefing methods and tools used in the process
   B. As an optional formative peer evaluative process
   C. As a summative self and quality improvement tool
   D. To assist them to participate more effectively in the process

3. A standardized patient (SP) would like to participate in debriefing with the simulation educator. The simulation educator understands that:

   A. Every SP has been educated in debriefing
   B. Debriefing is more difficult than communicating an assessment
   C. Debriefing is of more use than just giving feedback
   D. Debriefing is a complex activity for SPs to master

4. The reason standardized patients (SPs) provide feedback on communication is because:

   A. They are in the best position to judge learner communication
   B. It is easier to evaluate communication than the physical assessments
   C. They are trained and practiced to provide feedback
   D. They are trained to assess therapeutic communication

5. The simulation educator is debriefing a student after the student performed a physical examination on a standardized patient (SP). The MOST productive debriefing methods include:

   A. Telling the learner directly what they need to improve
   B. Showing the learner how the physical exam should be performed
   C. Asking the candidate to retry the exam and correct as necessary
   D. Letting the SP debrief the learner after the physical exam

6. The advantage of using Pendleton's Rules for debriefing is that:

   A. It helps both the standardized patient (SP) and the learner prepare for debriefing by listing positive performance and tells the learner what to do differently
   B. It is an easy technique for SPs and simulation educators to remember and repeat as often as needed
   C. Research shows it is an effective debriefing process and produces immediate improved competencies in learners
   D. Learners like to get both positive and negative feedback in that order and build confidence in skill attainment

## 1. B) One tool of debriefing

Feedback is a debriefing tool that focuses on providing learners with information about what they did well and what competencies need improvement. It is not another term for debriefing and it is not usually provided by peers. Feedback is given by another person so it is not a process of self-reflection.

## 2. D) To assist them to participate more effectively in the process

Debriefing works best when learners are part of and engaged in the process. Learners do not need to know the difference between debriefing methods and it is not a peer preview process. Reflection and self-improvement are part of it, but students need to be prepared to participate in self-reflection and improvement.

## 3. D) Debriefing is a complex activity for SPs to master

Debriefing is a complex skill, and not all SPs are prepared to conduct debriefing. Not all SPs have debriefing education and it is just as valuable as feedback. Communicating assessments is also complex but is not the main objective of debriefing.

## 4. A) They are in the best position to judge learner communication

SPs are in the best position to judge learner communication since they are the recipient of the care and interaction. All assessments are difficult and SPs are educated and trained in their role, which can or cannot include scripted communication.

## 5. B) Showing the learner how the physical exam should be performed

Demonstrating the competency is the best way to ensure learning. Telling the learner directly or asking them to retry may not produce the correct competency. The SP is not the best person to debrief healthcare competencies because they are trained in feedback but not always in debriefing techniques.

## 6. A) It helps both the standardized patient (SP) and the learner prepare for debriefing by listing positive performance and tells the learner what to do differently

Pendleton's Rules helps prepare for debriefing and provides a debriefing process. The technique is not necessarily easy and does not produce immediate results. Learners usually do not like negative feedback.

7. The simulation educator can best ensure standardized patient (SP) debriefing quality by:

    A. Giving the SP feedback about the debriefing
    B. Asking the SP to self-assess their work after reviewing the videos
    C. Questioning the SP about their knowledge of debriefing
    D. Using a debriefing quality assurance checklist to note SP behaviors

8. An affective attribute of healthcare providers is empathy, which can be demonstrated in simulation by:

    A. The standardized patient (SP) understanding the learner's frame of reference
    B. The SP acting warm and caring toward the provider
    C. Creating a psychologically safe space and culture for the learner
    D. An adult learning approach where the SP holds the learner accountable

9. The simulation educator promotes a reflective debriefing model in order to:

    A. Promote positive learning
    B. Provide appropriate feedback
    C. Promote self-assessment
    D. Provide the standardized patients (SPs) time to reflect

10. The novice simulation educator needs additional understanding when they state that using the sandwich style of feedback:

    A. "Makes learners active participants."
    B. "Can work well as reflective feedback."
    C. "Is congruent with physical examination debriefing."
    D. "Places the debriefer in charge of what to discuss."

## 7. D) Using a debriefing quality assurance checklist to note SP behaviors

A checklist ensures consistency and is a good method to audit the SP's interactions. Feedback helps, as does self-assessment, but a checklist can standardize correct debriefing techniques. Questioning the SP directly does not assess the debriefing behavior.

## 8. A) The SP understanding the learner's frame of reference

The SP can understand the learner's perspective and role-model empathy for the learner. Empathy is more than caring. Creating a positive learning environment is part of empathy. It is not an attribute specifically of adult learning theories.

## 9. C) Promote self-assessment

Promoting self-reflection in learners will assist them in their lifelong profession to continue to grow and refine competencies. It does promote positive learning and provide feedback, but this is not the main goal. It does not necessarily promote time for the SP to reflect.

## 10. A) "Makes learners active participants."

The sandwich type of feedback is passive learning, not active. It can work well with competencies and reflection, but it does place the debriefer in control of the conversation.

# REFERENCES

Adamo, G. (2003). Simulated and standardized patients in OSCEs: Achievements and challenges 1992–2003. *Medical Teacher, 25*(3), 262–270. https://doi.org/10.1080/0142159031000100300

Archer, J. C. (2010). State of the science in health professional education: Effective feedback. *Medical Education, 4*(1), 101–108. https://doi.org/10.1111/j.1365-2923.2009.03546.x

Barrows, H. S. (1993). An overview of the uses of standardized patients for teaching and evaluating clinical skills. *AAMC Academic Medicine, 68*(6), 443–451. https://doi.org/10.1097/00001888-199306000-00002

Barton, S. M., Calhoun, A. W., Bohnert, C. A., Multerer, S. M., Statler, V. A., Bryant, K. A., Arnold, D. M., Felton, H. M., Purcell, P. M., Kinney, M. D., Parrish-Sprowl, J. M., & Marshall, G. S. (2022). Standardized vaccine-hesitant patients in the assessment of the effectiveness of vaccine communication training. *Journal of Pediatrics, 241*, 203–203. https://doi.org/10.1016/j.jpeds.2021.10.033

Bartone, P. T., & Adler, A. B. (1995). Event-oriented debriefing following military operations: What every leader should know. *US Army Pamphlet, 95*(2), 1–12. https://doi.org/10.21236/ada300953

Berger-Estilita, J., Luthi, V., Greif, R., & Abegglen, S. (2021). Communication content during debriefing in simulation-based medical education: An analytic framework and mixed-methods analysis. *Medical Teacher, 43*(12), 1381–1390. https://doi.org/10.1080/0142159X.2021.1948521

Boulet, J. R., & Errichetti, A. (2008). Training and assessment with standardized patients. In R. H. Riley (Ed.), *Manual of simulation in healthcare* (pp. 185–207). Oxford University Press.

Chowdhury, R. R., & Kalu, G. (2004). Learning to give feedback in medical education. *Obstetrician and Gynaecologist, 6*, 242–247. https://doi.org/10.1576/toag.6.4.243.27023

Department of the Army. (1993). *A leader's guide to after-action reviews* [Training circular] (pp. 25–20). Author.

Dewey, J. (1933). *How we think: A restatement of the relation of reflective thinking to the educative process.* D. C. Heath.

Dillon, G. F., Boulet, J. R., Hawkins, R. E., & Swanson, D. B. (2004). Simulations in the United States Medical Licensing Examination (USMLE). *Quality & Safe Health Care, 13*(Suppl. 1), i41–i45. https://doi.org/10.1136/qhc.13.suppl_1.i41

Foley, D. M., & Robinson, J. (2021). Yes. . .and! Actor improvisation enhances psychiatric-mental health nursing education. *Nursing Education Perspectives, 42*(1), 59–60. https://doi.org/10.1097/01.NEP.0000000000000546

Goleman, D. (2006). *Social intelligence: The new science of human relationships.* Bantam Dell.

Hatcher, J. A. (1997). The moral dimensions of John Dewey's philosophy: Implications for undergraduate education. *Michigan Journal of Community Service Learning, 4*(1), 22–29. http://hdl.handle.net/2027/spo.3239521.0004.103

Itin, C. M. (1999). Reasserting the philosophy of experiential education as a vehicle for change in the 21st century. *Journal of Experiential Education, 22*(2), 91–98. https://doi.org/10.1177/105382599902200206

Knopp, A., Graham, A., Stowell, S., & Schubert, C. (2022). Using simulation to assess nurse practitioner education. *Nursing Education Perspectives, 43*(2), 137–138. https://doi.org/10.1097/01.NEP.0000000000000824

Kolb, D. A. (1984). *Experiential learning theory: Experience as the source of learning and development.* Prentice Hall.

Lewis, K. L., Bohnert, C. A., Gammon, W. L., Hölzer, H., Lyman, L., Smith, C., Thompson, T. M., Wallace, A., & Gliva-McConvey, G. (2017). The association of standardized patient educators (ASPE) standards of best practice (SOBP). *Advances in Simulation, 2*, 10. https://doi.org/10.1186/s41077-017-0043-4

Lopreiato, J. O. (2016, October). *Healthcare simulation dictionary.* Agency for Healthcare Research and Quality. AHRQ Publication No. 16(17)-0043.

Mayer, J. D., & Salovey, P. (1997). What is emotional intelligence? In P. Salovey & D. Sluyter (Eds.), *Emotional development and emotional intelligence: Implications for educators* (pp. 3–31). Basic Books.

Pendleton, D., Schofield, T., Tate, P., & Havelock, P. (1984). *The consultation: An approach to teaching and learning*. Oxford University Press.

Rudolph, J. W., Simon, R., Rivard, P., Dufresne, R. L., & Raemer, D. B. (2006). There's no such thing as non-judgmental debriefing: A theory and method of debriefing with good judgment. *Simulation in Healthcare*, 1(1), 49–55. https://doi.org/10.1097/01266021-200600110-00006

Rudolph, J. W., Simon, R., Rivard, P., Dufresne, R. L., & Raemer, D. B. (2007). Debriefing with good judgment. *Anesthesiology Clinics*, 25(2), 361–376. https://doi.org/10.1016/j.anclin.2007.03.007

Schön, D. (1983). *The reflective practitioner*. Basic Books.

Society for Simulation in Healthcare. (2021). *Certified healthcare simulation educator handbook*. https://www.ssih.org/Portals/48/Certification/CHSE_Docs/CHSE%20Handbook.pdf

Thorndike, E. L. (1920). Intelligence and its use. *Harper's Magazine, 140*, 227–235.

Vygotsky, L. (1978). Interaction between learning and development. In M. Cole, V. John-Steiner, S. Scribner, & E. Souberman (Eds.), *Mind in society* (pp. 79–91). Harvard University Press.

# Evaluation of Simulation Activities

Maryanne Halligan and Marilynn Poe Murphy

*One of the great mistakes is to judge policies and programs by their intentions rather than their results.*

*—Milton Friedman*

**This chapter addresses Domain III: Educational Principles Applied to Simulation (Society for Simulation in Healthcare [SSH], 2021).**

## ▶ LEARNING OUTCOMES

- Describe the basic components of performance and activity evaluation.
- Explain the importance of evaluation of simulation activities.
- Identify current practices for individual learner evaluation, team evaluation, and activity evaluation in simulation-based learning experiences (SBLEs).
- Discuss the future of evaluation in SBLE.

## ▶ INTRODUCTION

The healthcare world continues to evolve at an amazing speed with increasing individual and organizational accountability at the forefront. Experts agree that simulation is a valuable tool for healthcare education learning and for determining clinical competency (Armenia et al., 2018; Cant & Cooper, 2017; Kiernan, 2018). However, the question remains as to how one determines the effectiveness of simulation at the individual, team, organizational, and system levels. Assessing learner outcomes, whether for students or practicing healthcare professionals, individually or in teams, requires valid and reliable tools to ensure that instructional goals are achieved (Griswold et al., 2018). Although a variety of simulation-based learning experience (SBLE) and simulation-based team training (SBTT) evaluation tools exist, there continues to be a need to establish the validity and reliability of both the simulator and the tools (Bryant et al., 2020; Cantrell et al., 2017; Watts et al., 2021). In addition to accurately evaluating learners, outcome data are needed to determine the overall effectiveness of SBLE, including demonstration of translation to practice within organizations and the overall healthcare system.

This chapter begins with a brief discussion of evaluation and its importance in SBLE, both today and in the future. Next, the chapter focuses on evaluation of the individual learner, including the differences between formative and summative evaluation and a discussion of self and peer evaluation, followed by an overview of the evaluation of team members during SBTT. A summary of selected SBLE and SBTT evaluation instruments is presented. The chapter concludes with a discussion of methods and current tools available for evaluating the simulation activity itself.

## ▶ EVALUATION IN SIMULATION-BASED LEARNING EXPERIENCES

There are many essential elements when planning evaluation in SBLE: whether the evaluation should be formative, summative, or high-stakes, and when the evaluation should occur in the simulation; which tool will best measure the learning and how the evaluator will be trained in using the tool; and how the results of the evaluation will be communicated to the learners.

High-quality simulation design must begin with a clear understanding of the learning objectives. The International Nursing Association for Clinical Simulation and Learning (INACSL) Standards Committee defines *objective* as the "expected goal of a curriculum, course, lesson or activity in terms of demonstrable skills or knowledge that will be acquired by a student as a result of instruction" (INACSL Standards Committee, 2021b, p. 41). These objectives focus on what is to be evaluated. For example, is the focus on individual performance or is it on the teamwork displayed during the simulation? Is the outcome (patient safety) to be the sole focus, or should the process by which the outcome occurred also be considered worthy of note? (Webster et al., 2020). Actual behaviors within SBL are often divided into knowledge, skills, and attitudes (KSAs). These relate to the recognized learning domains, that is, cognitive (knowledge), affective (attitude), and psychomotor (skills). The instrument chosen for assessment or evaluation should not only reflect the appropriate domain in which the learning has occurred or an integration of all three if appropriate, but should also be a valid and reliable tool (Higham et al., 2019).

Of course, the ultimate goal of simulation is to achieve level 4 of Kirkpatrick's levels of evaluation (Kirkpatrick, 1998), when a change in practice will positively impact patient outcomes. Much attention has been given to how best to ensure that knowledge gained in simulation translates to practice (goes from Kirkpatrick's level 2 to level 4). This translation should be evident at several levels: the individual, the team, the organization, and the system. Despite the importance being placed on translation from simulation to practice, valid and reliable tools to measure this remain an ongoing challenge (Hanshaw & Dickerson, 2020).

## ▶ LEARNER SIMULATION-BASED LEARNING EXPERIENCE EVALUATION

The SBLE learner evaluation focuses primarily on the individual's performance and outcomes. Learner evaluation is recognized within the SBLE community as an essential component of an effective simulation experience. The INACSL requires all simulation-based experiences adhering to their published standards for best practice, Healthcare Simulation Standards of Best Practice™: Simulation Design (HSSOBP™), to include participant evaluation. They cite the following elements as necessary for conducting an authentic evaluation: (a) determine the type of evaluation for the SBLE; (b) design the SBLE to include timing of the evaluation; (c) use a valid and reliable evaluation tool; (d) provide evaluator training; and (e) complete the evaluation, interpret the results, and provide feedback to the learners (INACSL Standards Committee, 2021c).

The INACSL further cites potential consequences for failure to engage in authentic participant evaluations, including:

- inaccurate evaluation
- learner dissatisfaction
- failure to achieve learning outcomes
- inappropriate selection of tools
- assessment bias (2021c, p. 55)

In evaluating learners, it is important to determine the desired specific learning outcomes, maintain consistency, and apply standardization in order to be fair and objective with feedback (So et al., 2019). All evaluations of learners begin with the development of clear, measurable objectives for the SBLE. Evaluations should always be tightly aligned with the learning objectives. The appropriate choice of the evaluation tool is specific to the measurement of the learning outcomes, whether the activity is an individual or a group activity. The outcome of the evaluation may be formative, summative, or high stakes, which will be a major consideration when selecting the desired tool. A few of the more well-known SBLE evaluation tools are listed in Table 19.1 with brief descriptions. These tools have been used in a variety of studies; the references listed reflect the psychometrics that measure validity and reliability.

**Table 19.1** Validated Tools for Simulation Evaluation

| Selected Citations | Name of Instrument | Characteristics | Requirements | Measures | Other |
|---|---|---|---|---|---|
| **Tools For Evaluating Team Performance** | | | | | |
| AHRQ (2014) | TPOT | Observational measurement of team performance | Each specified team behavior is ranked on a 5-point Likert scale: very poor: 1; poor: 2; acceptable: 3; good: 4; excellent: 5, for an averaged team performance rating | Team structure, communication, leadership, situation monitoring, and mutual support | |
| Lyk-Jensen et al. (2016) | N-ANTS | Observational checklist of team performance | Evaluator rates four categories on a 4-point scale: good: 4; acceptable: 3; marginal: 2; poor: 1; not observed: 0 | Task management, teamworking, situation awareness, and decision-making | |
| Cooper and Cant (2013) | TEAM | Designed to assess resuscitation events in the hospital, either live or simulated | 5-point Likert scale measuring 10 items in 3 categories | Team leadership, teamwork, and task management | |

*(continued)*

Table 19.1 Validated Tools for Simulation Evaluation (*continued*)

| Selected Citations | Name of Instrument | Characteristics | Requirements | Measures | Other |
|---|---|---|---|---|---|
| Reid et al. (2011) | STAT | Used to evaluate pediatric resuscitations in a simulated environment | 94 items that were rated on a behavioral scale of 0–2: 2: complete and timely; 1: incomplete and untimely; 0: not necessary | Tool evaluated four domains: basic assessment skills, airway/ breathing, circulation, and human factors | |
| Thistlethwaite et al. (2016) | iTOFT | Tool for formative assessment specifically for students and novice health professionals | Observable behaviors: inappropriate, appropriate, and responsive | Tool with 11 observable behaviors under 4 categories: shared decision-making, working in a team, leadership, and patient safety | |
| **Individual Student Performance** | | | | | |
| Hayden et al. (2014) | C-CEI | A rating tool designed for evaluation of nursing students using simulation | Evaluator scores either a 0 or a 1 for 22 specific criteria; (e.g., "Responds to abnormal findings appropriately") | Assessment, communication, clinical judgment, and patient safety | Derived from the C-CEI |
| Ashcraft et al. (2013) | Lasater Clinical Judgment Rubric Modified | A validated tool used to measure clinical judgment, with the modified version including numeric grading and more clarity regarding clinical expectations | 11 dimensions in 4 columns of beginning, developing, accomplished, and exemplary Scoring items added from 0 to 3 | Effective noticing, effective interpreting, effective responding, and effective reflecting | |

(continued)

**Table 19.1** Validated Tools for Simulation Evaluation (*continued*)

| Selected Citations | Name of Instrument | Characteristics | Requirements | Measures | Other |
|---|---|---|---|---|---|
| **Facilitator Evaluation Tools** | | | | | |
| Simon et al. (2010) | DASH | Evaluates strategies and techniques used for debriefing and examines concrete behaviors | 6 elements with a 7-point rating scale: 1 is extremely ineffective and 7 is extremely effective | Dimensions and behaviors associated with debriefing, including prebrief | |
| Leighton et al. (2018) | Facilitator Competency Rubric | Designed to assess simulation facilitator competency | 21 items that are measured using a 5-point scale that follows Benner's novice-to-expert model | Five major constructs measured using subcontents: preparation, prebriefing, debriefing, facilitation, and evaluation | |
| **Student Evaluation of Simulation Experience** | | | | | |
| Leighton et al. (2015) | SET-M | Developed originally as a simulation effectiveness tool to document how effective the simulation experience was for the student and to assist with improving the simulation experiences, and was modified as new terminology was identified | 19-item questionnaire using a Likert scale of do not agree, somewhat agree, and strongly agree | Created to assess the experience of the simulation from the student perspective; items added include prebriefing and debriefing evaluation | |

AHRQ, Agency for Healthcare Research and Quality; C-CEI, Creighton Competency Evaluation Instrument; DASH, Debriefing Assessment for Simulation in Healthcare; iTOFT, Individual Teamwork Observation and Feedback Tool; N-ANTS, Nurse-Anesthetists' Nontechnical Skill; SET-M, Simulation Effectiveness Tool—Modified; STAT, Simulation Team Assessment Tool; TEAM, Team Emergency Assessment Measure; TPOT, Team Performance Observation Tool.

**Simulation Teaching Tip 19.1**

When choosing a means to evaluate a simulation, it is important to keep in mind the learning objectives and the students' level of knowledge and skill. A single simulation scenario cannot encompass all aspects of a case study; this means that it is crucial that the desired learning outcomes or assessment measures be clearly defined before beginning the evaluation process. The type of evaluation will also affect the tool and the process used. A formative assessment can be used to assist the students in knowledge acquisition. A summative evaluation requires that there be no cues or assistance, which would be an unfair advantage.

# ▶ FRAMEWORKS FOR EVALUATION STRATEGIES

There are several applicable frameworks that support the evaluative process in SBLE. These include Kirkpatrick's levels of evaluation, translational science research (TSR) phases, and Miller's pyramid (Prion & Haerling, 2021).

## KIRKPATRICK'S LEVELS OF EVALUATION

- Level 1 is *reaction*. What were the learners' perceptions of the activity? As the most basic level of evaluation, it is usually reflected by self-reporting on surveys, observations, or verbal feedback: "It was fun" or "I didn't like it."
- Level 2 is *learning*. How much did the participants learn? This level reflects a change in attitudes, skills, or knowledge.
- Level 3 is *behavior*. Did the learner's behavior change as a result of this activity? This level relates to a change in behavior and application of what has been learned.
- Level 4 is *results*. This relates to how learning changes practice. This level helps improve patient outcomes and safety (Adamson, 2014; Johnson et al., 2018; Johnston & Fox, 2020; Kirkpatrick, 1998).

## TRANSLATIONAL SCIENCE RESEARCH PHASES

The evaluation of the transfer of the KSAs learned with simulation to patient care and outcomes is appropriate for translational research (Cantrell et al., 2017; Griswold et al., 2018). TSR provides three levels of evaluation:

- T-1 is the lowest level in relation to simulation activities. It consists of learning in the simulation lab.
- T-2 is the carryover to patient care.
- T-3 is that the results of the simulation activity improve patient outcomes. As the name implies, evidence is required to prove the translation to practice, and this requires measurable outcomes at every level. Research design and data collection for the highest level of TSR continue to be a challenge in simulation education (So et al., 2019).

## MILLER'S PYRAMID

Miller's pyramid provides a visual model with "Knows" as the base of the pyramid, followed by "Knows how" and "Shows how." "Does" is the top level of the pyramid (Figure 19.1). The "Shows how" level relates to a demonstration of learning, for example, in objective simulated clinical examinations (OSCEs) or with simulations. The highest level, "Does," again relates to transfer to practice in the workplace (Miller, 1990).

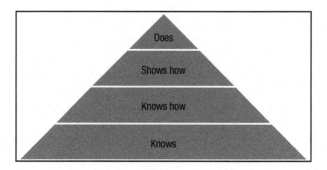

**Figure 19.1** Miller's pyramid.

*Source:* Adapted from Miller, G. E. (1990). The assessment of clinical skills competence performance. *Academic Medicine, 65*(9), 63–67. https://doi.org/10.1097/00001888-199009000-00045

A comparison of the levels, phases, and features of these frameworks confirms that the lowest level of learner evaluation relates to assessing learner response and if information was obtained. The highest level involves translation to practice and improving health outcomes. The intermediate levels, or phases, contain the observation of the learned behavior, that is, performance. Most learner evaluations during SBLE, whether formative or summative, are recognized as falling into these "in-between" levels (Figure 19.2).

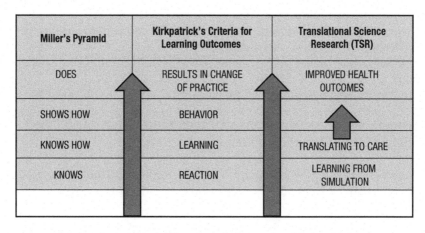

**Figure 19.2** Selected frameworks for evaluation strategies.

## ▶ FORMATIVE EVALUATION

Formative evaluation is one tool used in simulation-based assessment and is designed to measure students' grasp of material during the course (Arrogante et al., 2021). Generally, formative evaluation does not result in a recorded grade or assessment score. Rather, it provides the learners with important feedback to guide them in obtaining appropriate KSAs relative to the study topic. This type of assessment accomplishes multiple goals. It allows the educator to both identify and to improve student deficiencies. It also encourages self-reflection and assessment on the part of the students so that they may have a more accurate picture of their strengths and weaknesses before a final evaluation (Arrogante et al., 2021; INACSL Standards Committee, 2021a). These tools can be self-assessing questionnaires or behavioral assessments (Santomauro et al., 2020).

## ▶ SUMMATIVE EVALUATION

Summative evaluation, unlike formative assessment, is designed to measure the level of knowledge or skill acquisition that has been achieved at the conclusion of learning. According to the HSSOBP™, summative evaluation "focuses on the measurement of outcomes or achievement of objectives at a discrete moment in time, for example, at the end of a program of study" (INACSL Standards Committee, 2021, p. 54). The third type of evaluation, called "high-stakes" evaluation, refers to a simulation designed as an assessment tool that carries with it significant implications, such as a grade or progression through a program (INACSL Standards Committee, 2021a). An example of a high-stakes evaluation could be the commonly known objective structured clinical evaluation or OSCE, which can be used as formative, summative, or high-stakes evaluation (García-Mayor et al., 2021). There is increasing interest in using simulation not only for training, but also as the basis for learner evaluation. Because a high-stakes evaluation has the potential to lead to significant consequences for the learner, it is essential that the following required elements of best practice be included:

- to determine competence, gaps in knowledge, skills, and behaviors, and/or to identify safety issues
- based on specific learner objectives
- after the potential implications have been explained to the learners
- with predetermined learner actions that would result in the conclusion of the SBLE
- after the SBLE has been pilot-tested
- by formally trained evaluator(s)
- after the learner has had the opportunity for multiple exposures to various SBLEs, including those with summative evaluations
- use an evaluation instrument previously tested with similar and/or comparable populations
- if using an observation-based instrument, consider using more than one rater or evaluator for each learner, either directly observed or through video recording
- the evaluator be formally trained using a tool that has been previously tested for validity and reliability (INACSL Standards Committee, 2021a, p. 55)

The need remains for future research on reliable and valid tools to assess simulation, whether from a formative, summative, or high-stakes standpoint.

### Evidence-Based Simulation Practice 19.1

Brackney et al. (2017) studied simulation evaluation for senior-level bachelor of science in nursing (BSN) students ($N = 41$) in a capstone course and the National Council Licensure Examination for Registered Nurses (NCLEX-RN™) first-time passing rates. The faculty evaluated students' performance in simulation and the faculty evaluations were strongly correlated with NCLEX-RN success. Specifically, students who were evaluated as "lacking confidence" and who had "flawed skills" were less likely to pass the NCLEX-RN on the first attempt.

## ▶ SELF-EVALUATION

Self-evaluation commonly occurs in debriefing after SBLE, but can also occur during SBLE in which structured feedback is provided. Effective debriefing provides the opportunity to participate in critical reflection and is a valuable learning experience that occurs individually during the experience of the simulation and during debriefing (Lee et al., 2020). Self-evaluation may be enhanced by recording the simulation activities. Previous self-efficacy studies with nursing students and medical students indicate that abilities may be overrated (Hawker et al., 2022; Leighton et al., 2021; Massoth et al., 2019).

One tool that has been validated with undergraduate nursing students is the Simulation Effectiveness Tool (SET). This tool allows students to evaluate the SBLE as well as the facilitator. The evaluation includes questions that also allow the student to critically reflect on the experience and perform a self-assessment of performance. The INACSL Board of Directors (2013) clarified the terminology and described other items such as prebriefing to be included as part of the evaluation. As a result of this clarification by the INACSL, the SET was modified (SET-M). This validated tool measures students' perceptions of the SBLE (Leighton et al., 2015, p. 323).

## ▶ PEER EVALUATION

Adding participants' evaluation of each other has some benefits. Practitioners or students working collaboratively can learn from each other and develop the ability to make judgments and give and receive constructive criticism. Peer evaluation must be well designed to limit the possibility of "a sense of incompetence, anxiety and a hostile learning environment" (Tornwall, 2018, p. 266). Well-designed collaborative learning and assessment has proven effective in assisting nursing students with learning both theoretical information and clinical skills (Zhang & Cui, 2018).

## ▶ EVALUATION IN SIMULATION-BASED TEAM TRAINING

There are significant challenges to evaluating both the performance and the effectiveness of SBTT. Healthcare teams are complex entities, often comprising ever-changing members in a high-stress environment. The Agency for Healthcare Research and Quality (AHRQ; 2017) defines a *team* as:

- consisting of two or more individuals
- having specific roles, performing specific tasks, and interacting to achieve a common goal or outcome
- making decisions
- possessing specialized knowledge and skill and often functioning under conditions of high workload
- differing from small groups in that teams embody a collective action arising out of task interdependence

One of the most significant challenges in SBTT evaluation is the need to assess the KSAs of the team members within the context of the team. Team performance and effectiveness must also be considered. If individual team members do not have the KSAs needed to perform the tasks associated with their respective roles, the effectiveness of the team may be impacted. Most of the existing SBTT evaluation tools are observational checklists that focus primarily on the "soft skills" and overall team characteristics rather than the outcomes. For example, one of the most used team frameworks is the Team Strategies and Tools to Enhance Performance and Patient Safety™ (TeamSTEPPS™), developed by the AHRQ. (Although not technically an evaluation tool, TeamSTEPPS has been used as the foundation for many SBTT evaluation tools.) The following are the four key skills emphasized in TeamSTEPPS:

- leadership
- communication

- situational monitoring
- mutual support (TeamSTEPPS 2.0, 2019)

TeamSTEPPS provides a Team Performance Observation Tool (TPOT) that may be used in the evaluation of a team simulation activity. The TPOT uses a 5-point Likert scale to measure team structure, communication, leadership, situation monitoring, and mutual support, and provides a summative team performance rating that is useful in providing feedback (AHRQ, 2014). Other SBTT tools available evaluate the nontechnical skills that are part of team behaviors, including the Team Emergency Assessment Measure (TEAM), the Simulation Team Assessment Tool (STAT), and the Individual Teamwork Observation and Feedback Tool (iTOFT). All of these tools have been utilized in a number of different studies and with many different interprofessional education (IPE) simulations. Research has confirmed the existence of medical errors that occur due to the communication and nontechnical skills associated with teams (Neilsen et al., 2021). Utilization of validated tools to evaluate these behaviors during SBTT can help inform practice improvement initiatives.

## ▶ EVALUATING THE SIMULATION ACTIVITY

Another topic within the simulation community involves evaluating the simulation activity itself as well as the facilitator conducting the SBLE. Evaluation of the simulation activity is an important part of continuing quality improvement (INACSL Standards Committee, 2021). Since the debriefing process is a vital part of the learning process in simulation, it is crucial for the facilitator to also be evaluated (Leighton et al., 2018). There are many ways to evaluate simulation activities, from direct observation by peers to formal and informal surveys and questionnaires. It is important to consider instruments or tools with established validity and reliability instead of attempting to develop a new instrument (Adamson, 2014). There are a handful of SBLE assessment tools that address facilitator and activity effectiveness. The Simulation Design Scale (SDS) allows the participant not only to self-assess participation, but also to assess the effectiveness of the simulation activity. Another tool, the Educational Practices in Simulation Scale (EPSS), contains elements that assess for best practices in SBLE, including active learning, high expectations, diversity in learning, and collaboration (Jeffries, 2012). The Debriefing Assessment for Simulation in Healthcare© (DASH©) is a tool aimed at evaluating the debriefing experience following simulation (Center for Medical Simulation, 2014). Another validated tool is the Facilitator Competency Rubric (FCR). This tool has five measured constructs and follows Benner's novice-to-expert model (Leighton et al., 2018). This is a validated and reliable tool.

## ▶ EVALUATION INSTRUMENTS

Instruments for evaluating individual and team SBLE performance continue to be developed and tested. There is ongoing need for reliable and valid tools to evaluate simulation, as well as standardization in how selected tools are used (Higham et al., 2019).

- *Validity* relates to the degree that the instrument or tool measures what it is intended to measure, for example, communication skills.
- *Reliability* is the consistency and dependability of the measurement of a particular attribute by the instrument or tool (Polit & Beck, 2021).
- More multisite studies are needed to establish the validity and reliability of many tools, and choosing a tool that is already developed supports this initiative (MacLean et al., 2018).

■ Simulation evaluation instruments vary in design and levels of measurement. As noted in Table 19.1, these may include Likert scales with rankings from 0 to 5, scoring rubrics outlining expected behaviors linked to a score, or dichotomous scales of 0 to 1 (did not meet or met). In deciding the most appropriate tool to use, the most recently reported reliability and validity should be considered in addition to the objective of the evaluation (MacLean et al., 2018).

## ▶ SUMMARY

This chapter has explored concepts and tools for evaluating the performance and effectiveness of SBLE at the individual and team levels, with some discussions related to the need to move to the higher levels of organizational and system impact. Although a variety of SBLE, SBTT, and simulation activity evaluation tools exist, the need remains for valid and reliable tools that will measure organizational impact, as it relates to patient safety and translation from simulation to the practice setting (Armenia et al., 2018; Lewis et al., 2019). Data measuring outcomes are needed to determine the overall effectiveness of the SBLE, including demonstration of translation to practice within organizations and the overall healthcare system.

## ● CASE STUDY 19.1

An academic medical university is planning an interdisciplinary professional education simulation activity involving medical students, nursing students, physician assistant students, and pharmacology students. The simulation will consist of teams of four, with one from each discipline. The scenarios are designed for specific behaviors, such as effective communication, teamwork and collaboration, procedural skill, and critical thinking. Evaluations consist of facilitator input at debriefing and self-assessment of performance and the activity with an online questionnaire. Results are positive, but the facilitators are determined to improve the evaluative results with peer evaluation and measurement of the achievement of the learning outcomes of effective communication, teamwork and collaboration, procedural skill, and critical thinking.

## ● CASE STUDY DISCUSSION

There are several ways that the facilitators can most effectively evaluate students' performance. The choice of a rubric could be time-intensive and should involve an expert from each discipline observing the simulation either in real time, remotely, or on video. Establishing interrater reliability by requiring another faculty member to review the simulation independently is desirable, especially if this type of activity may be used in the future for high-stakes or summative assessments. Programmed menu items allow for assessment while running the simulation and can be assimilated with data retrieval to evaluate the learning for the course as a whole, to identify knowledge gaps, and to improve curriculum development. Simulation offers opportunities to evaluate learning in the cognitive, affective, and psychomotor domains, not just participants' reactions to the activity itself.

1. A faculty member is planning a formative simulation activity. When is the BEST time for this activity to occur?

   A. At the beginning of the course before any learning has occurred
   B. Near the end of the course, but before the final evaluations
   C. Shortly after the content has been taught in class
   D. As part of the final evaluation and grading process

2. A faculty member plans to evaluate simulation participants according to Kirkpatrick's levels of evaluation. In order to determine that the participant has reached level 4, what should be the focus of the evaluation?

   A. The participant's satisfaction with the simulation experience
   B. The participant's perception of their learning following the simulation
   C. The change noted in the participant's behavior following the simulation
   D. The change in outcomes noted in patient care following the simulation

3. A faculty member has asked where to begin in creating an effective learner evaluation for their planned simulation-based learning experience (SBLE). Which of the following would you say is the first step in this process?

   A. Use an evaluation that has been used successfully before
   B. Identify the learning objectives to be evaluated
   C. Assess the background and knowledge level of the learners
   D. Conduct statistical item analysis to determine reliability

4. Which situation would be MOST appropriate to use a checklist-type evaluation instrument?

   A. Summative assessment of a nursing student inserting a urinary catheter
   B. Summative assessment of a staff nurse's ability to recognize an unstable patient
   C. Formative assessment of a resident's ability to achieve an accurate differential diagnosis
   D. High-stakes evaluation of a medical student's ability to empathically communicate with a patient

5. A simulation educator is setting up a new summative evaluation and wants to ensure interrater reliability. The BEST method to ensure interrelated reliability would be:

   A. Two students evaluating each other
   B. A checklist of summative evaluation
   C. Two facilitators evaluating a simulation using the same instrument
   D. Two facilitators evaluating a simulation using different instruments

6. Additional rigorous research and evidence-based practice appraisals are needed to ensure:

   A. Students are satisfied with the simulation learning experiences
   B. Faculty are competent in providing simulation learning experiences
   C. Simulation is meeting learners' outcomes
   D. Simulation is impacting safe patient care

## 1.  C) Shortly after the content has been taught in class

Formative learning and evaluations are not the final grade and are best done after the content has been taught in order to reinforce the knowledge. It should not be done at the beginning before there is adequate grasp of the knowledge.

## 2.  D) The change in outcomes noted in patient care following the simulation

The fourth level of Kirkpatrick's learning achievement theory is application in the clinical area or translation to practice. The first level of Kirkpatrick's levels of learning is reaction to the simulation, which would be satisfaction. The second level is learning and the third level is change in behavior.

## 3.  B) Identify the learning objectives to be evaluated

Start with the learning outcomes that need to be accomplished. Using a reliable and previously used evaluation may work if the evaluation aligns with the student learning outcomes. The SBLE should be at the right level for student learning, but the student learning outcomes should be leveled so that is known.

## 4.  A) Summative assessment of a nursing student inserting a urinary catheter

Inserting a Foley is a procedure that lends itself to a checklist. The ability to recognize a deteriorating patient condition is clinical reasoning and does not lend itself to a checklist. Differential diagnoses are done using clinical judgment or an algorithm, not a checklist. Communication is an affective skill and is difficult to categorize on a checklist.

## 5.  C) Two facilitators evaluating a simulation using the same instrument

Interrater reliability can be confirmed by two evaluators looking at the same scenario and evaluating the scenario with a single evaluative form and then comparing the results. Students are usually not responsible for summative evaluations. A checklist can still be subjective if it is not validated. Using different instruments does not assist with interrelator reliability.

## 6.  D) Simulation is impacting safe patient care

Long-term studies are needed to ensure that simulation is positively impacting patient care. Evidence demonstrates that students' perceptions are positive and that the faculty is competent and meeting student learning outcomes.

7. An expert simulation educator understands that a high-quality simulation learning experiences should begin with:

   A. Resource management
   B. Clear learning objectives
   C. Participants in mind
   D. Secure technology needs

8. When choosing an evaluation tool for a simulation learning experience, it should reflect:

   A. The students involved
   B. The technology used
   C. The faculty's expertise
   D. The learning domain

9. Needed simulation research should be focused on which level of evaluation?

   A. Reaction
   B. Learning
   C. Behavior
   D. Results

10. An educator wants to evaluate learning that ultimately impacts patient care. What level of translational research should be the focus of the evaluation?

    A. T-1
    B. T-2
    C. T-3
    D. T-4

*(See answers next page.)*

## 7. B) Clear learning objectives

Starting with the student learning outcomes provides guidance to the learning activities and the type of simulation being used. Resource management, participants, and technology needs are important but not the first considerations needed.

## 8. D) The learning domain

The tool should reflect what the purpose of the learning is and this includes the domains of learning such as cognitive, psychomotor, or affective. The technology is chosen after the learning domain has been identified; faculty expertise is then considered.

## 9. D) Results

The results and the application to patient care are the ultimate outcomes of simulation learning. Reaction, learning, and behavior all lead up to results.

## 10. C) T-3

T-3 is that the results of the simulation activity improve patient outcomes. As the name implies, evidence is required to prove the translation to practice, and this requires measurable outcomes at every level. T-1 is translation to humans, T-2 is translation to patients, and T-4 is not a level.

# REFERENCES

Adamson, K. A. (2014). Evaluation tools and metrics for simulations. In P. R. Jeffries (Ed.), *Clinical simulations in nursing education: Advanced concepts, trends, and opportunities* (pp. 145–163). Wolters Kluwer, Lippincott Williams & Wilkins.

Agency for Healthcare Research and Quality. (2012). *Advancing Patient Safety.* https://www.ahrq.gov/patient-safety/reports/advancing/index.html

Agency for Healthcare Research and Quality. (2014). *Team performance observation tool.* https://www.ahrq.gov/teamstepps/instructor/reference/tmpot.html

Agency for Healthcare Research and Quality. (2017). *Simulation in education: Defining terms.* https://www.ahrq.gov/professionals/quality-patient-safety/patient-safety-resources/research/simulation-dictionary/index.html

Armenia, S., Thangamathesvaran, L., Caine, A. D., King, N., Kunac, A., & Merchant, A. M. (2018). The role of high-fidelity team-based simulation in acute care settings: A systematic review. *The Surgery Journal, 4*(03), e136–e151.

Arrogante, O., Gonzalez-Romero, G. M., Lopez-Torre, E. M., Carrion-Garcia, L., & Polo, A. (2021). Comparing formative and summative simulation-based assessment in undergraduate nursing students: Nursing competency acquisition and clinical simulation satisfaction. *BMC Nursing, 20,* 92. https://doi.org/10.1186/s12912-021-00614-2

Ashcraft, A. S., Opton, L., Bridges, R. A., Caballero, S., Veesart, A., & Weaver, C. (2013). Simulation evaluation using a modified Lasater clinical judgment rubric. *Nursing Education Perspectives, 34*(2), 122–126. https://doi.org/10.5480/1536-5026-34.2.122

Brackney, D. E., Hayes, L. S., Dawson, T., & Koontz, A. (2017). Simulation performance and National Council Licensure Examination for Registered Nurses outcomes: Field research perspectives. *Creative Nursing, 23*(4), 255–265. https://doi.org/10.1891/1078-4535.23.4.255

Bryant, K., Aebersold, M. L., Jeffries, P. R., & Kardong-Edgren, S. (2020). Innovations in simulation: Nursing leaders' exchange of best practices. *Clinical Simulation in Nursing, 41*(C), 33–40. https://doi.org/10.1016/j.ecns.2019.09.002

Cant, R. P., & Cooper, S. J. (2017). The value of simulation-based learning in pre-licensure nurse education: A state-of-the-art review and meta-analysis. *Nurse Education in Practice, 27,* 45–62.

Cantrell, M. A., Franklin, A., Leighton, K., & Carlson, A. (2017, December). The evidence in simulation based learning experiences in nursing education and practice: An umbrella review. *Clinical Simulation in Nursing, 13*(12), 634–667. http://doi.org/10.1016/j.ecns.2017.08.004

Center for Medical Simulation. (2014). *Debriefing assessment for simulation in healthcare (DASH).* https://harvardmedsim.org

Chappell, K., & Koithan, M. (2012). Validating clinical competence. *Journal of Continuing Education in Nursing, 43,* 293–294. https://doi.org/10.3928/00220124-20120621-02

Cooper, S. J., & Cant, R. P. (2013). Measuring non-technical skills of medical emergency teams: An update on the validity and reliability of the team emergency assessment measure (TEAM). *Resuscitation, 85*(1), 31–33. https://doi.org/10.1016/j.resuscitation.2013.08.276

García-Mayor, S., Quemada-González, C., León-Campos, Á., Kaknani-Uttumchandani, S., Gutiérrez-Rodríguez, L., del Mar Carmona-Segovia, A., & Martí-García, C. (2021). Nursing students' perceptions on the use of clinical simulation in psychiatric and mental health nursing by means of objective structured clinical examination (OSCE). *Nurse Education Today, 100,* 104866. https://doi.org/10.1016/j.nedt.2021.104866

Griswold, S., Fralliccardi, A., Boulet, J., Moadel, T., Franzen, D., Auerbach, M., Hart, D., Goswami, V., Hui, J., & Gordon, J. A. (2018). Simulation-based education to ensure provider competency within the health care system. *Academic Emergency Medicine, 25*(2), 168–176.

Hanshaw, S. L., & Dickerson, S. S. (2020). High fidelity simulation evaluation studies in nursing education: A review of the literature. *Nurse Education in Practice, 46,* 1–9.

Hawker, C., Gould, D., Courtenay, M., & Edwards, D. (2022). Undergraduate nursing students' education and training in aseptic technique: A mixed methods systematic review. *Journal of Advanced Nursing, 78*, 63–77.

Hayden, J., Keegan, M., Kardong-Edgren, S., & Smiley, R. A. (2014). Reliability and validity testing of the Creighton competency evaluation instrument for use in the NCSBN national simulation study. *Nursing Education Perspectives, 35*(4), 244–252. https://doi.org/10.5480/13-1130.1

Higham, H., Greig, P. R., Rutherford, J., Vincent, L., Young, D., & Vincen, C. (2019). Observer-based tools for non-technical skills assessment in simulated and real clinical environments in healthcare: A systematic review. *BMJ Quality & Safety, 28*, 672–686. https://doi.org/10.1136/bmjqs-2018-008565

International Nursing Association for Clinical Simulation and Learning Board of Directors. (2013). Standards for best practice: Simulation. *Clinical Simulation in Nursing, 9*(6 Suppl), Si–S32. https://doi.org/10.1016/j.ecns.2013.05.008

International Nursing Association for Clinical Simulation and Learning Standards Committee, McMahon, E., Jimenez, F. A., Lawrence, K., & Victor, J. (2021a, September). Healthcare simulation standards of best practice™ evaluation of learning and performance. *Clinical Simulation in Nursing, 58*, 54–56. https://doi.org/10.1016/j.ecns.2021.08.016

International Nursing Association for Clinical Simulation and Learning Standards Committee, Miller, C., Deckers, C., Jones, M., Wells-Beede, E., & McGee, E. (2021b, September). Healthcare simulation standards of best practice™ outcomes and objectives. *Clinical Simulation in Nursing, 58*, 40–44. https://doi.org/10.1016/j.ecns.2021.08.013

International Nursing Association for Clinical Simulation and Learning Standards Committee, Watts, P., I., McDermott, D. S., Alinier, G., Charnetski, M., & Nawathe, P. A. (2021c, September). Healthcare simulation standards of best practice™ simulation design. *Clinical Simulation in Nursing, 58*, 14–21. https://doi.org/10.1016/j.ecns.2021.08.009

Jeffries, P. R. (2012). *Simulation in nursing education: From conceptualization to evaluation* (2nd ed.). National League for Nursing.

Johnson, S., Coyer, F. M., & Nash, R. (2018). Kirkpatrick's evaluation of simulation and debriefing in health care education: A systematic review. *Journal of Nursing Education, 57*(7), 393–398.

Johnston, S., & Fox, A. (2020). Kirkpatrick's evaluation of teaching and learning approaches of workplace violence education programs for undergraduate nursing students: A systematic review. *Journal of Nursing Education, 59*(8), 439–447.

Kiernan, L. C. (2018). Evaluating competence and confidence using simulation technology. *Nursing, 48*(10), 45.

Kirkpatrick, D. L. (1998). *Evaluating training programs* (2nd ed.). Berrett-Koehler.

Lee, J., Lee, H., Kim, S., Choi, M., Ko, S., Bae, Y., & Kim, S. H. (2020). Debriefing methods and learning outcomes in simulation nursing education: A systematic review and meta-analysis. *Nurse Education Today, 87*, 104345. https://doi.org/10.1016/j.nedt.2020.104345

Leighton, K., Kardong-Edgren, S., McNelis, A. M., Fosey-Doll, C., & Sullo, E. (2021). Traditional clinical outcomes in prelicensure nursing education: An empty systematic review. *The Journal of Nursing Education, 60*(3), 136–142. https://doi.org/10.3928/01484834-20210222-03

Leighton, K., Mudra, V., & Gilbert, G. E. (2018). Development and psychometric evaluation of the facilitator competency rubric. *Nursing Education Perspectives, 39*(6), E3–E9.

Leighton, K., Ravert, P., Mudra, V., & Macintosh, C. (2015). Updating the simulation effectiveness tool: Item modifications and reevaluation of psychometric properties. *Nursing Education Perspectives, 36*(5), 317–323. https://doi.org/10.5480/15-1671

Lewis, K., Ricks, T., Rowin, A., Ndlovu, C., Goldstein, L., & McElvogue, C. (2019). Does simulation training for acute care nurses improve patient safety outcomes: A systematic review to inform evidence base practice. *Worldviews on Evidenced Based Nursing, 16*(5), 389–396.

Lioce, L. (Ed.), Lopreiato, J. (Founding Ed.), Downing, D., Chang, T. P., Robertson, J. M., Anderson, M., Diaz, D. A., Spain, A. E. (Assoc. Eds.), & the Terminology and Concepts Working Group. (2020, September). *Healthcare simulation dictionary* (2nd ed.). Agency for Healthcare Research and Quality. AHRQ Publication No. 20-0019. https://doi.org/10.23970/simulationv2

Lyk-Jensen, H. T., Dieckmann, P., Konge, L., Jepsen, R. M., Spanager, L., & Østergaard, D. (2016). Using a structured assessment tool to evaluate nontechnical skills of nurse anesthetists. *American Association of Nurse Anesthetists Journal, 84*(2), 122–127. PMID: 27311153

MacLean, S., Geddes, F., Kelly, M., & Della, P. (2018). Simulated patient training: Using inter-rater reliability to evaluate simulated patient consistency in nursing education. *Nurse Education Today, 62*, 85–90.

Massoth, C., Röder, H., Ohlenburg, H., Hessler, M., Zarbock, A., Popping, D. M., & Wenk, M. (2019). High-fidelity is not superior to low-fidelity simulation but leads to overconfidence in medical students. *BMC Medical Education, 19*(29). https://doi.org/10.1186/s12909-019-1464-7

Miller, G. E. (1990). The assessment of clinical skills competence performance. *Academic Medicine, 65*(9), 63–67. https://doi.org/10.1097/00001888-199009000-00045

Neilsen, R. P., Nikolasjen, L., Paltved, C., & Aagaard, R. (2021). Effect of simulation-based team training in airway management: A systematic review. *Anaesthesia, 76*, 1404–1415. https://doi.org/10.1111/anae.15375

Polit, D., & Beck, C. (2021). *Nursing research: Generating and assessing evidence for nursing practice* (11th ed.). Lippincott Williams & Wilkins.

Prion, S., & Haerling, K. A. (2021). Evaluation of simulation outcomes. *Annual Review of Nursing Research, 39*(1), 149–180. https://doi.org/10.1891/0739-6686.39.149

Reid, J., Stone, K., Brown, J., Caglar, D., Kobayashi, A., Lewis-Newby, M., Partridge, R., Seidel, K., & Quan, L. (2011). The simulation team assessment tool (STAT): Development, reliability and validation. *Resuscitation, 83*, 879–886. https://doi.org/10.1016/j.resuscitation.2011.12.012

Santomauro, C., Hill, A., McCurdie, T., & McGlashan, H. (2020). Improving the quality of evaluation data in simulation-based healthcare improvement projects. *Simulation in Healthcare: The Journal of the Society for Simulation in Healthcare, 15*(5), 341–355. https://doi.org/10.1097/SIH.0000000000000442

Simon, R., Raemer, D. B., & Rudolph, J. W. (2010). *Debriefing assessment for simulation in healthcare (DASH)© rater's handbook.* Center for Medical Simulation. https://harvardmedsim.org/wp-content/uploads/2017/01/DASH.handbook.2010.Final.Rev.2.pdf

So, H. Y., Chen, P. P., Wong, G. K. C., & Chan, T. T. N. (2019). Simulation in medical education. *Journal of the Royal College of Physicians of Edinburgh, 49*(1), 52–57. https://doi.org/10.4997/JRCPE.2019.112

Society for Simulation in Healthcare. (2021). *Certified healthcare simulation educator handbook.* https://www.ssih.org/Portals/48/Certification/CHSE_Docs/CHSE%20Handbook.pdf

TeamSTEPPS 2.0. (2019). *Content last reviewed June 2019.* Agency for Healthcare Research and Quality. https://www.ahrq.gov/teamstepps/instructor/index.html

Tornwall, J. (2018). Peer assessment practices in nurse education: An integrative review. *Nurse Education Today, 71*, 266–275.

Watts, P., Smith, T. S., Currie, E. R., Knight, C., & Bordelon, C., (2021). Simulating telehealth experiences in the neonatal care environment: Improving access to care. *Neonatal Network, 40*(6), 393–401. https://doi.org/10.1891/11-T-710

Webster, K. L. W., Tan, A. C., Unger, N., & Lazzara, E. H. (2020). Considerations and strategies for assessing: Simulation-based training in interprofessional education. In J. T. Paige, S. C. Sonesh, D. D. Garbee, & L. S. Bonanno (Eds.), *Healthcare simulation: Interprofessional team training and simulation* (pp. 121–134). Springer International Publishing. https://doi.org/10.1007/978-3-030-28845-7

Zhang, J., & Cui, Q. (2018). Collaborative learning in higher nursing education: A systematic review. *Journal of Professional Nursing, 34*(5), 378–388.

# Fostering Professional Development in Healthcare Simulation

Mary Ellen Smith Glasgow

*A mentor is someone who allows you to see the hope inside yourself.*

—Oprah Winfrey

> This chapter addresses Domain III: Educational Principles Applied to Simulation (Society for Simulation in Healthcare [SSH], 2021).

## ▶ LEARNING OUTCOMES

- Discuss the necessity of professional development in simulation education.
- Describe the roles and responsibilities of a simulation leader in an organization.
- Identify methods to disseminate simulation evidence for a wider audience.
- Review the role of a simulation educator mentor for novice educators.

## ▶ THE CONTEXT OF PROFESSIONAL DEVELOPMENT

Considering that members of any given profession maintain their professional status at the will of the society they serve, continuous professional expertise development is essential. To maintain professional status, a Certified Healthcare Simulation Educator® (CHSE®) needs to understand their service in the broader context of society.

Sullivan (2005) differentiates professionals from other workers by their responsibility to provide public goods such as healthcare. Called *civic professionals* (Sullivan, 2005), these individuals' work provides added value to the public and they are concerned with public values and identity. This then creates a social contract between the profession and the public, where the public grants status and authority to the profession for the service it provides within the society. A profession holds the trust of the society by maintaining civic contributions that remain current and beneficial through the profession's efficient and legitimate self-regulation (Sullivan, 2005). Opportunities for dialogue and scrutiny of the profession by society are expected; thus, the profession is compelled to continue to develop and grow in its civic contributions to society. This is accomplished by members of the profession engaging in professional development activities.

As professionals, faculty and clinicians in a simulation environment develop and maintain specified standards of practice in the provision of simulation healthcare education to healthcare providers through their professional organizations and societies. These standards are developed through ongoing critical analysis of best practices in the field of healthcare simulation and are continuously updated through rigorous scrutiny of the discipline. Such updates are then communicated to members of the profession through professional development activities that allow CHSEs to remain current in the discipline and meet their obligations to society as civic professionals.

Professional development is rooted in social learning, situated learning, and community of practice theories (Socolovsky et al., 2013; Zhou et al., 2016). The social learning theory proposes that for effective learning to occur individuals must believe that the benefits outweigh the costs of undertaking a new behavior and that they must have confidence in their ability to perform the new behavior. The new behavior must also be reinforced by other significant individuals (Bandura, 1977a). The situated learning theory asserts that learners should be provided with opportunities to develop, extend, and even simplify their skills and knowledge. Communities of practice, also referred to as professional communities and learning communities, are social structures where members update their knowledge, with an emphasis on person-to-person interaction, and which provide opportunities for professional development and networking across organizational boundaries (Brooks, 2010; Wenger et al., 2002). Simulation classes or cohorts can serve as such learning communities.

## ▶ STAYING CURRENT AND USING EVIDENCE IN HEALTHCARE SIMULATION

With an understanding of the importance of CHSEs' engagement in professional development, it is possible to explore how this can be accomplished by members of the profession. Staying current in practice is a matter of desire and curiosity. As professionals, CHSEs maintain a desire to provide the most effective educational experiences to healthcare providers who have a variety of learning styles. This desire is motivated by a curiosity that propels CHSEs to search for the most current evidence in the practice of their specialty. Keep in mind that evidence supporting the development of current professional practice takes a variety of forms, including the development of techniques, interpersonal and intrapersonal skills, and leadership and management skills. Most significant to the professional development of CHSEs is the importance of maintaining communication and support among other CHSEs. Independent, isolated professional development strategies must be further discussed among CHSEs well after the development event. With ongoing collegial support, through professional networking, professional development will directly impact the knowledge and practice of CHSEs (Margolis & Parboosingh, 2015).

The science of virtual simulation is just beginning to emerge and increased dramatically in use during the COVID-19 pandemic. The literature reveals a range of products, potential uses, and pilot studies related to virtual simulation; however, the learning outcomes have not been thoroughly established. Initial evidence indicates that virtual simulation improves learning outcomes; however, more evidence is needed to substantiate best practices in its development, methodology, and evaluation (Foronda et al., 2020).

Evidence of this is noted by Guillemin et al. (2009), who recognized the importance of desire and curiosity in stimulating professional development, particularly in health professions due to the ever-changing healthcare environment. They note that continuing professional development (CPD) provides development of necessary skills for success as a professional in the healthcare environment. Also, as health professionals gain expertise within their discipline, there is a need for CPD in areas such as leadership and management. These authors focused specifically on the use of CPD in helping health professionals develop ethically (Guillemin et al., 2009).

Yet focusing on the professional development of professionals may be limited, as discovered by Heller et al. (2012). These authors examined the relationships among professional development, teacher knowledge, practice, and learner achievement in a randomized study of 270 elementary school teachers and 7,000 students in six states. What the authors found was that professional development experiences may provide better educational outcomes when there is integration of learning content, student learning, and teaching. With this understanding, CHSEs are likely to benefit best from professional development activities that go beyond focusing solely on developing the professional, but rather include exploration of knowledge acquisition and learner experiences.

An example of utilization of evidence specific to the practice of the CHSE is provided by Brink et al. (2012). These authors provided an example of a simulated situation and the use of group supervision as a method of learning in the simulation environment. This was a qualitative study that explored participants' perceptions of the simulated, group supervision experience. Brink et al. found that participants had a sense of security in their engagement of the process, a positive response with collegial dialogue, a direct impact on values and attitudes, and a desire to further develop professional skills. Understanding this evidence, CHSEs can utilize the interventions used by Brink et al. to enhance their own practice in the development and provision of simulation scenarios.

Providing another example of the use of evidence to support the professional development of CHSEs, Roche et al. (2009) explored the need and use of workforce training in developing the skills of health professionals. Although their work focused on drug and alcohol care, the concepts they presented are transferable to the professional development needs of CHSEs, specifically the need for development to include acquisition of knowledge, attitudes, and skills. As CHSEs, it is important to utilize educational skills that are flexible enough to assess, develop, and adjust to any number of individual factors that influence learners' ability to grow from a simulation experience.

Ricketts and Fraher (2013) recognized the need for the training of healthcare professionals to be in line with reforms in healthcare delivery systems, as well as the need for an interprofessional workforce. Thus, it is important for CHSEs to develop understanding of organizational structures, systems, and culture, as well as the influence of policies and strategies on working conditions. This knowledge will help CHSEs in identifying opportunities to enhance their success within their organizations.

## ▶ PROMOTING AND LEADING EVIDENCE-BASED HEALTHCARE SIMULATION IN AN ORGANIZATION

As mentioned earlier, professional development includes a variety of topics. Understanding that healthcare simulation practices are most likely to occur within organizational systems, it is prudent for the CHSE to take advantage of professional development opportunities that enhance understanding of the context within which they practice. It has been noted that organizations can be considered social entities involving the interplay of individuals in order to reach specified goals (Scott, 2002). In order for CHSEs to succeed within the structures of their organizations, it is important for them to develop skills to navigate the elements of healthcare organizations.

Mulvey (2013) provided a perspective on the unique interplay among professional practitioners, their professional entities, and the employer as a triad in CPD. The CHSE needs to understand the tensions of all of these in order to effectively obtain and maintain resources, meet professional and organizational accrediting needs, and recruit and engage health professionals. An example of this is provided by Mulvey; the employer's focus is on finance, including the cost of training the employees, their time away from work, and the coverage needed when the employees are in simulation training. Their other concerns are the financial investment and the risk of training an employee who then leaves the organization (Mulvey, 2013). The CHSE needs to understand this fiscal perspective and be prepared to present a cost–benefit analysis within the organizational system, shifting the employer's perspective to "what if they stay and they are not trained?" (Mulvey, 2013).

An example of the importance of CHSEs' professional development in organizational leadership is provided by Kubitskey et al. (2012). Their study identified that the attrition among teacher participants fell under three general categories:

- a teaching assignment change
- organizational challenges
- personal challenges

Understanding these challenges upfront provides the CHSE an opportunity to take a leadership role to address these during the development of proposals for organizational implementation. Further, this is an example of utilization of evidence in the development of the CHSE. This study could be easily replicated to provide evidence on the positive outcomes of simulation education, thus supporting the cost–benefit analysis necessary for program sustainability within an organization.

Simmons et al. (2011) provided an example of the impact of an interprofessional educational program. The authors examined the use of five modules in teaching different topics and utilizing a variety of learning methods and teaching strategies. The authors noted the important role of immersion and experiential learning, interprofessional development to support practice, and anticipating change in educational and clinical practices. With an understanding of the evidence provided by Simmons et al., the CHSE can articulate to organizational leaders the significant role they can play in providing cost-effective educational programming, making a broader impact on patient care.

Foronda et al. (2020) noted that further evidence is needed in the emerging area of virtual simulation, with special attention to (a) examining its effects when integrated throughout the curriculum; (b) examining its effects when used in conjunction with manikin-based simulation; (c) determining the appropriate time and intervals of virtual simulation; (d) examining the retention of learning with virtual learning as opposed to other methods; and (e) examining if virtual simulation can be used as an alternative to a select number of clinical hours.

## ▶ CULTIVATING AND COMMUNICATING ONE'S PROFESSIONAL DEVELOPMENT EXPERTISE

Continuous self-improvement and learning is essential to improve national health. In order to acquire the requisite competencies, professional development competencies need to be integrated into all levels of health professions' curricula, along with appropriate experiential experiences and mentoring, as professional development is critical to advancing health. Healthcare providers need to learn to advocate for patients and engage in *crucial conversations* on behalf of patients in many instances. Crucial conversations are focused on tough issues, the conversations that people normally shy away from. In the professional realm, these conversations concern such issues as safety, productivity, diversity, and quality (Patterson et al., 2011). Healthcare simulation is an ideal forum to practice crucial conversations.

*Professional development* refers to a "positive change process" that healthcare providers experience in role performance, job roles, and better relationships with colleagues (Ismail & Arokiasamy, 2007). Safety, quality, and excellence underscore the need for healthcare providers to keep their skills and competencies current through ongoing professional development and career advancement (Adeniran et al., 2013). The influence of mentorship and self-efficacy on professional development deserves careful consideration. Mentors provide their protégés access to social networks that include sources of knowledge and professional contacts not available through normal channels. Self-efficacy influences how healthcare providers set career goals, influencing not only the initiation of behavior, but also the persistence of behavior in the presence of adversity. Moreover, self-efficacious individuals accept their roles as protégés with greater receptivity and willingness to engage in professional development activities, enhancing their capabilities and competencies (Adeniran et al., 2013).

Self-efficacy as a concept evolved from Albert Bandura's social cognitive theory (SCT) of behavior (Bandura, 1977b). SCT contends that individuals learn from the observation of others in a shared social environment. *Learning occurs if the role model is relevant, credible, and knowledgeable.* In the context of mentoring, protégés benefit from mentors who have the expert knowledge, social reference, credibility, and authority, leading to empowerment (Bandura, 1977b). Self-efficacy is considered one of the most powerful motivational predictors of success in one's career (Spurk & Abele, 2014).

In the context of healthcare simulation, the organizational leader in simulation needs to utilize best practices and maintain currency in the field, as well as serve as a role model. These can be accomplished in a variety of ways:

- conferences
- professional organizations
- continuing education
- literature on simulation
- mentors
- portfolio development

A list of resources, although not exhaustive, would include:

- International Nursing Association for Clinical Simulation and Learning (www.inacsl.org)
- Society for Simulation in Healthcare (www.ssih.org)
- International Meeting on Simulation in Healthcare (www.simulationinformation.com/ events/international-meeting-simulation-healthcare-imsh-2012)
- *Simulation in Healthcare* (www.journals.lww.com/simulationinhealthcare/pages/default .aspx)
- *Clinical Simulation in Nursing* (www.journals.elsevier.com/clinical-simulation-in-nursing/)
- *Journal of Simulation* (www.palgrave-journals.com/jos/journal/v3/n3/full/jos200910a .html)

In addition, there are simulation conferences associated with academic health centers and universities and experts in simulation who can provide consultation. Specific attention to one's professional development in simulation can lead to increased knowledge, skill, and confidence in leading simulation scenarios in an organization. Once mastery is obtained, the simulation expert has the responsibility to share their expertise via conferences and journal articles and by playing a mentoring or consultant role.

# ▶ THE MENTORING ROLE

Mentors support protégés to gain new competencies in a broad spectrum of skills, providing them challenges and opportunities to grow (Lombardo & Eichinger, 2009). Mentors promote learning and competencies that contribute to healthcare providers' vitality and success in their careers. Koberg et al. (1998) found that those who received mentoring reported higher levels of self-esteem and confidence than nonmentored healthcare professionals. Further, mentoring facilitates critical thinking, a connection to practice supporting professional development that can influence healthcare. This is especially true in the faculty/student role with respect to simulation. Further, Walton et al. (2011) noted that the faculty who, in their respective roles, function as role models and mentors also need to use evidence-based teaching in their simulation activities to effectively convey the art and science of simulation. Walton et al. (2011) argued that the faculty do not have adequate evidence-based resources on how students learn through simulation. Walton et al. suggested the use of a midrange conceptual model, negotiating the role of the professional nurse, as this particular model of professional socialization assists faculty in facilitating students' development during simulation learning activities, addressing such concepts as:

- feeling like an imposter
- trial and error
- taking the role seriously
- transference
- professionalization

Faculty strategies for each concept phase range from "[v]alidating students' feelings, debriefing with gentleness, role modeling expectations, asking questions about self-improvement and assisting students with visualizing goals" (Walton et al., 2011, p. 301).

Benner et al. (2010) supported a three-pronged approach needed in the professional role. These three attributes (Figure 20.1) are vital to the development of critical reasoning and professional development.

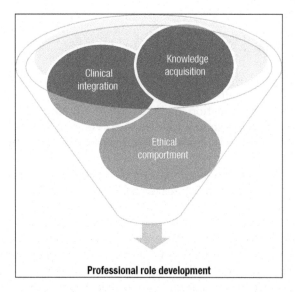

**Figure 20.1** Benner et al. (2010) three-pronged approach needed in the professional role.

In addition, fostering the professional development of healthcare providers requires experiential and situated learning, best conducted in a simulated environment, as these individuals must be prepared for the actual clinical situations or crucial conversations marked by uncertainty in the real world (Crider & McNiesh, 2011).

## ▶ MENTORING AND SUPPORT DURING COVID-19

The COVID-19 pandemic has projected the society into an unprecedented era characterized by feelings of helplessness and loss of control. Among healthcare providers, these feelings are magnified. COVID-19 has strained organizational resources to provide support to nurses and other clinicians. Even hospitals with built-in support systems for clinicians experiencing moral distress may be hard-pressed to provide this support during the pandemic. In a pandemic, resources are allocated to lifesaving treatments, and many of these programs are disrupted. In some cases, during the COVID-19 pandemic, visitation polices have been restricted to minimize the risk of spreading the disease over the interests of patients' need for emotional support. Frontline workers have experienced and witnessed intense suffering as a result, which not only have caused moral distress, but the constant barrage of traumatic events has resulted in nurses experiencing posttraumatic stress disorder (PTSD) and other mental health disorders. Support that is readily available and offered without judgment will be an important intervention at this critical time. Ethics consultations can also help healthcare providers reconcile their feelings of moral distress. Many organizations also offer a peaceful place in their institutions for nurses to decompress, listen to music, or meditate. These short quiet breaks are certainly helpful during a busy shift; however, healthcare providers will need to engage in self-care and to support each other. Colleagues can be a huge source of support by encouraging others to express emotion, verbalize feelings, and offer reassurance. In these instances, "Are you okay?" is an important intervention.

In its most basic form, mentorship addresses *relationship building*. Mentorship builds a supportive relationship that is developed by the experienced healthcare provider and novice clinician or student to assist them in acclimating to the practice environment. During the COVID-19 pandemic, mentoring resources were and are strained as leaders in the education and practice environments focus on organizational needs. Times of crisis may require a different form of mentoring to build and sustain relationships (Krofft & Stuart, 2021). Future simulations may focus on knowledge and experience gained during the pandemic.

## ▶ DEVELOPMENT OF THE PORTFOLIO

Packaging one's self to effectively communicate and capture one's work is very important to advancing one's career. The professional portfolio or dossier is one vehicle to display one's work when applying for appointments, certifications, promotions, and tenure. A portfolio or dossier should include sample publications, grant submissions, awards, syllabi, evaluations, simulation scenarios, photos, and recommendation letters. A portfolio or dossier is also a practical way to reflect upon and document one's work with respect to teaching, research, and service. The value of self-reflection of one's work cannot be underscored. The process lends itself to deep self-analysis—it provides a lens for the individual and the reviewer to analyze one's accomplishments in the area of simulation (Seldin & Miller, 2009). In recent years, electronic portfolios have come into use in institutions as a means for students to display their work and demonstrate competency related to writing, clinical objectives, and so on. The portfolio should involve the efforts of the candidate and the advice of their mentor in order to showcase their work in the best possible light, in addition to providing the reviewers with insight into the candidate's strengths, accomplishments, and work. Many institutions have requirements for the portfolio in terms of format and content. Typically, a philosophy, one's objectives, examples of work, reflections, and so on are required at some level (Wittmann-Price, 2012).

## ▶ SUMMARY

The process of professional development is best conducted in the formative years of one's education so healthcare providers can have maximum impact on the profession and health. It is also known that professional development is largely contextual—different settings will require different expectations and different practices. Therefore, a variety of professional development experiences are recommended in one's educational journey. Simulation provides a *dress rehearsal* for *real* leadership concerns, crucial conversations, ethical dilemmas, and advocacy issues.

**Simulation Teaching Tip 20.1**

Prebriefing should be conducted by a qualified simulation facilitator who is knowledgeable of best practices.

An essential element of a productive simulation is presimulation preparation time since better prepared learners are more effective. The prebriefing should encourage reflective practice in the debriefing. In essence, "the better the pre-brief-the better the debrief and that equals more learning" (McDermott, 2016, p. 224).

 ## CASE STUDY 20.1

**Colleague Who Is Unprepared for Class/Lab**

You are coteaching with Dr. Smith, a part-time adjunct faculty member. Dr. Smith is frequently unprepared for the class, Simulation Healthcare Experiences, which they are providing to physician assistant students. You have worked with Dr. Smith for less than a year but this level of preparation is unacceptable. Dr. Smith always has an excuse for their lack of preparation and frequently bluffs.

*Note: This case can be adapted for any work setting.*

**Case Study Objective:**

Engage in a crucial conversation with your colleague regarding their lack of preparation.

**Checklist:**

▪ Objectively state personal experience with concrete examples in a clear, concise manner.
▪ Address personal feelings.
▪ Use "I" statements.
▪ Remain calm.
▪ Listen actively.
▪ Summarize a crucial conversation indicating that you would no longer rearrange your schedule.
 ● Set firm boundaries with Dr. Smith regarding class preparation.
 ● Report to the chair or dean if not corrected.

 ## CASE STUDY 20.2

**Mentor and Faculty Colleague for a Graduate Certified Healthcare Simulation Educator (CHSE)**

You are participating in a skills simulation session with your colleague, Dr. Reilly, who teaches another section. You note that Dr. Reilly becomes sarcastic with male learners when they ask what you believe to be appropriate questions. Dr. Reilly is especially openly hostile with two male diverse students. You have witnessed this behavior before. You are concerned.

**Case Study Objective:**

Engage in a crucial conversation with your colleague regarding their defensive and sarcastic behavior.

*(continued)*

**Checklist:**
- ▪ Objectively summarize observations in a private setting.
- ▪ Explicitly address unprofessional behavior.
- ▪ Use "I" statements.
- ▪ Remain calm.
- ▪ Listen actively.
- ▪ Role-model the appropriate way to respond to questions.
- ▪ Offer faculty development resources.
- ▪ Summarize crucial conversation indicating that they must maintain a professional demeanor and open/trusting learning environment for students and explain the consequences if not maintained.
  - ● Report repeated unprofessional behavior to the chair or dean.
  - ● Report the observations to a Title IX officer for further investigation.

1. The expert healthcare simulation educator understands the governing principle of simulation education when they state:

   A. "Simulation is routine learning for health professionals."
   B. "Simulation assists society at large."
   C. "Simulation's goal is better learning outcomes."
   D. "Using simulation assists in procedural practice."

2. A simulation educator would like to develop a social contract with learners and should include:

   A. Students understanding their roles
   B. Society supporting the students' role
   C. Society trusting the works of the student
   D. Students being concerned with public values

3. Simulation educators understand that they are responsible for maintaining standards of practice by:

   A. Ensuring experts teach simulation to novice educators
   B. Critical analysis of best practice
   C. Solidifying practices used successfully
   D. Maintaining a specific set of skills

4. In academia, simulation educators understand that continuous professional development (CPD) in simulation assists professionals to improve in:

   A. Career advancement
   B. Debriefing techniques
   C. Effective communication
   D. The art of moulage

5. A simulation educator asks their mentor what method would be best to advance from an assistant to an associate professor of healthcare simulation. The mentor should advise the simulation educator to:

   A. Participate in continuous professional development (CPD)
   B. Take online teaching courses from another university
   C. Use higher fidelity when teaching advanced students
   D. Perform critical analysis of teaching outcomes

6. The novice simulation educator needs additional mentoring about continuous professional development (CPD) for healthcare simulation educators when they state that CPD:

   A. "Increases knowledge about systems, structures, and organizational cultures."
   B. "Addresses basic knowledge skills, and attitudes."
   C. "Increases engagement in the learning processes."
   D. "Promotes learning outcomes for teachers and students."

## 1.  C) "Simulation's goal is better learning outcomes."

The goal of simulation education is to reach the learning outcomes of healthcare students. Simulation may assist society because professionals learn well through simulation, but the goal is learning. Simulation is not just for procedures and is not routine.

## 2.  C) Society trusting the works of the student

Society entrusts the service work of individuals and credentials them. Students do need to understand their roles and public values in all aspects, and society should support the student's role of becoming a healthcare professional; however, the major issue is trust.

## 3.  B) Critical analysis of best practice

Critically analyzing best practices for simulation is the best method for simulation educators to keep using best practices in teaching students, not just novice simulation educators. Expert teachers may or may not be using best practices. Solidifying practices used successfully does not analyze those practices for more up-to-date techniques. Having a specific skill set means that those skills may need to be updated when new evidence is produced.

## 4.  A) Career advancement

CPD assists in career advancement. Learning new debriefing techniques, effective communication, and increasing moulage skills are all good competencies, but career advancement is the most valuable outcome for academic simulation educators.

## 5.  A) Participate in continuous professional development (CPD)

Participating in CPD will increase the networking and opportunity for scholarship and provide examples of simulation teaching excellence. Online courses may assist in promotion if they contribute to a degree. Analyzing outcomes is always good for process improvement. Fidelity should be used in relationship to the student learning outcomes.

## 6.  B) "Addresses basic knowledge skills, and attitudes."

CPD addresses more than basic knowledge, skills, and attitudes. CPD addresses knowledge about systems, structures, and organizational cultures. CPD promotes learning and increases engagement.

7. An expert simulation educator understands that for simulation development they should consider their organization's:

   A. Financial burden and employee compensation
   B. Career trajectory and professional growth
   C. Future organizational structure and changes
   D. Agendas of management and leadership

8. The simulation educator is choosing to practice crucial conversations in professional healthcare situations with advanced learners. A common issue to highlight in the scenario is:

   A. Promotion
   B. Diversity
   C. Compensation
   D. Leadership

9. The simulation educator understands that the graduate student needs further understanding when they list which of the following attributes in developing self-efficacy in simulation?

   A. Relevancy
   B. Credibility
   C. Knowledge
   D. Critical thinking

10. The simulation educator understands that the third step of negotiating a professional role that can be fostered in a simulation scenario is:

    A. Feeling like an imposter
    B. Taking the role seriously
    C. Trial and error
    D. Transference

## 7. C) Future organizational structure and changes

The future of the organization will affect the simulation programming. Financial issues are important to maintain a simulation program. Career trajectory and professional growth of simulation educators are important but must be supported by the organization in which they are employed. Agendas of leadership and management are important in the development of simulation programs, but people can easily change. Future considerations will position the simulation program well to thrive.

## 8. B) Diversity

Diversity is a common issue that comes to light in crucial conversations. Promotion, compensation, and leadership are other issues that possibly can be part of a crucial conversation but are usually not as sensitive.

## 9. D) Critical thinking

Critical thinking is not a listed attribute of self-efficacy, while relevancy, credibility, and knowledge are listed as attributes.

## 10. B) Taking the role seriously

Taking the role seriously is the third step. Feeling like an imposter is the first, trial and error is the second, transference is the fourth, and professionalism is the fifth.

# REFERENCES

Adeniran, R., Smith Glasgow, M. E., Bhattacharya, A., & Xu, Y. (2013). Career advancement and professional development in nursing. *Nursing Outlook, 61*(6), 437–446. https://doi.org/10.1016/j.outlook.2013.05.009

Bandura, A. (1977a). Self-efficacy: Toward a unifying theory of behavioral change. *Psychological Review, 84*, 191–215. https://doi.org/10.1037/0033-295x.84.2.191

Bandura, A. (1977b). *Social learning theory*. Prentice Hall.

Benner, P., Sutphen, M., Leonard, V., & Day, L. (2010). *Educating nurses: A call for radical transformation*. Jossey-Bass/Carnegie Foundation for the Advancement of Teaching.

Brink, P., Back-Pettersson, S., & Sernert, N. (2012). Group supervision as a means of developing professional competence within pre-hospital care. *International Emergency Nursing, 20*(2), 76–82. https://doi.org/10.1016/j.ienj.2011.04.001

Brooks, C. F. (2010). Toward "hybridised" faculty development for the twenty-first century: Blending online communities of practice and face-to-face meetings in instructional and professional support programmes. *Innovations in Education and Teaching International, 47*(3), 261–270. https://doi.org/10.1080/14703297.2010.498177

Crider, M., & McNiesh, S. (2011). Integrating a professional apprenticeship model with psychiatric clinical simulation. *Journal of Psychosocial Nursing & Mental Health Services, 49*(5), 42–49. https://doi.org/10.3928/02793695-20110329-01

Foronda, C. L., Fernandez-Burgos, M., Nadeau, C., Kelley, C. N., & Henry, M. N. (2020). Virtual simulation in nursing education: A systematic review spanning 1996 to 2018. *Simulation in Healthcare, 15*(1), 46–54.

Guillemin, M., McDougall, R., & Gillam, L. (2009). Developing "ethical mindfulness" in continuing professional development in healthcare: Use of a personal narrative approach. *Cambridge Quarterly of Healthcare Ethics, 18*, 197–208. https://doi.org/10.1017/S096318010909032X

Heller, J. I., Daehler, K. R., Wong, N., Mayumi, S., & Miratrix, L. W. (2012). Differential effects of three professional development models on teacher knowledge and student achievement in elementary science. *Journal of Research in Science Teaching, 49*(3), 333–362. https://doi.org/10.1002/tea.2100

Ismail, M., & Arokiasamy, L. (2007). Exploring mentoring as a tool for career advancement of academics in private higher education institutions in Malaysia. *Journal of International Social Research, 1*(1), 135–148.

Koberg, C. S., Boss, R. W., & Goodman, E. (1998). Factors and outcomes associated with mentoring among health-care professionals. *Journal of Vocational Behavior, 53*(1), 58–72. https://doi.org/10.1006/jvbe.1997.1607

Krofft, K., & Stuart, W. (2021). Implementing a mentorship program during a pandemic. *Nursing Administration Quarterly, 45*(2), 152–158.

Kubitskey, B. W., Vath, R. J., Johnson, H. J., Fishman, B. J., Konstantopoulos, S., & Park, G. J. (2012). Examining study attrition: Implications for experimental research on professional development. *Teaching and Teacher Education, 28*(3), 418–427. https://doi.org/10.1016/j.tate.2011.11.008

Lombardo, M. M., & Eichinger, R. W. (2009). *FYI for your improvement: A guide for development and coaching* (5th ed.). Lominger International: A Korn/Ferry.

Margolis, A., & Parboosingh, J. (2015). Networked learning and network science: Potential applications to health professionals' continuing education and development. *Journal of Continuing Education in the Health Professions, 35*(3), 2011–2019. https://doi.org/10.1002/chp.21295

McDermott, D. S. (2016). The prebriefing concept: A Delphi study of CHSE experts. *Clinical Simulation in Nursing, 12*, 219–227.

Mulvey, R. (2013). How to be a good professional: Existentialist continuing professional development (CPD). *British Journal of Guidance & Counseling, 41*(3), 267–276. https://doi.org/10.1080/03069885.2013.773961

Patterson, K., Grenny, J., McMillan, R., & Switzer, A. (2011). *Crucial conversations: Tools for talking when the stakes are high* (2nd ed.). McGraw-Hill.

Ricketts, T. C., & Fraher, E. P. (2013). Reconfiguring health workforce policy so that education, training, and actual delivery of care are closely connected. *Health Affairs, 32*(11), 1874–1880.

Roche, A. M., Pidd, K., & Freeman, T. (2009). Achieving professional practice change: From training to workforce development. *Drug and Alcohol Review, 28*(5), 550–557. https://doi.org/10.1111/j.1465-3 362.2009.00111.x

Scott, W. R. (2002). *Organizations: Rational, natural, and open systems* (5th ed.). Prentice Hall.

Seldin, P., & Miller, J. E. (2009). *The academic portfolio: A practical guide to teaching, research, and service.* Jossey-Bass.

Simmons, B., Oandasan, I., Soklaradis, S., Esdaile, M., Barker, K., Kwan, D., & Wagner, S. (2011). Evaluating the effectiveness of an interprofessional education faculty development course: The transfer of interprofessional learning to the academic and clinical practice setting. *Journal of Interprofessional Care, 25*(2), 156–157. https://doi.org/10.3109/13561820.2010.515044

Society for Simulation in Healthcare. (2021). *Certified healthcare simulation educator handbook.* https:// www.ssih.org/Portals/48/Certification/CHSE_Docs/CHSE%20Handbook.pdf

Socolovsky, C., Masi, C., Hamlish, T., Aduana, G., Arora, S., Bakris, G., & Johnson, D. (2013). Evaluating the role of key learning theories in ECHO: A telehealth educational program for primary care providers. *Progress in Community Health Partnerships, 7*(4), 361–368. https://doi.org/10.1 353/cpr.2013.0043

Spurk, D., & Abele, A. E. (2014). Synchronous and time-lagged effects between occupational self-efficacy and objective and subjective career success: Findings from a four-wave and 9-year longitudinal study. *Journal of Vocational Behavior, 84*(2), 119–132. https://doi.org/10.1016/j.jvb.2013 .12.002

Sullivan, W. M. (2005). *Work and integrity: The crisis and promise of professionalism in America* (2nd ed.). Jossey-Bass.

Walton, J., Chute, E., & Ball, L. (2011). Negotiating the role of the professional nurse: The pedagogy of simulation: A grounded theory study. *Journal of Professional Nursing, 27*(5), 299–310. https://doi .org/10.1016/j.profnurs.2011.04.005

Wenger, E. C., McDermott, R. A., & Snyder, W. (2002). *Cultivating communities of practice: A guide to managing knowledge.* Harvard Business School Press.

Wittmann-Price, R. A. (2012). *Fast facts for developing a nursing academic portfolio.* Springer Publishing Company.

Zhou, C., Crawford, A., Serhal, E., Kurdyak, P., & Sockalingam, S. (2016). The impact of Project ECHO on participant and patient outcomes: A systematic review. *Academic Medicine, 91*(10), 1439–1461. https://doi.org/10.1097/ACM.0000000000001328

# The Role of Research in Simulation

**21**

Crystal L. Murillo, Colette Townsend-Chambers, Sevilla Bronson, and Karen Worthy

*Research is formalized curiosity. It is poking and prying with a purpose.*

*—Zora Neale Hurston*

This chapter addresses Domain III: Educational Principles Applied to Simulation (Society for Simulation in Healthcare [SSH], 2021).

## ▶ LEARNING OUTCOMES

- Discuss the importance of research in simulation for healthcare educators.
- Identify the current state of simulation research.
- Identify gaps in simulation research.
- Discuss research knowledge via case study and practice questions.

## ▶ INTRODUCTION

Simulation in the education of healthcare practitioners is not a new concept. As the use of simulation in health profession programs increases, the simulation literature grows. While there are still things that we do not know, simulation science continues to advance at an astounding rate. Results of a groundbreaking empty systematic review identified that we know more about learning outcomes in simulation than traditional apprenticeship models used in undergraduate nursing education (Leighton et al., 2021). This chapter discusses the importance of research in simulation, provides a summary of the current state of research on simulation, identifies gaps in the literature, and provides teaching tips and application exercises.

At the time of the previous edition of this review manual, one of the hot topics debated was how many clinical hours or what percent of clinical time can be substituted with simulation. While there is more research to be done regarding dosing in simulation, there is empirical evidence supporting a 2:1 ratio of clinical to simulation time (Sullivan et al., 2019). The results of this study do not answer the dose–response question but do provide an excellent beginning to revealing the intense, efficient learning environment of simulation.

A current hot topic in simulation is how to effectively use stimulation as a means to reduce implicit bias and advance health equity. Additionally and as a result of the shift in educational modalities in health profession programs during the COVID-19 pandemic, hot topics also include can virtual and screen-based learning be used to replace traditional clinical hours and simulation dosing.

To determine its efficacy, additional questions must be answered, and the simulation modality needs to consider the level of the participant, the concepts being taught, and the theoretical knowledge required (Roberts et al., 2019). At this point, we still do not know the best dose of simulation needed to get the best response from the participants. The need to answer these questions will be a driving force in simulation research as empirical evidence supports the use of simulation, its effectiveness, and its relationship to patient safety. For this review, the current state of research on simulation is divided into three components of simulation: prebriefing, simulation, and debriefing.

# ▶ PREBRIEFING

According to the Healthcare Simulation Standards of Best Practice™ (HSSOBP™) Prebriefing: Preparation and Briefing of the International Nursing Association for Clinical Simulation and Learning (INACSL; 2021b), *prebriefing* provides an opportunity for participants to complete educational activities before the simulation as a means of preparation, while also briefing participants on the ground rules and specifics of the simulation-based experience. HSSOBP™: Prebriefing: Preparation and Briefing (INACSL et al., 2021b) developed the latest criteria and guidelines for facilitators. Dividing them into three categories (general, preparation, and briefing), the nine criteria provide a succinct and structured approach to prebriefing that are informed by the HSSOBP™(INACSL et al., 2021b).

The committee further purports that at minimum the facilitator must be knowledgeable regarding the concept of prebriefing and have the ability to develop the SBE based on the determined learning objectives. This new delineation may make it easier for facilitators to utilize this standard. When preparing the participant for success, activities should help them review content via assignments such as concept maps or care plans and case studies, which can include relevant medications and anticipated interventions. To ensure participants are prepared, requiring them to complete a "Ticket to Sim" before entering the simulation lab may be considered (INACSL et al., 2021b).

In addition to providing participants with prescenario assignments to prepare them to assimilate the educational content, providing a psychologically safe container by laying ground rules is paramount. Yockey and Henry (2019) found that high participant anxiety related to simulation was associated with the roles given, the fear of making mistakes, and knowing that their peers are watching. To compound that anxiety, consider participants who have cultural or linguistic differences, and the challenges that can occur with the increasingly larger number of globally and ethnically diverse body of participants (Kelly et al., 2018). When experiencing SBE, nursing participants of color reported feeling more pressure to perform, a sense of isolation, and a need to keep the peace as a means of avoiding retaliation or being ignored by their white counterparts. These participants also described being treated in a manner that makes them feel inadequate or overlooked by white faculty (Graham & Atz, 2015). As a result, facilitators are encouraged to self-evaluate for unconscious bias and how it may impact participant outcomes.

Prebriefing is essential to set the tone and to focus participants on the main objective, which is learning. Healthcare professionals tend to focus on performance outcomes rather than learning. Participants are disappointed if they do not meet their performance expectations. To this end, creating a "fiction contract" which holds all participants accountable for professionalism and confidentiality can bolster the psychologically safe container. To maintain this psychological safety and reduce anxiety, facilitators can promote the expression "what happens in simulation, stays in the simulation." Orienting participants to their environment, roles, equipment, and evaluation tools, including orientation time with the manikin's technology, is an equally important aspect of prebriefing. Briefing participants on the scenario's content and client information and connecting this to the objectives may help ensure successful learning outcomes. Incorporating all criteria from the standard can also promote a more reflective and effective debriefing session (INACSL et al., 2021a).

Preparation during prebriefing is critically important to build confidence in simulation. Some additional recommendations to decrease anxiety are limiting the number of observers and having them observe in areas separate from the SBE, providing private remediation if needed.

> **Simulation Teaching Tip 21.1**
>
> Enhancing participants' practice readiness, providing safe care, and improving patient outcomes are some of the reasons for utilizing clinical simulation (Kelly et al., 2018). However, with the increased globalization of healthcare, have you considered the learning expectations of culturally diverse participants? Is avoiding eye contact or not seeking clarification indicators of an "unprepared" participant or perhaps a cultural norm? Being cognizant of embedded cultural nuances or norms is critical in ensuring all participants can have a meaningful simulation-based education (SBE; Kelly et al., 2018).

## ▶ SIMULATION

Simulation is an educational strategy in which a particular set of conditions is created or replicated to resemble authentic situations that are possible in real life. The SBE is the entire set of actions and events from initiation to termination of an individual simulation event; in the learning setting, this is often considered to begin with the prebriefing and end with the debriefing (Lioce et al., 2020).

Previously known as the National League for Nursing (NLN) Jeffries Simulation Framework, the NLN Jeffries Simulation Theory (2015) identifies contextual factors as the starting point in designing or evaluating simulation. Situated within this context, the theory posits the background as goals of the simulation and specific expectations or benchmarks that influence design. The NLN Jeffries Simulation Theory identifies events outside of and preceding the actual simulation experience as specific elements that make up the design. In this theory, simulation has four important components:

- simulation experience
- facilitator and educational strategies
- participant (previously learner)
- outcomes

The SBE is characterized by a learner-centric environment that is experiential, interactive, and collaborative. The theory posits trust as a shared responsibility of both the facilitator and the participant that ensures psychological fidelity within the experience (Jeffries et al., 2015). Within the simulation experience is a dynamic interaction between the facilitator and the participant (Jeffries et al., 2015). Of particular importance to the facilitator and educational strategies is the acknowledgment of characteristics that each facilitator brings to the experience and how these might impact simulation outcomes. The facilitator and educational strategies relationship requires that the facilitator responds to emerging needs during the simulation experience to include but not be limited to cues (during) and debriefing (toward the end) of the simulation. The NLN Jeffries Simulation Theory posits that the facilitator must be able to adjust the educational strategies based on participant needs. Participant attributes such as age, gender, level of anxiety, and self-confidence can affect the simulation learning experience. There is a growing body of research signaling the need to explore whether race is a participant attribute that also impacts learner outcomes (Graham & Atz, 2015; Graham et al., 2016; Graham et al., 2018; Fuselier et al., 2016). Finally, the theory identifies outcomes by participants, patients, or systems.

Kirkpatrick's evaluation model (Kirkpatrick & Kirkpatrick, 2006) is used to present examples of research on evaluation. In Kirkpatrick's model, the four levels of evaluation consist of the following:

1. reaction
2. learning
3. behavior
4. results

Evaluations in level 1 are determined as the degree to which participants find the simulation experience favorable, engaging, and/or relevant. Level 2 constitutes the evaluation of experiences designed to measure improvements in knowledge, skills, attitude, and/or confidence. When measuring learning in the cognitive domain, it is important to design the simulation so that participants will be able to demonstrate learning by applying knowledge to make decisions in the scenario. There is an overlap between the cognitive and psychomotor domains because one must have the knowledge to complete the skill (Adamson et al., 2012). Studies in the psychomotor domain of learning measure a range of skills from basic to complex. Evaluation in the affective domain is more subjective. Affective learning and Kirkpatrick's reaction (level 1) overlap. Kirkpatrick's last two levels, behavior (level 3) and results (level 4), have not been evaluated as extensively as satisfaction (level 1) and learning (level 2). Evaluation of the degree to which participants apply what they have learned to future practice is level 3. Level 4 focuses on the evaluation of results of patient outcomes because of participation in the simulation experience. Behavior measures the change in future performance resulting from the learning process, whereas results measure the tangible outcome of the learning process in relation to cost, quality, and efficiency. Collectively, levels 3 and 4 are directly focused on improving healthcare processes and outcomes, which are considered translational science (Brazil, 2017).

Many authors have developed both quantitative and qualitative instruments to evaluate Kirkpatrick's level 1, participants' perceptions of simulation, and level 2, learning outcomes in simulation. While there is still more to be known about simulation, there are several systematic and integrative reviews that provide meaningful evaluation data supporting simulation as a learning pedagogy. Participant satisfaction (level 1), a reaction to participation in simulation, and self-confidence (level 2) and critical thinking (level 2) have been the most heavily researched. The evaluation of Kirkpatrick's reactions and learning has been highlighted in an integrative review that included 101 studies identifying five major themes, namely confidence/self-efficacy (level 2), satisfaction (level 1), anxiety/stress (level 1), skills/knowledge (level 2), and interdisciplinary experiences (Foronda et al., 2013). In the category of skills/knowledge (level 2), the authors included 29 studies, reporting that the preponderance of evaluation findings supporting simulation to be effective in teaching knowledge and skills. A systematic review conducted to identify the effectiveness of using whole-body, high-fidelity manikins to teach clinical reasoning identified evaluation of Kirkpatrick's level 2 and found that simulation improved critical thinking, performance of skills, and knowledge of the subject matter, and increased clinical reasoning in certain areas (Lapkin et al., 2010). In 2020, the results of a comprehensive review of the literature were published with the following research question: What is the state of the science on the evidence of learning outcomes in high-fidelity simulation in undergraduate nursing education? (Hanshaw & Dickerson, 2020). The time frame of the search was from 2010 to 2018. After inclusion and exclusion criteria, 20 studies were included in the review. The studies included reported the outcomes of high-fidelity simulation for a total of 1,787 participants. The data available from this synthesis of the literature support that the use of high-fidelity simulation as an educational intervention (compared with teaching methods without the use of high-fidelity simulation) increases higher level thinking knowledge (level 2), critical thinking (level 2), self-efficacy (level 1), self-confidence (level 1), clinical judgment (level 2), and motivation (level 2).

The largest study ever conducted in nursing education, the National Council State Board of Nursing's (NCSBN's) longitudinal, randomized, controlled trial, was conducted to explore whether simulated clinical experiences can be substituted effectively for traditional undergraduate clinical experiences (Hayden et al., 2014). Evaluation measures included participants' knowledge (level 2), clinical competency (level 2), critical thinking (level 2), and perceptions of how well their learning needs were met (level 1). The second arm of this study determined the long-term impact of substituting traditional clinical with SBE and therefore captured measures from Kirkpatrick's level 3. Second-phase level 3 measures included clinical competency, critical thinking, and readiness for practice. The results of this landmark study support simulation as an equivalent, although not superior, alternative to traditional clinical experiences. For reasons yet to be identified, the members of a minority population demonstrated the highest attrition rate in the study and were randomized to the group experiencing 50% substitution with simulation. This incidental finding further supports the need to explore race as a participant attribute that may impact outcomes in simulation (Graham et al., 2018).

The results of another integrative review identified that Kirkpatrick's reactions and learning have been measured and that, overall, participants' reaction to repeated SBE demonstrates satisfaction (level 1) and self-confidence (level 2; Al Gharibi & Arulappan, 2020). This review also identified evaluation results indicating that a range of simulation fidelity enhanced participants' self-confidence (level 2), competence (level 2), knowledge (level 2), and critical thinking (level 2). The use of low-, mid-, and high-fidelity simulation with repeated experiences was found to be the teaching practice most attributed to these increases. More specifically regarding the learning domains, Kirkpatrick's level 2 evaluation of learning has been measured and a synthesis of the findings has been published in multiple high-level reviews to include the cognitive (Al Gharibi & Arulappan, 2020; Lee & Oh, 2015), affective (Cantrell et al., 2017; Kim et al., 2016; Lee & Oh, 2015), and psychomotor domains (Kim et al., 2016).

Examples of valid and reliable instruments measuring Kirkpatrick's levels include but are not limited to a rubric developed by Lasater (2007) to measure clinical judgment (level 2) by scoring participants on a scale that rated the following:

- noticing
- interpreting
- responding
- reflecting

Participants were rated as beginning, developing, accomplished, or exemplary on this tool. Radhakrishnan et al. (2007) developed the Clinical Simulation Evaluation Tool (CSET), a clinical performance tool, to measure the following:

- basic and problem-based assessment (level 2)
- prioritization (level 2)
- delegation (level 2)
- communication (level 2)
- interventions and safety (level 2)

The INACSL has developed a repository of valid and reliable simulation evaluation instruments for use in SBE based on the NLN Jeffries Simulation Theory. This comprehensive list is further categorized to include evaluation tools designed to measure learning outcomes in the cognitive, psychomotor, and affective domains.

Valid and reliable instruments to measure the performance of medical participants and residents were developed by Rosen et al. (2008) and Murray et al. (2007). Both instruments were specifically designed for performance measurement in simulation (level 2). Although these psychomotor tools are specific to medical skills, the American Heart Association Basic Life Support (BLS) and Advanced Cardiac Life Support (ACLS) performance tools may be used for research across professions. In a revisit to the originally published critical review of simulation-based medical education (SBME), McGahie et al. (2016) highlight unequivocal research synthesis demonstrating SBME with deliberate practice to be superior to traditional clinical education for clinical skills acquisition among participants (level 2). The authors continue to support SBME as a viable alternative to traditional clinical medical education. In this critical review, the authors also identify that simulation was the highest rated area of importance for medical education research.

Historically, the goals of outcomes of healthcare simulation have focused on Kirkpatrick's levels 1 and 2. Extant literature highlights that the transfer to practice outcomes (levels 3 and 4) is difficult to design and execute as outcomes are much more difficult to measure. Examples of simulation evaluation leading to improvement of patient outcomes (levels 3 and 4) include lower central line infection rates and reduction in perinatal asphyxia (Bailey, 2020). There is also emerging evidence that participation in simulation may not translate to improvements in patient outcomes. The results of an open, multicenter, parallel, cluster-randomized controlled trial demonstrated that a 1-day simulation-based obstetric team training of hospital teams in a simulation center focusing on 80% teamwork skills did not improve a composite of obstetric complications (Fransen, 2018). The global simulation community supports the need for more work in translational simulation science.

In 2020, a meta-analysis was conducted to highlight the effectiveness of different scaffolding types and technology in facilitating complex skills in simulation-based higher education learning environments. The results include robust findings from 145 empirical studies highlighting simulations as among the most effective means to facilitate learning of complex skills across domains and that different scaffolding types can facilitate simulation-based learning during the different phases of development of knowledge and skills (Chemikova et al., 2020).

In summary, some of the gaps in simulation research include but are not limited to the need to identify if race is a participant attribute that influences simulation outcomes. Additionally, gaps include the need for more rigorous multisite studies that focus on participant and/or patient outcomes (Mariani & Doolen, 2016) and the effectiveness of virtual and screen-based learning in health profession programs.

## ▶ DEBRIEFING

The 2021 INACSL HSSOBP™ describes debriefing as an intentional and adaptable process that is planned to occur at designated points of the simulation, immediately following the activity, or both (INACSL et al., 2021a). The debriefing process is a learning strategy that assists participants in improving general nursing knowledge, psychomotor and critical thinking skills, professional attitudes, and communication while improvements in individual, team, and system performance are recognized and solutions are developed (Edwards et al., 2021). The purpose of the debriefing process is to support reflection on major learning points, engage in real-world thinking for future performance, and incorporate the application and integration of learning into future practice (Edwards et al., 2021; INACSL et al., 2021a). Reflective thinking, referred to as "conscious consideration or reflection," is essential to learning and making connections between the actions performed and the actual practice (INACSL, 2014, p. 1).

The debriefing process consists of three strategies or techniques that are referred to as feedback, debriefing, and/or guided reflection activities (INACSL et al., 2021). Deployment of one strategy or a combination of either is determined by the level of the participant. It is particularly important to ensure that the process for debriefing is derived from theory and/ or evidence-based concepts and that the participants' psychological safety is maintained (Cheng et al., 2020). Psychological safety allows the participant to fully engage without being ridiculed, blamed by others, or forced to speak during the debriefing process.

The simulation activity promotes learning primarily during the debriefing process. A sure way of implementing the debriefing is unknown (Kim & Yoo, 2020). However, in utilizing existing frameworks as well as the strategies of feedback, debriefing, and/or guided reflection activities, participants are facilitated through discussions on various aspects of the simulation to ensure the established learning objectives and goals are met (Cheng et al., 2020). In addition, structured and unstructured debriefing should be determined by an experienced facilitator to maintain the participants' motivation and self-esteem throughout the process (Frandsen

& Lehn-Christiansen, 2020). A variety of debriefing frameworks are available to complete the debriefing process, including but not limited to the following:

- debriefing with good judgment *(RAS—reaction, analysis, summary*; Rudolph et al., 2006)
- debriefing for meaningful learning (DML; Dreifuerst, 2015)
- promoting Excellence and Reflective Learning in Simulation (PEARLS; Eppich & Chang, 2015)
- plus delta debriefing (Cheng et al., 2021)

Videotaped recordings of simulation activities and video-assisted debriefing have also been found to benefit participant learning during the debriefing process (Dreifuerst et al., 2021; Zhang et al., 2020). Participants who engaged in video-assisted debriefing viewed their facilitators as being more prepared for the activity (Zhang et al., 2020). Reviewing critical points instead of the full video was more beneficial, and stress or performance levels did not differ from that of oral debriefing. Although stress levels among participants decreased with repeated simulations, repetition may not effectively evaluate participants' ability to understand and correct the performed actions (Dreifuerst et al., 2021). Moreover, the proliferation of video-assisted debriefing that emerged due to the coronavirus pandemic led to rapid adaptation to develop guidelines and platforms for simulated learning (Cheng et al., 2020). Keeping with maintaining a safe learning environment, their communities of inquiry conceptual framework supporting the three core elements of facilitator, social, and cognitive presence provides structure and guidance for remote learning and video-assisted debriefing.

Facilitation of the debriefing process should be designed to promote reflective thinking and can be implemented by "expert facilitators with significant experience in reflective inquiry strategies" (Edwards et al., 2021, p. 1) or through the construction and design of electronic debriefing programs (INACSL et al., 2021a). Facilitating reflection can occur in three phases: reflection-before-action, which occurs during the prebriefing activity; reflection-in-action, which takes place when barriers are recognized, strategies are developed, and "learners pause, think-out-loud, collaborate, and/or change the course of their actions"; and reflection-on-action, which takes place during the debriefing process (Mulli et al., 2022, p. 1). Reflection-in-action enhances learning when expressed thoughts are addressed early, barriers are eliminated (e.g., appropriate simulation design, facilitator interest and preparation, and psychological safety for participant anxieties and fear), and elements of nursing practice are realized through collaboration, critical thinking, and increased self-confidence. According to Kim and Yoo (2020), facilitators may determine the debriefing method based on staffing and available resources that will best fit the educational and cultural needs of the participants. Their study found that the debriefing process occurring outside of the simulation room/lab provides an environment that is comfortable and more relaxing for the participants, thereby promoting reflection as well as flexibility in the length of time for the debriefing process.

Studies on simulation debriefing have addressed a plethora of topics. However, gaps in the literature concerning the debriefing process continue to exist. Suggestions for continued research may include formal versus informal structure and learning goals, management of participant and facilitator cognitive load, cultural considerations in safe debriefing environments, and development of a gold standard for debriefing. Identifying what is best may ensure continuity in simulation education that is efficient for both the participant and the facilitator.

## ▶ RESEARCH

Research is a process that is used to explain, expand, and develop knowledge in any discipline. Engaging in this process requires the use of paradigms that aid in interpreting assumptions, experiences, beliefs, and values to understand our relationship to the world around us.

Paradigms are patterns of beliefs and practices that regulate inquiry within a discipline by providing lenses, frames, and processes through which investigation is accomplished (Weaver & Olsen, 2006). The research approach of quantitative and qualitative methods flows from the established foundation of the paradigm. Each method evaluates phenomena differently. In brief, quantitative research examines numerical and statistical data to test a hypothesis, while qualitative research seeks to understand phenomena through an individual's perspective.

Although this section does not include a detailed review of paradigms and a discussion of research frameworks, a basic review of both methods will allow readers to evaluate the benefits of how the synthesis of research enhances our understanding of phenomena. Table 21.1 provides a simplified overview of each method.

### Table 21.1 Research Method

| Research Paradigm | Overview | Benefits | Challenges |
|---|---|---|---|
| Quantitative research method | It tests hypothesis through empirical evidence gathered through the senses and is rooted in a reality that is objective and measurable. It uses deductive reasoning rather than personal beliefs. | It evaluates with reliable and valid instruments (e.g., surveys, questionnaires, observations). Collection of numerical data is analyzed to test hypotheses and make generalizable conclusions of the population. | Validity and reliability of instruments with abstract phenomena may be difficult to measure. |
| Qualitative research method | It provides broad context of multiple realities that are subjective, differences among participants create variability, and values and biases are desirable. It uses inductive reasoning to seek an in-depth understanding of the phenomena. | Emerging design provides flexibility by focusing on human experiences that are holistic and nonquantifiable (e.g., interviews, focus groups, observations). Real-life experiences yield rich narrative information to identify concepts, variables, and themes that may influence research outcomes. | No research instruments are used; all data are obtained from human participants. Analysis of subjective data is more tedious than analysis of numerical data. It is difficult to replicate findings. Evidence is not as generalizable due to subjectivity. |

### Evidence-Based Simulation Practice 21.1

Dix et al. (2021) used a qualitative approach to examine undergraduate final semester nursing participants' ability to transfer clinical judgment skills to clinical practice. Participants exposed to clinical stressors and new experiences perceived that the simulation contributed to increasing their level of clinical judgment, clinical practice preparation, and emotional intelligence.

## Evidence-Based Simulation Practice 21.2

Padden-Denmead et al. (2016) investigated junior baccalaureate nursing degree participants' ($N =$ 23) critical thinking and clinical reasoning skills after clinical simulation with debriefing and guided reflective journaling. The Holistic Critical Thinking Scoring Rubric (Facione & Facione, 2009) and the level of reflection on action assessment (Padden, 2013) were used. Participants were able to achieve higher scores in critical thinking and journal entries with debriefing as opposed to hospital experiences without debriefing.

## Evidence-Based Simulation Practice 21.3

Baisden and Gray (2020) employed a mixed-methods approach using the Hearing Voices Simulation to measure empathy among preprofessional healthcare participants. Participants improved their knowledge of interventions and their level of empathy, as well as their understanding of voice-hearing experiences. Fears decreased and comfort increased as knowledge increased.

Simulation research can be examined through the utilization of a variety of design perspectives and methods. Whether inductive or deductive, the approach of the mixed-method design, which includes both qualitative and quantitative methods, adds richness to the data and enhances understanding of simulation on learning.

## Evidence-Based Simulation Practice 21.4

In a systematic literature review regarding the evaluation of teamwork assessment tools for interprofessional simulation, Wooding et al.'s (2020) initial search of 233 articles yielded only 24 articles that met the criteria for review. They concluded that a framework for reporting tool psychometrics of simulation studies assessing teamwork could improve the quality of the methodology in future studies and support the need for future research.

Ultimately, a review process looks at the evidence, regardless of the method used to examine the data. There are various forms of reviews, including but not limited to integrative, systematic, umbrella, critical, or scoping, that evaluate the current state of knowledge on a selected topic and identify gaps to generate future research.

# ▶ SIMULATION RESEARCH RESOURCES

## KEEPING CURRENT

One of the most important ways to keep up to date on the research in simulation is by joining one or more of the simulation societies. The two organizations that are frequently accessed for simulation research, accreditation, and developing standards of best practice are the INACSL and the Society for Simulation in Healthcare (SSH, 2021). Both organizations publish a monthly journal devoted to simulation. The journal articles are peer-reviewed and indexed in medical and nursing databases. Other associations that may be helpful include the Association of Standardized Patient Educators (ASPE) and the Simulation Learning, Education and Research Network (SimLEARN). The organizational mission or goals are listed in Table 21.2. Involvement in professional organizations can provide opportunities for active engagement in advancing similar goals, discussion of diverse opinions, and participation in educational offerings (Harris, 2017).

### Table 21.2 Simulation Organizations for Healthcare Educators

| Organization | Mission/Goals | Publication |
|---|---|---|
| **INACSL** (www.inacsl .org) | The INACSL's mission is to be the global leader in the art and science of healthcare simulation through excellence in nursing education, practice, and research (www.inacsl.org, 2022). Although started by a group of nursing educators in 1976, the INACSL promotes collaboration, discovery, and diversity of simulation practitioners in various disciplines. The INACSL envisions simulation and innovation transforming lives. This is accomplished by disseminating evidence-based practice standards for clinical simulation methodologies and learning environments. Each year, the INACSL convenes in a different city and is the catalyst for many burgeoning simulation educators. It is a community of practicing leaders, scholars, and service-oriented professionals. Novice and expert practitioners can network, share ideas, and learn from and with each other about the knowledge, skills, and attitudes necessary for best practices in the use of simulation. | *Clinical Simulation in Nursing* |
| **SSH** (www.ssih.org) | Established in 2004, the SSH's mission is to influence simulation practice to enhance the quality of healthcare globally, with the primary goal of improving performance and reducing errors in inpatient care. This is accomplished by informing ethics and standards, while championing the practice of simulation, and fostering education, research, and professional development. The SSH is a multidisciplinary, multispecialty, international society with ties to many medical specialties, nursing, allied health, paramedical personnel, and industry utilizing many modalities. The SSH promotes simulation-based modalities such as task trainers' virtual reality, human patient simulators, and standardized patients. Networking and educational opportunities abound at the annual IMSH. | *Simulation in Healthcare* |

*(continued)*

**Table 21.2** Simulation Organizations for Healthcare Educators (*continued*)

| Organization | Mission/Goals | Publication |
|---|---|---|
| **ASPE** (www .aspeducator.org) | The ASPE is the international organization of simulation educators that was formed in 2001. It comprises many fields, including dentistry, pharmacy, veterinary, and allied health professions. This organization is dedicated to "transforming professional performance through the power of human interaction" (https://www.aspeducators .org/about-aspe, 2022, para. 7). A *standardized patient* (*SP*) is the term to describe a person trained to realistically portray a patient, repeatedly and in a standardized manner. The promotion of best practices in the application and dissemination of SP methodology for education, assessment, and research, as well as fostering the advancement of professional knowledge and skills, is vital to the mission of the ASPE. The ASPE has evolved to include "hybrid" simulations, which include scenarios using SPs, task trainers, and manikins. The ASPE also convenes an annual international conference. | There are many web resources. The ASPE recently announced its collaboration with MedEdPORTAL to house SP cases. MedEdPORTAL is "[a] peer-reviewed, open-access journal that promotes educational scholarship and dissemination of teaching and assessment resources in the health professions" (Association of American Medical Colleges, 2018, p. 1). |
| **SimLEARN** | The SimLEARN is the VHA's program for simulation in healthcare training. Serving the largest integrated healthcare system in the world, VHA's SimLEARN provides an ever-growing body of curricula and best practices that improve healthcare for our nation's veterans. | SimLEARN newsletter |

ASPE, Association of SP Educators; IMSH, International Meeting for Simulation in Healthcare; INACSL, International Nursing Association for Clinical Simulation and Learning; SimLEARN, Simulation Learning, Education and Research Network; SP, standardized patient; SSH, Society for Simulation in Healthcare; VHA, Veterans Health Administration.

The SSH is the organization that provides the simulation certification examination and accredits simulation programs. Simulation facilitators can apply for various designations of certification, including the Certified Healthcare Simulation Educator® (CHSE®), the Certified Healthcare Simulation Operations Specialist® (CHSOS®), and the advanced certification for each (CHSE-A, and CHSOS-A). Programs that comply with core standards and fulfillment of standards applied to one or more of the areas of assessment, research, teaching/education, and/or systems integration are eligible for application. The SSH's goal is to lead in facilitating excellence in (multispecialty) healthcare education, practice, and research through simulation modalities.

On July 17, 2009, the acting undersecretary for health authorized the establishment of a national simulation training and education program for the Veterans Health Administration (VHA). Dubbed the "Simulation Learning, Education and Research Network" or SimLEARN, the program is improving the quality of healthcare services for America's veterans through the application of simulation-based learning strategies in clinical workforce development. The program operations and management are aligned with the VHA Employee Education System

(EES), in close collaboration with VHA's Office of Patient Care Services (PCS) and Office of Nursing Services (ONS). Although the use of simulation for healthcare training and education is not new to VHA, it has become critical for VHA to develop an integrated approach to better realize the maximum benefits of simulation for VHA staff and the veterans it serves.

Accessing these simulation communities can provide research and practice collaborations as well as mentoring opportunities. For those new to simulation, participation can decrease the learning curve, and for the experienced facilitator provide international dissemination platforms. Leaders and members of these organizations advance the science of simulation while providing trusted and invaluable professional and personal connections which can last a lifetime.

---

### Simulation Teaching Tip 21.2

I vividly remember my first International Nursing Association for Clinical Simulation and Learning (INACSL) conference. As a novice simulationist, I stood in awe at the sophisticated manikins and hundreds of excited participants. It is reputed once you are "bitten," by the simulation "bug," you become a passionate advocate for all things simulation. Since then, simulation organizations have grown exponentially, and I continue to glean from the valuable and seemingly limitless resources for academic and clinical practitioners alike.

—Colette R. Townsend-Chambers, DNP, MSN, CHSE

---

## ▶ SUMMARY

In summary, the organizations listed above are not all-encompassing of the simulation societies that currently exist. In addition, there are many independent blogs, podcasts, and online webpages available. Product manufacturers also provide valuable resources on the latest innovative technology, often supporting collaborative research. There is a plethora of recent literature closing the gap regarding prebriefing, facilitating, and debriefing. The literature on clinical reasoning, self-efficacy, and participant satisfaction is current with robust evidence which provides answers to the following questions:

- What are the best practices for prebriefing, facilitating, and debriefing simulations?
- What effects does simulation have on the self-efficacy and clinical reasoning of learners?
- What percentage of clinical hours can be replaced by simulation?
- What are the benefits of using simulation to teach cultural humility and sensitivity?
- What effect does simulation have on the knowledge, skills, and abilities of learners?

To remain current in research, simulation facilitators are encouraged to stay connected with simulation societies, attend simulation conferences, and read evidence-based simulation literature. As this heutagogy continues to spread through practice and academia, it is vital to continue research and learning to ensure the advancement of simulation.

 ## CASE STUDY 21.1

Shekita is an experienced nurse educator but is new to simulation. One of her participants confides that they recently lost a family member due to an opioid overdose. Shekita tells the participant that the simulation is essential to the course and that they must participate. Does this format follow the recommendations of simulation research? How would you counsel Shekita to improve her simulation educator skills?

## CASE STUDY DISCUSSION

Shekita's response does not follow the recommendations. As observers who are actively engaged get just as much out of the simulation as participants, Shekita should give the participant a choice to observe, using an observation guide, rather than participate in this emotionally charged simulation. To ensure psychological safety, Shekita should address the possibility of emotional triggers in the prebriefing. Participants should be given the choice to observe rather than participate in the simulation if they think that participation elicits an emotional response that impacts performance.

1. The novice simulation educator needs additional understanding when they state:

   A. "Prebriefing sets the stage for the scenario and assists participants in achieving learning objectives."

   B. "Prebriefing activities include creating a fictional contract and orienting participants to their roles, equipment, and scenario."

   C. "During prebriefing, it is important to emphasize that perfection is expected."

   D. "The main objective of prebriefing is to set the tone for learning."

2. The novice simulation educator needs additional understanding of the National League for Nursing (NLN) Jeffries Simulation Theory when they state one of the components is:

   A. "Educational practices"

   B. "Student learner"

   C. "Design characteristics"

   D. "Participant"

3. A skilled simulation educator plans time in the simulation to include which of the following?

   A. Flexibility in the length of time for the debrief

   B. 10-minute orientation and prebrief

   C. Time to watch the entire video

   D. Allow 10 minutes for participants to write a reflection paper during the debrief

4. The simulation educator understands that they are successful when their learners reach which level of Kirkpatrick's four-level learning theory of evaluation?

   A. Results

   B. Learning

   C. Reaction

   D. Behavior

5. Which is a participant reaction to simulation that has not been supported by research?

   A. Participants learn to think critically and problem-solve

   B. Participants are allowed to make mistakes

   C. Participants experience improved self-confidence

   D. Participants express a lack of anxiety

6. Which two learning domains overlap in simulation?

   A. Cognitive and psychomotor

   B. Affective and psychomotor

   C. Cognitive and affective

   D. Responding and cognitive

*(See answers next page.)*

### 1. C) "During prebriefing, it is important to emphasize that perfection is expected."

Perfection is not an expectation and this is an issue that can be addressed during prebriefing. Prebriefing does include a fictional contract and assist in staging and setting the tone for learning.

### 2. B) "Student learner"

Participants include all learners, not just students, and can include others taking roles during simulation. Simulations always include a design and educational practices.

### 3. A) Flexibility in the length of time for the debrief

Flexibility in debriefing time is needed because different groups may react differently to scenarios and it is important not to rush this learning phase of simulation. Writing a reflection paper, watching a video, and prebriefing do not need exact times because in some instances they may take longer than others, depending on the subject and the complexity of the scenario.

### 4. A) Results

Results in patient care is the ultimate learning goal. Reaction is the first stage, learning is the second stage, and behavior is the third stage that leads up to the results.

### 5. D) Participants express a lack of anxiety

Participants do experience some anxiety because they are expected to treat the situation as real and they may be unfamiliar with the condition being displayed in the simulation scenario. Simulation assists in critical thinking development and improved self-confidence. Participants are allowed to make mistakes and learn from their mistakes in simulation.

### 6. A) Cognitive and psychomotor

Cognitive and psychomotor overlap because learners need to know what they are doing in order to demonstrate the competency. Affective does not have to be part of skills attainment unless a standardized patient is present. Responding is not a learning domain.

7. Which learning method used during debriefing leads the participant to a higher level of critical thinking?

A. Responding
B. Reflection
C. Interpreting
D. Noticing

8. To maintain participant motivation and self-esteem during simulation, what is the BEST role for the debriefer to assume?

A. Advisor
B. Mentor
C. Coach
D. Facilitator

9. Which organization promotes competence, recognition, and development of healthcare facilitators through accreditation standards and processes for certification?

A. International Nursing Association for Clinical Simulation and Learning (INACSL)
B. Association of Standardized Patient Educators (ASPE)
C. Society for Simulation in Healthcare (SSH)
D. American Nurses Credentialing Center (ANCC)

10. What is the MOST effective component of simulation-based education and the corner-stone of the learning experience?

A. Prebriefing
B. Simulation
C. Debriefing
D. Lifesavers

### 7. B) Reflection

Reflection leads to critical thinking because it assists the learners in evaluating their own behavior and how they can improve their behavior. Responding, interpreting, and noticing do not necessarily promote reflection.

### 8. D) Facilitator

Facilitation assists in keeping the learners engaged and on task without spoon-feeding the information to students. Advising and mentoring provide a more learner passive role, and coaching provides learner engagement with more direction from the simulation educator than facilitating.

### 9. C) Society for Simulation in Healthcare (SSH)

The SSH is the organization that promotes simulation accreditation. The INACSL assists with nursing simulation development, and the ASPE is the organization for standardized patients. The ANCC credentials nurses.

### 10. C) Debriefing

Debriefing is important because it is where the learner reflects and uses the experience to improve competencies. Prebriefing and the simulation experience are important, but the majority of learning takes place in the debriefing phase. Lifesavers are part of a simulation experience and are needed to keep learners on track.

## ● REFERENCES

Adamson, K. A., Jeffries, P. R., & Rogers, K. J. (2012). Evaluation: A critical step in simulation practice and research. In P. Jeffries (Ed.), *Simulation in nursing education: From conceptualization to evaluation* (2nd ed., pp. 131–162). National League for Nursing Press.

Al Gharibi, K. A., & Arulappan, J. A. (2020). Repeated simulation experience on self-confidence, critical thinking, and competence of nurses and nursing students—An integrative review. *SAGE Open Nursing, 6*. https://doi.org/10.1177/2377960820927377

Association of American Medical Colleges. (2018). *Explore MedEdPORTAL*. https://www.mededport al.org/

Bailey, K. (2020, February 10). *Using translational simulation in healthcare to improve patient outcomes.* Healthy Simulation. https://www.healthysimulation.com/22544/translational-simulation -in-healthcare/

Baisden, P., & Gray, C. (2020). Hearing voices: An interprofessional education simulation to increase empathy among preprofessional healthcare students. *International Journal for Human Caring, 24*(4), 233–236. https://connect.springerpub.com/content/sgrijhc/24/4/233

Brazil, V. (2017). Translational simulation: Not 'where' but 'why?' A functional view of in situ simulation. *Advances in Simulation, 2*(1), 20. https://doi.org/10.1186/s41077-017-0052-3

Cantrell, M. A., Franklin, A., Leighton, K., & Carlson, A. (2017). The evidence of simulation-based learning experiences in nursing education and practice: An umbrella review. *Clinical Simulation in Nursing, 13*(12), 634–667. https://doi.org/10.1016/j.ecns.2017.08.004

Chemikova, O., Heitzmann, N., Stadler, M., Holzberger, D., Seidel, T., & Fischer, F. (2020). Simulation-based learning in higher education: A meta-analysis. *Review of Educational Research, 90*(4), 499–541. https://doi.org/10.3102/0034654320933544

Cheng, A., Eppich, W., Epps, C., Kolbe, M., Meguerdichian, M., & Grant, V. (2021). Embracing informed learner self-assessment during debriefing: The art of plus-delta. *Advances in Simulation, 6*(1), 1–22. https://doi.org/10.1186/s41077-021-00173-1

Cheng, A., Kolbe, M., Grant, V., Eller, S., Hales, R., Benjamin, S., Griswold, S., & Eppich, W. (2020). A practical guide to virtual debriefings: Communities of inquiry perspective. *Advanced Simulation, 5*(1), 1–18. https://doi.org/10.1186/s41077-020-00141-1

Dix, S., Morphet, J., Jones, T., Kiprillis, N., O'Halloran, M., Piper, K., & Innes, K. (2021). Perceptions of final year nursing students' transfer of clinical judgment skills from simulation to clinical practice: A qualitative study. *Nurse Education in Practice, 56*, Article 103218. https://doi.org/10.1016/j.nepr.2021.103218

Dreifuerst, K. T. (2015). Getting started with debriefing for meaningful learning. *Clinical Simulation in Nursing, 11*(5), 268–275. https://doi.org/10.1016/j.ecns.2015.01.005

Dreifuerst, K. T., Bradley, C. S., & Johnson, B. K. (2021). Using debriefing for meaningful learning with screen-based simulation. *Nurse Educator, 46*(4), 239–244. https://doi.org/10.1097/NNE.0000000000000930

Edwards, J., Wexner, S., & Nichol, A. (2021). *Debriefing for clinical learning. Patient Safety Network.* Agency for Healthcare Research and Quality (AHRQ). https://psnet.ahrq.gov/primer/debriefing-clinical-learning

Eppich, W., & Cheng, A. (2015). Promoting excellence and reflective learning in simulation (PEARLS). *Simulation in Healthcare, 10*(2), 106–115. https://doi.org/10.1097/SIH.0000000000000072

Facione, N. C., & Facione, P. A. (2009). *Insight assessment: Holistic critical thinking rubric.* The California Academic Press.

Foronda, C., Liu, S., & Bauman, E. B. (2013). Evaluation of simulation in undergraduate nurse education: An integrative review. *Clinical Simulation in Nursing, 9*(10), 409–416. https://doi.org/10.1016/j.ecns.2012.11.003

Frandsen, A., & Lehn-Christiansen, S. (2020). Into the black-box of learning in simulation debriefing: A qualitative research study. *Nurse Education Today, 88*, 104–373. https://doi.org/10.1016/j.nedt.2020.104373

Fransen, A. F. (2018). *Technology-enhanced team training in obstetrics: Design and evaluation* [Doctoral dissertation]. Eindhoven University of Technology.

Fuselier, J., Baldwin, D., & Chambers, C.T. (2016). Nursing students' perspectives on manikins of color in simulation laboratories. *Clinical Simulation in Nursing, 12*(6), 197–201. https://doi.org/10.1016/j.ecns.2016.01.011

Graham, C., Atz, T., Phillips, S., Newman, S., & Foronda, C. (2018). Exploration of a racially diverse sample of nursing students' satisfaction, self-efficacy, and perceptions of simulation using racially diverse manikins: A mixed-methods pilot study. *Clinical Simulation in Nursing, 15*, 19–26. https://doi.org/10.1016/j.ecns.2017.08.007

Graham, C. L., & Atz, T. (2015). Baccalaureate minority nursing students' perceptions of high-fidelity simulation. *Clinical Simulation in Nursing, 11*(11), 482–488. https://doi.org/10.1016/j.ecns.2015.10.003

Graham, C. L., Phillips, S. M., Newman, S. D., & Atz, T. W. (2016). Baccalaureate minority nursing students perceived barriers and facilitators to clinical education practices: An integrative review. *Nursing Education Perspectives, 37*(3), 130–137. https://doi.org/10.1097/01.nep.0000000000000003

Hanshaw, S. L., & Dickerson, S. S. (2020). High fidelity simulation evaluation studies in nursing education: A review of the literature. *Nurse Education in Practice, 46*, 102828. https://doi.org/10.1016/j.nepr.2020.102818

Harris, M. (2017). Benefits of membership in professional organizations. *Home Healthcare Now, 35*(2), 129–130. https://doi.org/10.1097/nhh.0000000000000488

Hayden, J. K., Smiley, R. A., Alexander, M., Kardong-Edgren, S., & Jeffries, P. R. (2014). The NCSBN national simulation study: A longitudinal, randomized, controlled study replacing clinical hours with simulation in prelicensure nursing education. *Journal of Nursing Regulation, 5*, S3–S64. https://doi.org/10.1016/S2155-8256(15)30062-4

International Nursing Association for Clinical Simulation and Learning. (2011). Standard VI: The debriefing process. *Clinical Simulation in Nursing, 7*(4S), s16–s17. https://doi.org/10.1016/j.ecns.2011.05.010

International Nursing Association for Clinical Simulation and Learning Standards Committee. (2021). Healthcare simulation standards of best practice™. *Clinical Simulation in Nursing, 58*, 66. https://doi.org/10.1016/j.ecns.2021.08.018

International Nursing Association for Clinical Simulation and Learning Standards Committee, Decker, S., Alinier, G., Crawford, S. B., Gordon, R. M., & Wilson, C. (2021a). Healthcare simulation standards of best practice™: The debriefing process. *Clinical Simulation in Nursing, 58*, 27–32. https://doi.org/10.1016/j.ecns.2021.08.011

International Nursing Association for Clinical Simulation and Learning Standards Committee, McDermott, D., Ludlow, J., Horsley, E., & Meakim, C. (2021b). Healthcare simulation standards of best practice™ prebriefing: Preparation and briefing. *Clinical Simulation in Nursing, 58*, P9–P13. https://doi.org/10.1016/j.ecns.2021.08.008

Jeffries, P., Rodgers, B., & Adamson, K. (2015). NLN Jeffries simulation theory: Brief narrative description. *Nursing Education Perspectives, 36*(5), 292–293. https://doi.org/https://doi.org/10.5480/1536-5026-36.5.292

Kelly, M., Balakrishnan, A., & Naren, K. (2018). Cultural considerations in simulation-based education. *The Asia Pacific Scholar, 3*(3), 1–4. https://doi.org/10.29060/taps.2018-3-3/gp1070

Kim, J., Park, J.-H., & Shin, S. (2016). Effectiveness of simulation-based nursing education depending on fidelity: A meta-analysis. *BMC Medical Education, 16*(152), 1–8. https://doi.org/10.1186/s12909-016-0672-7

Kim, Y.-J., & Yoo, J.-H. (2020). The utilization of debriefing for simulation in healthcare: A literature review. *Nurse Education in Practice, 43*, 102698. https://doi.org/10.1016/j.nepr.2020.102698

Kirkpatrick, D. L., & Kirkpatrick, J. D. (2006). *Evaluating training programs* (3rd ed.). Berrett-Koehler.

Lapkin, S., Fernandez, R., Levett-Jones, T., & Bellchambers, H. (2010). The effectiveness of using human patient simulation manikins in the teaching of clinical reasoning skills to undergraduate nursing students: A systematic review. *JBI Database of Systematic Reviews and Implementation Reports, 8*(16), 661–694. https://doi.org/10.11124/01938924-201008160-00001

Lasater, K. (2007). High-fidelity simulation and the development of clinical judgment: Students' experiences. *Journal of Nursing Education, 46*(6), 269–276.

Lee, J., & Oh, P. J. (2015). Effects of the use of high-fidelity simulation in nursing education: A meta-analysis. *Journal of Nursing Education, 54*(9), 501–507. https://doi.org/10.3928/01484834-20150814-04

Leighton, K., Kardong-Edgren, S. K., McNelis, A., Foisy-Doll, C., & Sullo, E. (2021). Traditional clinical outcomes in prelicensure nursing education: An empty systematic review. *Journal of Nursing Education, 60*(3), 136–142. https://doi.org/10.3928/01484834-20210222-03

Lioce, L., (Founding Ed.), Lopreiato, J., Downing, D., Chang, T. P., Robertson, J. M., Anderson, M., Diaz, D. A., Spain, A. E. (Assoc. Eds.) & the Terminology and Concepts Working Group. (2020, September). *Healthcare simulation dictionary* (2nd ed.). Agency for Healthcare Research and Quality. https://doi.org/10.23970/simulationv2

Mariani, B., & Doolen, J. (2016). Nursing simulation research: What are the perceived gaps. *Clinical Simulation in Nursing, 12*(1), 30–36. https://doi.org/10.1016/j.ecns.2015.11.004

McGahie, W. C., Issenberg, B., Petrusa, E. R., & Scalese, R. J. (2016). Revisiting a critical review of simulation-based medical education research: 2003-2009. *Medical Education, 50*(10), 986–991. https://doi.org/10.1111/medu.12795

Mulli, J., Nowell, L., Swart, R., & Estefan, A. (2022). Undergraduate nursing simulation facilitators lived experience of facilitating reflection-in-action during high-fidelity simulation: A phenomenological study. *Nurse Education Today, 109*, 105251. https://doi.org/10.1016/j.nedt.2021.105251

Murray, D. J., Boulet, J. R., Avidan, M., Kras, J. F., Heinrich, B., & Woodhouse, J. (2007). Performance of residents and anesthesiologists in simulation-based skill assessment. *Anesthesiology, 107*(5), 705–713. https://doi.org/10.1097/01.anes.0000286926.01083.9d

Padden, M. L. (2013). A pilot study to determine the validity and reliability of the level of reflection-on-action assessment. *Journal of Nursing Education, 52*(7), 410–415. https://doi.org/10.3928/01484834-20130613-03

Padden-Denmead, M. L., Scaffidi, R. M., Kerley, R. M., & Farside, A. L. (2016). Simulation with debriefing and guided reflective journaling to stimulate critical thinking in prelicensure baccalaureate degree nursing students. *Journal of Nursing Education, 55*(11), 645–650. https://doi.org/10.3928/01484834-20161011-07

Radhakrishnan, K., Roche, J. P., & Cunningham, H. (2007). Measuring clinical practice parameters with human patient simulation: A pilot study. *International Journal of Nursing Education Scholarship, 4*(1), 8. https://doi.org/10.2202/1548-923x.1307

Roberts, E., Kaak, V., & Rolley, J. (2019). Simulation to replace clinical hours in nursing: A meta-narrative review. *Clinical Simulation in Nursing, 37*, 5–13. https://doi.org/10.1016/j.ecns.2019.07.003

Rosen, M. A., Salas, E., Silvestri, S., Wu, T. S., & Lazarra, E. H. (2008). A measurement tool for simulation-based training in emergency medicine: The simulation module for assessment of resident targeted event responses (SMARTER) approach. *Simulation in Healthcare, 3*(3), 170–179. https://doi.org/10.1097/sih.0b013e318173038d

Rudolph, J. W., Simon, R., Dufresne, R. L., & Raemer, D. B. (2006). There's no such thing as "nonjudgmental" debriefing: A theory and method for debriefing with good judgment. *Simulation in Healthcare: Journal of the Society for Simulation in Healthcare, 1*(1), 49–55. https://doi.org/10.1097/01266021-200600110-00006

Society for Simulation in Healthcare. (2021). *Certified healthcare simulation educator handbook*. https://www.ssih.org/Portals/48/Certification/CHSE_Docs/CHSE%20Handbook.pdf

Sullivan, N., Swoboda, S. M., Breymier, T., Lucas, L., Sarasnick, J., Rutherford-Hemming, T., Budhathoki, C., & Kardong-Edgren, S. K. (2019). Emerging evidence toward a 2:1 clinical to simulation ratio: A study comparing the traditional clinical and simulation settings. *Clinical Simulation in Nursing, 30*, 34–41. https://doi.org/10.1016/j.ecns.2019.03.003

Weaver, K., & Olson, J. (2006). Understanding paradigms used for nursing research. *Journal of Advanced Nursing, 53*(4), 459–469. https://doi.org/10.1111/j.1365-2648.2006.03740.x

Wooding, E. L., Gale, T. C., & Maynard, V. (2020). Evaluation of teamwork assessment tools for inter-professional simulation: A systematic literature review. *Journal of Interprofessional Care*, 34(2), 162–172. https://doi.org/10.1080/13561820.2019.1650730

Yockey, J., & Henry, M. (2019). Simulation anxiety across the curriculum. *Clinical Simulation in Nursing*, 29, 29–37. https://doi.org/10.1016/j.ecns.2018.12.004

Zhang, H., Wang, W., Goh, S. H. L., Wu, X., V., & Morelius, E. (2020). The impact of a three-phase video-assisted debriefing on nursing students' debriefing experiences, perceived stress, and facilitators practices: A mixed methods study. *Nursing Education Today*, 90, 1–8. https://doi.org/10.1016/j.nedt.2020.104460

# PART V

**Simulation Resources and Environments**

# Operations and Management of Environment, Personnel, and Nonpersonnel Resources

Carolyn H. Scheese

*By failing to prepare, you are preparing to fail.*

—*Benjamin Franklin*

This chapter addresses Domain IV: Simulation Resources and Environments (Society for Simulation in Healthcare [SSH], 2021).

## ▶ LEARNING OUTCOMES

- Discuss basic managerial and operational principles associated with delivering simulation activities and effective and efficient management of personnel and nonpersonnel resources.
- Analyze ways in which the physical environment can be modified to maximize simulation-based learning, including the use of timelines and checklists to improve outcomes.
- Describe common policies, procedures, and practices of an efficient simulation program.
- Discuss effective ways to manage and respond to technical and material issues (e.g., video capture, simulator failures, and material supplies) that may occur in the simulation environment.
- Identify gaps and opportunities in staffing, policies, organizational structure, physical environment, and so on.
- Articulate how specific factors impact operations, that is, physical environment, staffing, scheduling, policies, leadership, and management.
- Apply risk management strategies to a simulation center or program.

## ▶ INTRODUCTION

This chapter focuses on the management and operations of a simulation center, including the management of personnel and nonpersonnel (space, supplies, equipment, technology, money, etc.) resources. Whether large or small, completely outfitted with the latest high-fidelity technology or an outdated space stocked mainly with task trainers and low- to mid-fidelity manikins, there are key operational principles that can apply to almost any setting. This chapter is divided into sections with multiple headings and is intended to serve as a guide and resource, not only to provide sufficient information to aid in passing certification examinations, but also as a resource that you can come back to from time to time so you can improve planning, organizing, managing, and executing simulations in your center.

# ▶ OPERATIONS MANAGEMENT: WHAT IS OPERATIONS?

Operations management is the process of managing and coordinating all resources—personnel and nonpersonnel—and coordinating and managing them in such a way that they are used efficiently and effectively to meet the goals and mission of the institution. Operations provides the support and infrastructure to get things done; it is considered the business side of simulation. Business operations usually includes four key areas:

- the physical space (location)
- equipment and supplies (tools)
- personnel (staff, standardized patients, all employees or volunteers of the center)
- policies, procedures and/or flowcharts, and processes (Pakroo, 2020)

Operations is the coordination and management of the many support pieces that are required to put a plan into place and then execute that plan. Identifying and addressing gaps in each of these key areas are critical to a smooth-running simulation center.

# ▶ SCHEDULING

Scheduling of the space, personnel, and equipment is one of the biggest challenges and headaches of a simulation center because scheduling events involves a complex set of rules and variables. Scheduling involves matching personnel (faculty, learners, volunteers, staff, information technology [IT] support, etc.) and nonpersonnel resources (space, technology, manikins, supplies, etc.) with dates and times. Throughout this section, you will note that scheduled items are referred to as "events." Events can include many things: a simulation scenario, an open house, or a very important person (VIP) tour; meeting with faculty/instructors; standardized patient (SP) training; an objective structured clinical examination (OSCE); skills lab training session; open lab time for learners; or center closures to install or maintain equipment. Each of these events is unique, yet all require the coordination of personnel and nonpersonnel resources within a date and time.

## METHODS TO TRACK SCHEDULING

Many different methods may be used to schedule and track simulation center activities. Paper-and-pencil office scheduling ledgers are available for a minimal cost and may meet the needs of a small center with just a few activities or events per day. Ideally, keep all various pieces related to an event in one location; having items in multiple locations can be frustrating and lead to lost or missing information critical to the event's success.

The advantages of pen-and-paper scheduling are that it is inexpensive, portable, and easy to use and update. The limitations to this method include the following:

- Limited access: Only one person has access to the ledger at a time.
- The ledger may get lost, making it difficult to reconstruct upcoming events.
- As the center grows, this system can be time-intensive to manage and maintain.
- Limited information can be written in the ledger, which may require additional support methods to manage event information, such as the final confirmed date and time, names of learners, scenario details, and other resources.

Schedules can be maintained through a variety of electronic methods, some of which are free or of very low cost, such as Google and Outlook calendars or homegrown methods, whereas other commercially available event managers and scheduling products may be very costly. The available features vary according to the product. Some advantages of commercial products may include:

■ Calendar sharing: These products provide greater access to information related to the simulation center-scheduled events as these can frequently be shared and may have varying levels of access and privilege for the audience who is viewing the calendar, such as view-only and full-scheduling rights.
■ They provide the ability to link communication/emails and event information to the scheduled event.
■ Some systems include the ability to track learners, personnel, space, supplies, and equipment to generate detailed invoices reflecting event and center costs.
■ Some systems house the prework and allow instructor access to learner and scenario information remotely.
■ Some systems allow self-registration and automatic event reminders and allow learners and faculty to sign into the center upon arrival.

Scheduling and maintaining the schedule so that the information is disseminated to the level needed for implementation can take a lot of time. So, although the cost of an electronic event manager may be high, it can potentially generate cost savings by saving time and decreasing frustration, as well as increasing quality and event consistency (Exhibit 22.1).

---

**EXHIBIT 22.1 THINGS TO CONSIDER WHEN SCHEDULING**

■ Mission of the center
■ Priorities of the center
■ Resource limits (time, personnel, faculty/instructors, space, etc.)
■ Personnel (support personnel, faculty, staff, learners/students, volunteers/SPs, etc.)
■ Knowledge and skills/skill level
■ Availability of personnel and nonpersonnel items
■ Physical space
■ Equipment/supplies

SP, standardized patient.

---

## THE SCHEDULER

The individual who is responsible for the scheduling calendar is potentially one of the most powerful individuals in the center. This individual is your public relations officer. The scheduler is often the first individual with whom your customers interact. The scheduler is the face of the business, a gatekeeper who can deter or encourage the use of the center by the very manner in which the scheduler interacts with those who contact the center. How the scheduler's power is used and managed will, to a large extent, determine the accessibility to the center. If someone is unable to schedule an event, or if the hassle factor is too high or negative in nature, customers will go elsewhere. It stands to reason that unless events are scheduled, you would not run events. Understanding your customers and providing good customer service from the very first encounter are essential to sustained success (Scheese, 2013).

A business absolutely devoted to service will have only one worry about profits. They will be embarrassingly large.

—Henry Ford

The schedule is a linchpin. The scheduling calendar holds all the information together so that a successful event can occur. A poorly managed schedule creates inefficiencies and frustration for those who use the center as well as those who support the events. An ideal scheduler is detail-oriented, good at organizing content and information, proactive, a good communicator, and willingly accepts direction.

## BLOCK SCHEDULING

Block scheduling has been used for many years in operating rooms (ORs) and surgical centers to provide predictability for the end user and the facility (Lee et al., 2018). Simulation centers have many common elements with these facilities and may benefit from this method of scheduling events. Block scheduling consists of providing/setting aside a block of days or times for an end user. In this situation, an *end user* could refer to a faculty member, course, class, or pass-off/exam where there is predictability in the need for resources. For example, medical students in your center may have OSCEs every 6 weeks. Scheduling these events out even as far as 1 year in advance makes sense, if supporting the education of medical students is consistent with the center's mission. Using block scheduling, SPs, space, staff, and faculty/instructor support may also be scheduled out into the future and made predictable.

The greater the predictability in the schedule, the easier it is to adjust for minor changes and challenges that come along. Block scheduling is based on the principle that if you schedule your highest priority customers first, you can work the lower priority customers into the vacancies that exist.

First, determine what groups have priority and why. This determination can be made by an oversight committee and should be consistent with the center's mission, vision, and values. One method is to classify users into three groups, according to definitions of priority—A, B, and C—and to schedule As first and Bs second, followed by Cs.

Sharing space and other available resources can be challenging. Distribution of resources takes negotiation and open communication. Like filling a jar with various sizes of rocks, pebbles, and sand, if you put the rocks in first, starting with the largest, followed by the pebbles and last of all the sand, then the jar can hold the maximum amount of material. This principle can be applied to scheduling. Fill the schedule with the largest (priority) users first, then fit your other users around them to maximize the capacity of the center.

### DISADVANTAGES

This system can be abused and needs a check-and-balance system to be most effective. You may have some users who schedule block time and then do not use it, especially ones who do not cancel with sufficient notice to schedule other users. Users in the C group may feel frustrated at not getting their first choice or prime slots. Again, ensuring that the scheduling process reflects the mission, vision, and values of the center will help in the decision-making process related to this challenge. One way to deal with this dilemma is to reassess your users at regular intervals and reprioritize groups as needed. Clearly established policies, including any noncancellation fees that may be assessed, will help all parties understand expectations.

## FIRST COME, FIRST SCHEDULED

First come, first served is another philosophy that can be used when scheduling events. Simply put, customers and events are prioritized and scheduled in accordance with when the request is received. Using a hybrid or a combination of both block scheduling and first come, first served is another way to manage the schedule. Regardless of the method chosen, it should be consistent with the mission, vision, and values of the center; clearly communicated to the "communities of interest" or "stakeholders"; and supported by the policies and procedures of the center.

# ▶ PREPARING FOR DELIVERY OF A SIMULATION EVENT

Preparation and organization are essential to the successful outcome of a simulation experience. Templates may be useful in scheduling events and writing scenarios. Timelines and checklists can be helpful in outlining expectations and organizing events, from conception to implementation and final evaluation. Tracking and organizing scenarios can be done electronically, with a physical hard copy, or by a combination of both electronic and hard copies.

Clearly establish timelines and expectations with those who schedule events so that there is sufficient time for all to prepare for the event (Exhibit 22.2).

---

**EXHIBIT 22.2 TIMELINE AND CHECKLIST FOR A NEW SIMULATION EVENT**

**3–6 Months Prior to the Event**
- Determine goals/learners/instructor support (overarching concept of the event determined).
- Schedule space and use of any major equipment and supplies needed to support the event.
- Schedule learners/instructors and support personnel.
- Write scenarios/OSCEs.
- Order the needed equipment and supplies.

**6–8 Weeks Prior to the Event**
- Finalize the number and begin to schedule SPs.
- Verify the request for ordering of any special supplies.

**4 Weeks Prior to the Event**
- Finalize the event/scenario.
- Review plan with those who will be implementing and modify as needed.

**2 Weeks Prior to the Event**
- Do a "walk-through": Facilitators/instructors and support staff meet together in the space where the simulation will occur and review the scenario and identify and resolve areas of question or concern or that need to be clarified or modified.
- Train SPs 5 to 10 days prior.

**Week of the Event**
- Send reminders to participants and instructors.
- Review the need for and last-minute changes by facilitators/instructors.
- Pre-event evaluation/survey and prework should be sent out and completed by learners.

**Day Prior/Day of the Event**
- Arrive early.
- Set up the room.
- Conduct team huddle/preprocedure checklist, verify room setup, and modify as needed.
- Complete learner postsimulation evaluation and other postwork as assigned.

**Following the Event**
- Debrief all team members: Meet to discuss what went well and what can be improved.
- Revise the scenario and document changes as needed.
- Get feedback from the customer on user experience. Review for quality improvement.

OSCE, objective structured clinical examination; SP, standardized patient.

Events themselves can also have timelines to aid in keeping the event on time and focused on what matters most. Both simple and complex events can benefit from timelines.

Checklists can be used just prior to when the simulation starts to verify that all items are set up and ready to go, much like the OR uses a checklist for a "time-out" prior to surgery, or the airlines use a preflight checklist (Exhibit 22.3). This checklist can be part of the "huddle" some centers use. The "huddle" is a short meeting that occurs just prior to starting the simulation to ensure that everyone is ready to go, to ensure a common understanding of the sequence of events, and to answer any questions any member of the team may have (Table 22.1).

---

## EXHIBIT 22.3 PRESCENARIO CHECKLIST

**Simulation Event**
- Scenario duration and number
- Sequence of events
- Anticipated end time
- Anticipated breaks/setup changes
- Simulation room number
- Debriefing room number

**Technical Issues**
- Video/camera setup
- Video debriefing needs
- Electronic files and location
- Smart board needs

**Virtual Reality Equipment and Supplies**

**Manikin**
- Type
- Preprogrammed/on-the-fly programming
- Position/location
- Moulage
- Fluids
- Name and allergy band

**Standardized Patient**
- Training/instructions
- Moulage/clothing/attire
- Waiting/staging area
- Props/name and allergy band
- Two-way radio/walkie-talkie
- Time cards/parking validations/meals

**Room Setup**
- Equipment
- Supplies
- Electronic health record/bedside computer needs
- Props
- Bed type/gurney/crib
- Special needs?

**Medications**
- Label
- Name

■ Dose
■ Planned med error?
■ Location: medication refrigerator
■ Medication dispenser programming

**Roles and Responsibilities**
■ Technical roles/responsibilities
■ Faculty roles/responsibilities
■ Confederate (a supportive actor used in some simulations) role needed?
■ Adequate resources?

**Other?**

*Source:* Adapted from Lassche, M., & Scheese, C. (2013). *Effective team work—More than a game of chance* [Poster presentation]. 12th Annual International Nursing Simulation/Learning (INACSL) Resource Centers Conference: Hit the Jackpot with Evidence Based Simulation, Las Vegas, Nevada, United States.

### Table 22.1 Simulation Event Timeline

| Timeline | Sequence of Events | Resources: Facilitator and Roles |
|---|---|---|
| 20 min | Orientation to environment<br>Overview and expectations<br>Prework<br>Division of roles | Orient learners to simulation room<br>Collect consent from learners<br>Review prework, discussion, and articles<br>Use PowerPoints with prescenario videos<br>Determine roles<br>Review chart contents/divide into roles |
| 10 min | Scenario 1: Patient needs blood<br>Group B participates in the scenario | Group A observational engagement |
| 20 min | Debrief | All facilitators debrief |
| 15 min | Scenario 2: Patient develops acute blood transfusion reaction<br>Group A participates in the scenario | Group B observational engagement |
| 20 min | Debrief | All facilitators debrief |
| 5 min | Wrap-up | Closing remarks, handouts, reminder to do postsurvey, and confidentiality |
| Total time = 1.5 hours | | |

## ▶ TRACKING CENTER ACTIVITIES

Simulation is expensive. Those who support simulation financially or by other means will want to know how their contributions made a difference. In business, this is referred to as *return on investment* (*ROI*). In other words, what was the benefit of the time, energy, and resources put into this event or center as a whole? In order to provide this information to those who invest in the center, it is important to track the usage, productivity, and costs associated with the center. The following are just a few items that can be tracked for each event: number of learners, number of instructors, length of simulation (time/hours), supply costs, equipment and space usage, time required for event setup and breakdown, administrative and support time, and so on. This information can be tracked by individual events and then compiled at the end of the year as a portion of the annual report. Data are invaluable when it comes to asking for continued or additional financial support. It is also important in tracking expenses and depreciating equipment.

## ANNUAL AND PERIODIC REPORTS

Preparing and publishing annual and periodic reports is a way to report on and evaluate accomplishments; ROI of the center; and opportunities and gaps, to the many communities of interest and stakeholders, and to measure and track progress on goals. Items that may be listed in an annual report include changes in leadership, instructors, or personnel; income and expense reports; purchases and needs of new equipment; grants received and processed; scholarship activities such as manuscripts submitted and published; type and number of presentations; center event utilization rates; and student/learner contact hours.

### Simulation Teaching Tip 22.1

The number of learners times the number of hours present for a learning activity equals learner contact hours.

## MISSION, VISION, AND VALUES

Businesses (yes, education and simulation can be considered businesses) often create a mission statement to define their purpose and priorities. Many times, but not always, a vision statement and values are also defined. A mission statement is a statement of purpose; it defines the institution's purpose for existence and its focus (Pakroo, 2020). Vision is the overarching view of purpose—where the company is headed. Key values may also be selected and defined. Examples of values include integrity, quality, collaboration, and so on. Mission, vision, and values help determine what projects to undertake and which ones to decline. Consider defining *why* your simulation center exists. Take time to understand how your simulation center fits into the goals, mission, and operational and strategic plans of the organization. A simulation center that is siloed is not going to be as successful as one that is closely aligned with the rest of the organization. Most likely, it is relatively easy to define *what* your center does and probably not too challenging to explain *how* your center functions and does what it does. However, businesses and individuals that start with *why* tend to be more innovative and flexible and attract a loyal customer base who support them in the long term (Sinek, 2009).

## BUSINESS PLAN

The business plan is like a road map or navigational chart that provides a plan and summaries of information related to that business. This information may include the purpose and organizational structure of the business, company strategy, the existing marketplace, a marketing plan, a review of finances, and action plans with a timetable. A business plan can be used not only to help establish a business, but also to help improve operations and efficiencies, or provide a new direction (Pakroo, 2020). It takes time and effort to develop a business plan, and it can be challenging because there are many difficult questions that must be addressed when putting this plan together. However, it is worth the effort and is one of the most important steps you can take for success. A written business plan can help a company stay focused on its purpose (Pakroo, 2020). Be realistic in creating a timetable when establishing a new center. Recognize that it takes about 18 months to get a simulation center fully operational. Even once a center has been established, the business plan should be revisited regularly and modified to meet changing needs. The U.S. Small Business Administration (www.sba.gov) has many resources for starting and managing small businesses.

## STRATEGIC PLAN

A strategic plan is a plan for the future that links present and future operations to the organization's mission, vision, and values. Strategic plans are commonly generated for 3 to 5 years into the future, but can be changed more frequently if the business climate is dynamic or in a rapidly changing environment. Annual and semiannual goals are generated to support and achieve the strategic plan. Strategic plans should be reviewed at least annually. Alterations in the marketplace and other factors, such as changes in an administration with a new direction or goals, may necessitate a change in the strategic plan. The simulation center's strategic plan must be congruent and align with the organization's strategic plan.

## BUDGET

A budget is a fiscal plan that includes estimated expenses and income for a predetermined amount of time, generally 1 year. Costs must be planned and tracked. However, it is important to realize that a budget is a forecast or plan for the future and will likely need some flexibility, reassessment, and revisions to account for unforeseen happenings (Marquis & Huston, 2021). Depending on the size of your center, you may have a budget of a few thousand dollars, or in a larger center your budget may be several million dollars or more. However, the principles of a budget remain the same. Revenue, or money coming in, must not exceed expenses, or money going out. All money coming in and going out must be tracked and accounted for. Costs are usually broken down into personnel and nonpersonnel cost or salary and nonsalary items.

One of the largest ongoing expenses is personnel costs in the form of salaries. Personnel may be paid in part or in full, from the organization's budget or from the simulation center's budget. Determine if personnel are expected to help offset the cost of their salary through generating business in the simulation center. Benefits generally account for about one-third of the wage. Cost of living raises may be given on an annual basis and can have a tremendous impact on a simulation center's budget and must be considered when planning future expenses.

A budget should take into account the depreciation of equipment and plan for the replacement of durable equipment. Other considerations include software licensing and upgrades, equipment repair and maintenance, office supplies, and so on. Computers and technology have a very short life span, about 3 to 6 years. A state-of-the-art center without a plan and budget to consistently and thoughtfully upgrade, repair, and replace old equipment will quickly become outdated and enter a state of disrepair.

When creating a budget, plan for both current and future costs and needs. Consider the items that you need to request to keep your center going, not just now, but in the future. Work with your finance administrator or chief financial officer (CFO) to see how your institution can set aside money each year for anticipated purchases and to plan for the replacement of simulators, computers, and other technological devices and equipment. Consider the infrastructure; anticipate needs for growth and updates.

Determine the life span of the equipment in your center, then plan for its replacement. Staggering the replacement of some of these items over a few years can help level out the cost in the overall budget. For example, if you have 21 computers that are aging and need to be replaced within the next 3 years, you can budget for seven computers per year for 3 years.

This can help to even out the overall budget. Likewise, cameras, manikins/human patient simulators (HPSs), task trainers, and so on, and their life expectancy need to be considered and put into the budget accordingly.

Capital equipment is generally considered as durable equipment that has a life expectancy of greater than 1 year and exceeds a certain purchase amount. The amount is usually determined by the institution. For example, it might be defined by an institution as $5,000. So anything that costs more than $5,000 would be considered capital equipment and usually has to go through different channels and processes in order to make that purchase. Some institutions require that all capital purchases go out for bid or may require at least three quotes from competing vendors. In simulation, most HPSs fall into the capital equipment request category of the budget. Do not be shy about asking for what you need to run a good program. Recognize that it may take a few budget cycles to get the things you need. Do not give up. Prepare yourself to speak knowledgeably about the proposed purchase and do your research so that you know what features you need and the expected ROI for learners.

> Asking is the beginning of receiving. Make sure you don't go to the ocean with a teaspoon. At least take a bucket so the kids won't laugh at you.
>
> —Jim Rohn

One thing to keep in mind when considering approval of expenses is learning the restrictions on various funds/revenue accounts. For example, money donated to the center may be restricted to a specific purchase, such as a crib, task trainer, or manikin. Money from grants may also have strict limitations on how it can be spent. In academic institutions, there are many restrictions on what student fees, state funds, or tuition money can purchase. Tracking and accounting for each type of incoming revenue and the requisite expenses are very important. Misuse of funds may result in embarrassment, loss of trust, and even loss of employment.

Equipment and supplies can also be obtained by networking with those in your community who have access to outdated supplies and equipment. This can save a tremendous amount of money for programs that do not have a budget for these items (Massie, 2019). Some equipment can be rented; refurbished rather than new items can be purchased at a fraction of the cost.

Simulation centers can obtain their revenue in a variety of ways, such as student fees, tuition, grants, donors, usage fees, and so on. Some are for profit, whereas others are nonprofit. A cost recovery center or recharge center is a center that is able to recoup costs by charging fees to users such that it is able to compensate the cost of doing business. Other approaches are called *pay to play*. In order to use the center, you must first agree to pay. Often the payment is received upfront. No matter the source of the revenue stream, in order for a center to be viable it must be sustainable. Expenses cannot exceed revenue.

## ▶ PHYSICAL SPACE

As much as possible, organize the physical space of the center so that items are grouped according to similar supplies and convenient to the site or point of use. For example, locate all moulage supplies in the same area, and group all wound dressings or IV supplies together. Organizing the physical space increases efficiency, reduces frustration in not being able to find needed supplies and equipment, and facilitates the ease of tracking the inventory of supplies and equipment. Label everything (Figure 22.1). Supplies for specific scenarios or skills can be organized and placed in containers with their specific inventory sheets/required supply lists and instructions.

Keep reference materials, such as user manuals, policies and procedure manuals, simulation scenarios, skill equipment checklists, and so on, in a common area that can be accessed by all who may need these reference materials. Create logbooks to track capital equipment inventory, periodic maintenance, and repair histories that can be traced to a particular device/piece of equipment such as a specific HPS. This history and tracking information is necessary if a piece of equipment ever malfunctions or needs repairs covered by warranty.

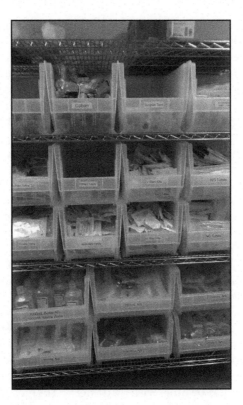

**Figure 22.1** Shelves of labeled supplies.

Quick setup guides can be created (or may be available from the manufacturer) and filed in a common area or attached to a device as appropriate. A short-list "quick setup"/"troubleshooting guide" can be written up in bullet points and attached to the equipment/device with clear waterproof tape or laminated and attached as appropriate for the end user. Be sure to include the sales representative's name, phone number, and the manufacturer's contact information.

## MODIFYING THE ENVIRONMENT

Assessing and modifying the physical environment is an important part of setting up a simulation. The physical space of a simulated environment can be modified to create realism. Our senses help us form memory. Sight, smell, sound, and temperature can all be part of an engaging physical setup for simulation. Moulage can be used to create a more realistic experience for the learner. It can be a wig, a fake scar, vomit, urine, blood, and so on. Moulage is an art that increases realism. Odors can enhance realism, too. For example, combining lemon juice and finely grated Parmesan cheese with food coloring can create not only the appearance of vomit, but also an odor associated with vomit. Sprays that simulate feces can be purchased, iron tablets can be added to fake blood to create odor, and a small amount of ammonia can be added to fake urine to create a realistic odor (Langford, n.d.). The presence of odors can enhance realism and emotionally engage the learner. A simple search on the internet brings up thousands of recipes and ideas for moulage and recipes.

A simulation room at the Winter Institute for Simulation, Education, and Research (WISER), the Peter Winter Institute for Simulation in Pittsburgh, Pennsylvania, has several sets of ceiling-to-floor curtains with various images from the environment they want to portray, such as a scene of a big city for a group of emergency medical technicians (EMTs) or a scene of an OR, to help immerse their learners in the physical environment.

The Center for Advanced Medical Learning and Simulation (CAMLS) in Tampa, Florida, has a trauma OR that projects images on the walls, using sights, sounds, and temperature changes in the environment they wish to recreate to increase realism.

HPSs can be dressed in expected attire, and a few pieces of furniture or relevant objects may be brought into the scenario room. For example, the realism of a disaster scenario may be improved with the use of strobe lights and a fog machine.

A balance between learner goals and costs should be considered. Reviewing the goals and learning outcomes of the simulated event can provide clear guidance as to what is required and what is an unnecessary expense. For example, if there is a scenario that includes a patient-controlled anesthesia (PCA) pump and the center does not own a pump (but could rent one with tubing for a month for $350), reviewing the scenario objectives may help determine whether it is worth the extra cost of renting the pump. If a key component of the scenario objectives includes the setup and use of the PCA pump, it may be worth the additional cost. If the pump plays a very minor role and the setup and use of the PCA pump are minor, then it may not be worth the extra costs. In its place, a mocked-up pump may work to achieve the learning objectives.

The greater the realism in sights, sounds, smells, and temperature, the easier it is for a learner to engage in the realism of the scenario. The use of prescenario video clips or briefs can be effective engagement tools. Of utmost importance is the willingness of the learner to engage and suspend disbelief; no amount of realism can overcome an unwilling participant. However, a highly realistic environment that takes into account all senses makes it easier to suspend disbelief than it would be otherwise (Muckler & Thomas, 2019).

## ▶ POLICIES, PROCEDURES, AND PRACTICES

A policy is a brief description of a plan or standard that is used in decision-making. A procedure is the step-by-step process or set of instructions outlining how to implement the policy. Procedures are usually used for complex procedures or for procedures that require detail and quality control. Processes are the manner in which things actually occur. Quality improvement assumes that there is a connection between processes and efficiency or quality care. Process audits can be done to evaluate current inefficiencies and to identify efficiencies (Marquis & Huston, 2021).

Every center should have formally written documents, including organizational structure and policies and procedures, to help establish an understanding of expectations for facility users, employees, and the communities of interest/stakeholders. Policies can be either formal (written and sanctioned by a formal authoritative body [governing board or perhaps a guidance or steering committee]) or informal, based on historical actions. Written policy is best as it allows for transparency and consistency. Writing policies can be very time-consuming and often requires many drafts before a final policy gains approval, is agreed on, and implemented (Exhibit 22.4).

### EXHIBIT 22.4 DEFINE AND CLARIFY PROCESSES

- What needs to be done?
- Who will do it?
- How will it be done?
- Are there any costs? How will these be covered?

Basic organizational documents include the following:

- mission, vision, and values
- organizational chart
- job descriptions with roles and responsibilities

Core polices should be consistent and support the mission of the facility whether it be research, education/teaching, assessment, or an integration of several of these (Marquis & Huston, 2021; SSH, 2021).

Basic policies, procedures, and processes include scheduling an event, managing tours, retention and access to video (how long video is retained/archived), resolving customer/communities of interest/stakeholder complaints, hours of operation, access to center and admittance criteria, loaning of equipment and supplies, costs/charges, and many others. Human resource policies and procedures may include dress code, payroll and attendance issues (clocking in, scheduling vacation, calling in sick, etc.), role and expectations, and so on (Marquis & Huston, 2021; SSH, 2021). Consider developing policies and procedures related to the accreditation requirements. It will provide a good foundation for your center, even if you choose not to go through the accreditation process (Exhibit 22.5).

---

### EXHIBIT 22.5 REQUIRED DOCUMENTATION FOR ACCREDITATION

- Mission and governance
- Organization and management
- Facilities, technology, simulation modalities, and human resources
- Evaluation and improvement
- Integrity
- Security
- Expanding the field
- Learning activities
- Qualified educators
- Curriculum design
- Learning environment
- Ongoing curriculum feedback and improvement
- Educational credit

*Source:* Adapted from the Society for Simulation in Healthcare. (2014b). *Council for accreditation of healthcare simulation programs accreditation standards self-study review.* http://www.ssih.org/Accreditation/Full-Accreditation

---

## PHYSICAL SECURITY: LOCKED UP

Simulation centers often contain hundreds of thousands of dollars' worth of equipment and supplies. In order to protect this investment, security systems with alarms should be put into place and policies adopted that can achieve a balance between protecting the valuable assets and allowing entry into the facility in a manner that is consistent with the mission of the center. Some centers allow access to specific users 24/7, whereas other centers greatly restrict access to standard operating hours. For example, medical residents, desiring to improve their skills with laparoscopic surgery, are among those who may want 24/7 access to the equipment and supplies. Their hours are unpredictable and ready access to the center may be required to meet the needs of the user/learner. Clearly established policies and procedures for access and expectations of cleanup, along with proper training on the care and use of the equipment, are essential to preserving the investment and preventing costly repairs or replacements.

## SEPARATION OF SIMULATED AND ACTUAL PATIENT MEDICATIONS, SUPPLIES, AND EQUIPMENT

Simulation in situ is a simulation done in the actual clinical setting, for example, within an actual OR, ED, or critical care unit at a functioning hospital or clinic. This allows for maximum realism as related to the environment. Simulation in situ is particularly valuable in examining processes.

---

### Evidence-Based Simulation Practice 22.1

**In Situ Simulation Can Improve Patient Safety**

An adult ICU used in situ simulation to identify latent safety issues due to a recent change in the location and storage of medications. Through this simulation, they were able to identify and correct medication labeling issues (Bapteste et al., 2020).

---

When using in situ simulation, there must be a clear separation among actual patient information, equipment, and supplies, and items used for simulation. Patient safety is of utmost concern. Fake medications and expired or unsterile supplies may be used in simulation and must be clearly identified "Not for patient use—for simulation use." All simulated medications, supplies, and equipment should be clearly labeled to prevent inadvertent use on an actual patient (Figure 22.2).

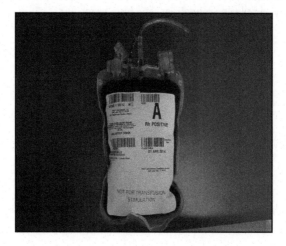

**Figure 22.2** Labeling props for simulation.

## PERSONNEL

*Personnel* or *human capital* are terms that may be used to identify anyone who is employed or volunteers for the simulation center. Personnel is a business' greatest resource because, while equipment, supplies, and space (nonpersonnel resources) may depreciate and decline in value over time, personnel can continually improve and increase in value. It is the individual and collective personnel's talents, skills, knowledge, attitudes, and abilities that create the unique nature of each center. Not only are personnel the most valuable asset, but they are also the most expensive.

Titles, roles, and responsibilities differ from center to center, but support of essential functions remain: Managing, planning and preparing, implementing, cleaning up, and evaluating are all required support activities of a simulation event. Each center determines how best to meet the various needs of its unique center accordingly. Some common titles and roles of simulation center personnel may include simulation technology specialists (STSs)/simulation technologists, information technologists, computer support, faculty/instructors, student workers/teaching assistants, administrative support/secretary, simulation coordinators, managers, program directors, operations directors, administration, SPs/patient actors, and so on.

Simulation centers are unique in many ways, which may make it difficult to find and hire personnel who have experience in simulation and which can result in gaps in training and knowledge of the culture or language, as well as gaps in knowledge and expertise of the unique technology of the simulation center. Often the best staff for a simulation center is a mix of individuals who have both clinical and technical expertise, and a desire to learn and innovate (Gantt & Young, 2016).

## STAKEHOLDERS AND COMMUNITIES OF INTEREST

Every simulation center has an impact on individuals and groups in their community. These individuals and groups are called *stakeholders*. Stakeholders can be internal or external. Internal stakeholders include people with a direct vested interest in the success of the center, whereas external stakeholders have an indirect interest in the success of the center due to the actual or potential impact of the center (Exhibit 22.6). Stakeholders can have a variety of goals and vested interests in the center (Marquis & Huston, 2021).

| EXHIBIT 22.6 EXAMPLES OF STAKEHOLDERS IN AN ACADEMIC HEALTHCARE SIMULATION CENTER | |
|---|---|
| **Internal Stakeholders** | **External Stakeholders** |
| Employees/staff<br>Administration<br>Financial donors/grantors<br>Learners/students<br>Instructors/faculty<br>Board of directors/governing board | Local businesses/hiring hospitals<br>Accrediting bodies<br>Certification agencies<br>Community leaders<br>Professional organizations<br>Alumni boards<br>Malpractice insurance companies |

Together (the combination of external and internal stakeholders), these groups are sometimes referred to as *communities of interest*. This term, *communities of interest*, is frequently used in accreditation criteria and by accrediting bodies. These groups are important because they can provide valuable information on how well the center is doing at meeting the expectations of the communities of interest and center goals.

## ▶ VARIOUS USERS OF A SIMULATION CENTER

Depending on the physical structure, equipment, and personnel, simulation centers have many opportunities to serve various groups and users. A center can specialize, or expand to fit, several audiences depending on its resources. In healthcare simulation, a center may develop a plan to focus on a wide variety of customer groups or users, including interprofessional education (IPE), continuing education, nurse residency programs, team training on patient safety (Dwyer et al., 2019), certification pass-offs, research, and medical student and resident training and subspecialty training fellowships.

IPE involves a simulated experience with one or more professions. SPs are individuals who are hired to portray a specific disease or condition with consistency, enabling learners to demonstrate their skills and knowledge of these conditions and diseases. Training, high-stakes testing, and a certification required to obtain or maintain employment are all activities that occur in a simulation center and are events that occur in addition to simulation. Centers may also be used to conduct research, not just research on simulations, but research on group therapy or equipment and how it interfaces with humans, that is, device testing, or as a bench-to-bedside innovation center. Some centers have successfully marketed and generated revenue by renting out their space for filming or for equipment training by healthcare companies. Fire departments have used centers to train EMT and paramedics on the latest protocols and psychiatric interventions. Consider ways you can market your center to encourage users, especially those who would benefit from using it when it would otherwise sit idle. Some lesser known ways to use a simulation center include designing, planning, and rehearsing for new programs or facilities and supporting a root-cause analysis or medicolegal defense (Gaba, 2021).

---

### Simulation Teaching Tip 22.2

Evolving to meet the needs of your community can include purchasing equipment and supplies that are representative of those in the clinical settings in which your learners practice. Such purchases will decrease reality shock and the amount of time required to transition to the work setting.

---

A good hockey player plays where the puck is. A great hockey player plays where the puck is going to be.

—Wayne Gretzky

## MANAGERS AND ADMINISTRATORS

Managers and administrators have many responsibilities that can keep them on the job and at the office for long hours, especially those who are involved in expansion projects, renovations, mergers, or if they are in the process of bringing an entire new center online. It is not easy to work long hours for extended amounts of time. This can result in fatigue and burnout. Recognize your limitations and ask for the help and support you need. Document your hours and activities and then review your accomplishments so that you can focus your time and strength on items that have the greatest ROI of time and energy.

Eliminate those items that are not valued and focus on what matters most. Align your goals and efforts with those of the administration or board of directors to avoid a mismatch of expectations and resultant conflict. As new projects are added, assess what can be handed off and delegated to others, simplified, eliminated, or negotiated so that workload and life can be brought back into balance. Learn to say "no." It is far better to focus time and energy on a few essential things than to divide your focus, time, and efforts into many things. Less can be more. Determine your priorities and what is truly essential. Letting go of the nonessential can help bring energy and balance back into your work and life. Take time to meditate, think, reflect, or read something uplifting each day. Put time and energy into your personal wellness. Invest in yourself, your mind, body, and spirit (Blount et al., 2020), and encourage and support your employees to do likewise through your visible and tangible support (Passey et al., 2018) As much as possible, use flexible work practices to help bring work–life balance into your center. Support your employees through your example and reduce turnover by supporting work–life balance (Ferdous et al., 2021).

Be like Switzerland; do not make enemies with anyone. It is a small world, and you never know when a critical and sensitive negotiation or partnership will depend on the relationships you have established and maintained. Do not view others as competitors. Figure out how you can help support the mission of your center. Look at "value added" by using the simulation center and consider it from the customers' or stakeholders' viewpoint; communicate positively and explore and speak to what motivates them to gain and maintain your stakeholders' and volunteers' support (Kramer et al., 2021).

## ▶ PERSONNEL AND NONPERSONNEL ISSUES

Personnel issues are any dealings that have to do with human beings. Nonpersonnel issues are concerned with anything that is not human, for example, equipment, supplies, hardware- or software-related items, and so on. Both personnel and nonpersonnel issues have their unique challenges.

Personnel issues may include the following:

- hiring
- orienting
- training
- coaching
- counseling
- termination

Most centers can tap into human resources to assist them in many of these aspects. It is especially important to involve human resources in the hiring, counseling, and termination of employees so as to ensure that the laws and rights of individuals are not violated anywhere in the process. Each region, state, and country can have varying laws and employee rights. Those in human resources generally have the expertise in this area to ensure compliance with local requirements.

The first 90 days of employment are the most important time in helping the new employee understand job expectations and receive orientation and training for their position, knowledge, attitudes, and skills. Opportunities for continuing education and personal development support will help keep the support staff energized about the role they play in supporting the facilitators and improving operations. Institutional review board (IRB) training for support staff involved in research may be necessary.

### EVIDENCE-BASED FEATURE: A LEADER'S EXAMPLE IN WELLNESS MATTERS

An integrative literature review of 21 articles between 1990 and 2016 found that a manager's support of onsite wellness programs was influenced by their organizational structure, support from senior managers, if they had training on health topics, and their own personal attitudes and beliefs about wellness. Specific and visible managerial support can influence an employee's perceptions of support, wellness behaviors, and the organizational culture. Implications: When implementing a workplace wellness program, target senior, midlevel, and frontline leaders for support (Passey et al., 2018).

### LEADERSHIP STYLES AND RETENTION

If you have a high turnover rate (you are not retaining your employees for at least 1–2 years), you are spending a lot of time, money, and energy on recruiting, hiring, orienting, and training employees. There are many hidden costs in turnover, including loss of knowledge and institutional memory. High turnover can result in poor quality and low morale and burnout in existing employees (Porter-O'Grady & Mallock, 2018; De Winne et al., 2019).

While paying an appropriate wage is important in retaining workers, it is not necessarily the thing that will motivate and engage workers. Hertzberg's motivation-hygiene theory (Herzberg et al., 1957) identifies minimum features that must be present in an environment, known as maintenance factors to retain employees, including salary, supervisor, status, personal life, positive working conditions, and job security. These hygiene factors are satisfiers and are necessary to recruit and retain employees. Motivation factors are important in long-term motivation of employees and include opportunities to be involved in meaningful work, to achieve, be recognized, and take on challenges and opportunity for growth (Marquis & Huston, 2021).

The frontline manager is in the best position to affect and implement motivational factors and is really key to retention and employee satisfaction. Transformational leaders have a tremendous impact on an employee's decision to stay in a position (Tian et al., 2020), whereas task-oriented, transactional, laissez-faire, and management by exception leadership styles are used by those who focus primarily on tasks and goal attainment and typically experience higher turnover rates (Cummings et al., 2010; Hughes, 2019).

The attitude leaders have regarding errors can set the tone for the team. Humans make errors. No one is perfect; we all may make mistakes. Some errors are the result of systems and outdated or poor processes. It is important that leaders take the time to review failures and errors with individuals and their team to determine the root cause of problems. Consider: Is this a onetime event, caused by human error? Or is there more? Support the well-intended worker with remediation. If the mistake is the result of deliberate carelessness, other steps, such as discipline, should be taken. Recognize that any time something new is tried, there is the potential for error. Error is essential to success. Embracing and recognizing the need to allow for responsible errors and failures as an opportunity to learn and grow is necessary for workers to have confidence that they can be innovative and creative without punishment (Porter-O'Grady & Malloch, 2018). There should be no tolerance of workplace bullying. Bullying and incivility are demoralizing and wrong. They can result in an increase in staff turnover and burnout (Simpson et al., 2020).

## COUNSELING AND TERMINATION

When counseling an employee or a learner, some common elements should be present. Meet when you are both calm and have sufficient time for the meeting with the employee/learner, clarify and establish expectations, document these expectations, and monitor and revisit as needed. If expectations continue to be met, no further action is required. If expectations are not met, set a meeting during which expectations are again clarified, with documentation of missed expectations/misbehaviors and possible consequences of continued noncompliance, including probable termination/failure. Take time to gain valuable communication skills and tools in difficult conversations by attending relevant workshops and reading leadership and communication books, such as *Crucial Conversations: Tools for Talking When Stakes Are High* by Grenny et al. (2021) and *Critical Confrontations: Tools for Resolving Broken Promises, Violated Expectations, and Bad Behavior* by Patterson et al. (2004). Talk with a trusted mentor. Be sure to include administration and human resources personnel in these crucial meetings. Do not meet alone with the individual who is hostile or angry. Halt and reschedule. Meetings that turn hostile rarely have a good outcome. Carefully document meeting events; otherwise it can turn into an anecdotal scenario that is difficult to prove. Involving another individual can help ensure the message is consistent, and the person can also be there as a neutral party, as protection, or as a witness (Exhibit 22.7).

| EXHIBIT 22.7 PROCESS OF PROGRESSIVE DISCIPLINE FOR RULE BREAKERS | | | | |
|---|---|---|---|---|
| Offense | First Infraction | Second Infraction | Third Infraction | Fourth Infraction |
| **Insubordination** | Written admonishment | Suspension | Dismissal | |
| **Use of intoxicants while on duty** | Dismissal | | | |
| **Theft or willful damage of property** | Written admonishment | Suspension | Dismissal | |
| **Falsehood** | Verbal admonishment | Written admonishment | Suspension | Dismissal |
| **Violation of safety rules** | Written admonishment | Suspension | Dismissal | |
| **Abuse of leave** | Verbal admonishment | Written admonishment | Suspension | Dismissal |

*Source:* Adapted from Marquis, B. L., & Huston, C. J. (2021). *Leadership roles and management function in nursing: Theory and application* (10th ed.). Lippincott Williams & Wilkins.

## MANAGING RISK

Risk is uncertainty and there is risk in almost everything. Often, risk is thought of as a negative event or threat, such as an equipment failure. However, risk can also be positive, an opportunity, such as a new donor to the center after a successful VIP tour. Some risks have little consequence, while others can have a lasting negative impact. When negative risk is managed well, it is scarcely noticed. When risk is managed poorly, it may require a tremendous effort to manage or overcome the impact. The important thing about risks is to identity and then manage each one intentionally. It is much better to manage risk upfront than to let risk manage you. Put together a risk management plan for your simulation center that can help you manage areas of vulnerability. This will be unique to each center and your given resources, equipment, staff, roles, and responsibilities. First, sit down with your team and brainstorm all those areas where you are at risk. Challenges your assumptions. Write down and list each risk by number. Then score each risk by putting it into a risk matrix (Table 22.2). Each risk should be scored low, medium, or high according to the probability of the event occurring and the impact of that event (Schwalbe, 2021).

### Table 22.2 Probability Impact Risk Matrix

| Probability | High | R1 | | R6 |
|---|---|---|---|---|
| | Medium | | | R3 |
| | Low | R4 | R2 | |
| | | Low | Medium | High |
| | | Impact | | |

*Source:* Adapted from Schwalbe, K. (2021). *Healthcare project management, predictive, agile and hybrid approaches* (3rd ed.). Schwalbe Publishing.

Once you have scored each risk, create a risk management plan by putting each risk into a risk register so you can see all the risks and begin to actively manage them. Finally, be intentional about how you will choose to deal with the risk. There are five ways to handle risk: (a) Choose to accept the risk, (b) mitigate the risk, (c) transfer the risk, (d) elevate the risk, and (e) avoid the risk (Schwalbe, 2021). If you choose to accept the risk, acknowledge this. Do not clutter your risk register with a lot of things that are low probability and low impact. Instead focus your attention on the other areas of the risk matrix. You can mitigate the risk by doing some action to lower the probability of it occurring or lower the impact if it does occur, such as building in redundancies, or ordering supplies that you think might be on backorder sooner and exploring other vendors. You can transfer risk. This is usually when you purchase an insurance policy to help cover an item or event that is very costly. Elevate the risk when the issue is outside your area of authority and beyond your scope to a higher level manager or administrator. Avoid the risk by getting rid of the risk all together, such as replacing a faulty electrical cord or battery.

The risk register shown in Table 22.3 is partially complete. What events or issues can you identify from your simulation center that would be scored the same as R2 and R4? How would you manage these risks? What other things would you plan for?

### Table 22.3 Sample Risk Register: Partially Completed

| No. | Risk | Probability | Impact | Plan | Status |
|-----|------|-------------|--------|------|--------|
| R1 | Manikins may fail and need minor or costly repairs. | High | High | Purchase extended warranty and help the simulation technician get training on fixing common problems. | Ongoing: warranty purchased |
| R2 | | Medium | Medium | Mitigate or transfer risk. | |
| R3 | A simulation technician is sick and cannot come in to cover the simulation. | Medium | High | Mitigate risk: Train team members so that there are redundancies, and every role is at least 2 deep. Cross-train. Document of duties and tips is available in a ready reference binder. | Ongoing: 1/3 positions x-trained 2 deep Working on binder |
| R4 | | Low | Low | Accept risk. | |
| R5 | Supplies do not come in on time. | Low | High | Mitigate risk: Order supplies with 2- to 3-week lead time. Check on shipment regularly. Locate alternate sources. | |
| R6 | | | | | |

## WHEN THINGS DO NOT GO AS PLANNED: UNDERSTANDING AND RESPONDING TO TECHNICAL AND MATERIAL ISSUES

There is little as unnerving as when you have spent hours preparing the "perfect" simulation only to have technical difficulties occur and completely throw you off the scenario. Blood pressure cuffs break, technology does not function correctly, HPSs turn off automatically or lose connection, IV pumps go on the blink, and computers or cameras need to be reset. In addition to technology, learners can respond in unexpected ways, misunderstanding the objectives of the scenario and having difficulty suspending reality (Muckler & Thomas, 2019). The scenario may be too easy or too complex, or a learner does something that is not in the scenario and changes the progress or the outcome of the scenario (Dieckmann et al., 2010).

> If you so choose, even the unexpected setbacks can bring new and positive possibilities. If you so choose, you can find value and fulfillment in every circumstance.
> —Ralph Marston

How one chooses to frame or view these situations that can occur from time to time and how one responds to them will have a tremendous impact on the learner and the learning that can take place. So what is the best way to respond to these unexpected events? It is important to consider this in two phases: immediate and long term. What is the best immediate response during the event and when the learners are present? First, consider the core learning objectives you have for the scenario, and as much as possible use the unexpected event to meet the goals.

Scenario lifesavers can be delivered from inside or outside the scenario. Inside-scenario lifesavers use things from within the scenario to influence the learners and the direction the scenario is headed so that they can return to the key learning objectives (Dieckmann et al., 2010).

Dieckmann et al. (2010) suggest that if the unexpected turn of events is a safety issue for the learners or the equipment, such as the possibility of someone being injured with the incorrect use of the defibrillator, you can intervene by making an overhead announcement. This is called a *lifesaver from outside the scenario*. Another approach is to come up with a plausible background story as to why something may have occurred. This is an example of an inside lifesaver because it is based on something that occurred inside the scenario.

If the scenario has gone way off course, or there are critical technology failures, consider stopping the scenario and then restarting it so that the core learner objectives can be met. Lifesavers are also discussed in Chapter 5, "Special Learning Considerations in Simulation."

As a debriefer or simulation instructor, take a deep breath and collect your thoughts before you return to debrief the learners. The learners will often mirror the response of the debriefer. If the debriefer is flustered and complains, the learners will quickly pick up on this and join in, and a teaching moment is lost. On the other hand, if the debriefer is composed and positive, the learners can still walk away with a positive learning experience.

> How we choose to see things and respond to others makes all the difference.
> —Thomas S. Monson

Normalize the feelings of the group—share what it is that groups frequently feel or how they respond in this given situation. Normalizing helps decrease the feelings of guilt and resistance.

During the debriefing session, as individuals point out the problems that occurred, agree with them quickly: Yes, there was a problem with item A. Then quickly bring it back to real life and ask: Could that ever happen in the actual clinical setting? Could item A stop working? What actions would be appropriate? What can be learned? Then redirect the group back to the learning objectives. Ways to defuse anger can include committing to keeping your cool, speaking softly and with a steady slow tone, calling the learner by name, stopping and focusing on the learner, respecting their right to be angry, and clarifying the issue—do not assume you know what the issue is, own the problem, and look for agreement. Actively listening to upset learners can quickly diffuse the emotion surrounding the situation (Hills, 2010). Once the emotion is defused, learning can take place.

What is the best long-term response to technical issues? Troubleshoot the item that caused the problem. Determine the cause and get the item repaired, or find a substitute or work around as quickly as possible so that this does not become a common occurrence. Reschedule other events if an acceptable solution is not possible. Include money for technology repairs in the budget. If the unexpected response comes from the learner, edit the scenario to prevent a recurrence.

## TROUBLESHOOTING EQUIPMENT: GENERAL INFORMATION

When dealing with technology, troubleshooting has some standard steps:

1. Ensure all cable connections are secure.
2. Ensure the device is plugged in/charged.
3. Shut down the device and start it back up again.
4. Refer to the owner's manual for troubleshooting.
5. Call the sales representative/manufacturer.
6. Repair or replace the defective item.

Create a notebook to log all major pieces of equipment: their purchase, service and repairs, and problems. Document everything: date of occurrence, details of event, actions taken, name(s) of individual contacted with number, expected resolution with date, any follow-up, and so on. This record will become particularly useful if you have to make claims on the warranty of an item. Ensuring that all individuals who use the equipment are adequately trained will decrease the problems and breakage of equipment. Again, be sure to budget sufficient funds to repair and replace the equipment.

## ▶ SUMMARY

Effective operation of a simulation center is based on principles of leadership, risk management, recognition of opportunities you can capitalize on and gaps to be reported and acted on, management of personnel and other resources, policies, procedures, and processes. Additional skills include effective troubleshooting when unexpected events occur and using good judgment in influencing the scenario from inside or outside sources.

## ● CASE STUDY 22.1

An event that uses standardized patients (SPs) will run all day long, 8 hours, for a total of 14 cases. What items should be considered when scheduling this event? Breaks, attire, length, complexity of the case, and the nature of the case—whether it is invasive or not. SPs have the right to be treated with respect and the right to refuse to continue a simulation experience. For example, if a learner is new to conducting a physical assessment exam and is having challenges seeing the SP's pupil reflexes or tonsils, the SP may find it uncomfortable for the learner to continue to repeat these portions of the physical examination. The SP has the right to tell the learner they cannot continue shining a light in their eyes or using a tongue depressor at the back of their throat. Be aware of SPs who may have sensitivity to certain simulation experiences.

## ● CASE STUDY 22.2

The human patient simulator (HPS) suddenly turns off; the monitor has flat lines. The learner notices this, interprets this as a cardiac arrest, and calls a code. What possible responses can you have? What responses can keep you consistent with the key learning objectives?

1. When managing supplies and equipment, it is critical to:

   A. Use the same equipment and supplies as utilized in your local hospitals and clinics
   B. Track equipment repairs and warranty and service agreement information
   C. Set up a cooperative with local simulation centers so you can share equipment and supplies
   D. Order capital equipment at the end of the budget cycle

2. A mission statement is:

   A. A statement of global plans and goals
   B. The road map of a simulation center
   C. The purpose for the existence of the center
   D. A comprehensive 3- to 5-year plan

3. Recommended policies and procedures for a simulation center include:

   A. Mission, vision, and value statements
   B. Collection of prepackaged scenarios with debrief guide and checklist
   C. Video retention, archiving, and access guidelines
   D. Income and expense reports and marketing plans

4. Depreciation is:

   A. The part of a budget that refers to capital equipment
   B. The sudden loss in value of a piece of equipment
   C. The calculated loss of value based on the projected lifetime
   D. Used to represent supply inventory and losses

5. Purchasing an extended warranty on high-fidelity human patient simulator (HPS) is an example of:

   A. Risk transference
   B. Risk acceptance
   C. Risk mitigation
   D. A positive risk

*(See answers next page.)*

## 1. B) Track equipment repairs and warranty and service agreement information

Setting up a system for tracking equipment repairs and service information is critical to understanding and managing operational costs. Using the same equipment and supplies as those utilized in local hospitals and clinics is good for the learner as this might help with familiarity, but it is not of critical importance. Setting up a cooperative with other simulation centers may be helpful, but not essential to running a simulation center. Capital equipment is very costly and is usually best ordered at the beginning of the budget cycle when there is the most amount of money available.

## 2. C) The purpose for the existence of the center

A mission statement describes the purpose of the center. A statement of global plans and goals is a vision statement. The road map is known as a business plan. A comprehensive 3- to 5-year plan is a strategic plan.

## 3. C) Video retention, archiving, and access guidelines

How to retain and store materials that are vital to the history and/or the functioning of the simulation center should be guided by policy and procedure. A collection of prepackaged scenarios with debrief guide and checklist are considered teaching resources, not policies and procedures. Mission, vision, and value statements are usually part of the business plan. There may be policies and procedures regarding the format, content, and frequency of income and expense reports and marketing plans, but the actual reports are all outside of policies and procedures.

## 4. C) The calculated loss of value based on the projected lifetime

Depreciation is used in accounting to help describe the impact of wear and tear and loss of value of an asset, such as a piece of equipment, over time. Capital equipment is usually set up on a depreciation scale, where the initial purchase price and the expected lifetime of the asset are used to decrease and value of the equipment over time. Capital equipment is commonly depreciated and is commonly a line item in a budget; however, depreciation is not a part of the budget that refers to capital equipment. Depreciation refers to a planned and calculated loss of value, not a sudden loss. Depreciation is used for durable equipment, not consumable supplies and inventory losses.

## 5. A) Risk transference

The risk of the high costs of repairing and replacing the HPS is transferred to the company that offered the extended warranty on the HPS. Risk acceptance would be accepting the risk and not doing any intervention—not purchasing an extended warranty and accepting the HPS as the company offers it. An example of mitigating risk might include doing extensive testing on the HPS to identify any weaknesses and to try and detect any issues in the HPS prior to expiration of the initial warranty. A positive risk might be an influx of new clients because your center purchased a new HPS.

6. The stakeholder asks the simulation educator how to make the "simulation real." What should the simulation educator tell them is the most important to increasing realism and learner engagement in a simulation?

   A. Inclusion of actor (standardized patient [SP]) and confederates in the scenario
   B. Willingness of the learner to engage in the learning process
   C. Realistic smells, sounds, and images within the simulation center
   D. High-fidelity human patient simulators with voice modulators

7. When setting up the room for a scenario, the simulation educator notices a piece of equipment is not working correctly. Select the item with the best sequence for troubleshooting and correcting this problem.

   A. Call the sales representative or manufacturer helpline, ensure the device is plugged in/charged, refer to the owner's manual for troubleshooting, shut down the device, and start it back up again
   B. Refer to the owner's manual for troubleshooting, check to see whether the device is plugged in/charged, ensure all cable connections are secure, shut down the device and start it back up again, and call the sales representative or manufacturer helpline
   C. Ensure all connections are secure, shut down the device and start it back up again, refer to the owner's manual for troubleshooting, and call the representative or manufacturer helpline
   D. Shut down the device and start it back up again, ensure the device is plugged in/charged, ensure all cable connections are secure, refer to the owner's manual for troubleshooting, and call the sales representative or manufacturer helpline

8. During a simulation, it is noted that some of the requested supplies and equipment are not in the room and available for learner use as expected. What is the BEST initial step to take toward addressing this issue?

   A. Stop the simulation and ask the simulation technology specialist (STS) why the supplies are not available. Restart the simulation once the proper supplies have been obtained
   B. Continue the simulation with the STS introducing the supplies and equipment into the scenario stating, "These supplies have just arrived from central supply for this patient"
   C. Continue the simulation observing how the learners adapt to the lack of supplies and equipment
   D. Stop the simulation and begin the debrief explaining to the participants that this is a common occurrence and that they are the unfortunate victims of a poorly managed center

## 6. B) Willingness of the learner to engage in the learning process

Confederates, smells, sounds, images, and high-fidelity simulators are all very beneficial, but unless a learner is willing to suspend disbelief these other environmental enhancements will be of limited benefit.

## 7. B) Refer to the owner's manual for troubleshooting, check to see whether the device is plugged in/charged, ensure all cable connections are secure, shut down the device and start it back up again, and call the sales representative or manufacturer helpline

The best initial step to take is to check all cords and electrical plugs to ensure the connections are secure. Many problems can be corrected by doing this step first. Next, shutdown and then restart the human patient simulator. Consult the troubleshooting section of your user's manual. Last, call your sales representative or manufacturer. These steps are recommended in this sequence from most probable and easiest and quickest to fix to the most time-consuming and resource-intensive. Some centers find it helpful to put a short troubleshooting checklist on or near the piece of equipment or device so that it can be readily referred to in times of need.

## 8. B) Continue the simulation with the STS introducing the supplies and equipment into the scenario stating, "These supplies have just arrived from central supply for this patient"

Using an "outside" lifesaver, such as having the STS introduce the supplies into the scenario in a somewhat realistic manner, can help the scenario progress and stay on target with the scenario objectives. Keep your focus on the learners and the scenario objectives. Stopping the simulation and asking the STS why the supplies are not available and then restarting the simulation once the proper supplies have been obtained can break the suspension of reality that has been established and change the focus of the simulation. Maintain realism during a simulation for best learner outcome. Stick to the scenario objectives. Complete the simulation event first and then go back and resolve the issues related to why the supplies were not there. The response to continue the simulation observing how the learners adapt to the lack of supplies and equipment is not correct because this would change the scenario objectives; it is best to stay with the objectives. Lastly, it is never appropriate to stop the simulation and begin the debrief by explaining to the participants that this is a common occurrence and that they are the unfortunate victims of a poorly managed center. This would be a poor response as marginalizing other team members is inappropriate. Issues of this nature should be dealt with privately and not in front of the learners.

9. During a simulation, the Wi-Fi connection to the baby human patient simulator is lost and the baby becomes unresponsive. The learners believe that the baby has gone into cardiac arrest and begin CPR. As a facilitator, what is the BEST initial course of action?

A. Stop the simulation and attempt to reestablish the Wi-Fi connection while you give the learners a break

B. Continue the simulation and modify the scenario on the fly as the learning outcomes can be met within this evolving scenario

C. Stop the simulation and debrief the scenario based on the objectives the learners have met

D. Announce to the students that the Wi-Fi connection was lost again and continue the simulation with modified objectives

10. A recently purchased high-fidelity human patient simulator (HPS) does not function as intended for the third time this week. Each time this occurs, the HPS is turned off and then restarted, after which it begins to work properly. What action should be taken?

A. Review the troubleshooting section in the HPS manual

B. Report your problems and frustrations with this HPS on Facebook

C. Accept the fact that this is a normal challenge when working with this HPS

D. Call the sales representative or manufacturer customer service

**9. B) Continue the simulation and modify the scenario on the fly as the learning outcomes can be met within this evolving scenario**

If the learning objectives can be met, then the evolving scenario is a good solution to this challenge. Stopping the simulation and attempting to reestablish the Wi-Fi connection while you give the learners a break may waste valuable time and interrupt the suspension of reality that the learners have established. Stopping the simulation and debriefing the scenario based on the objectives the learners have met will result in incomplete learning. Announcing to the students that the Wi-Fi connection was lost again and to continue the simulation with modified objectives is not desirable as this will not meet the initial learning objectives.

**10. D) Call the sales representative or manufacturer customer service**

Report this problem and work with the company for resolution. Determining that this is a normal challenge when working with this HPS and not reporting the problem and only documenting it in your HPS equipment logbook are helpful for historical data but will not resolve the issue. Simply documenting incidents will not bring the problem toward a resolution. Reporting the problem early can help resolve this issue. Although you may feel justified in reporting your problems and frustrations on Facebook, this will not resolve the issue with the HPS.

# REFERENCES

Bapteste, L., Bertucat, S., & Balanca, B. (2020). Unexpected detection of latent safety threats by in situ simulation: About two cases in an adult intensive care unit. *Clinical Simulation in Nursing, 47,* 6–8. https://doi.org/10.1016/j.ecns.2020.07.001

Blount, A. J., Dillman Taylor, D. L., & Lambie, G. W. (2020). Wellness in the helping professions: Historical overview, wellness models, and current trends. *Journal of Wellness, 2*(2), 6. https://doi.org/10.18297/jwellness/vol2/iss2/6

Cummings, G. G., MacGregor, T., Davey, M., Lee, H., Wong, C. A., Lo, E., Muise, M., & Stafford, E. (2010). Leadership styles and outcome patterns for the nursing workforce and work environment: A systematic review. *International Journal of Nursing Studies, 47,* 363–385. https://doi.org/10.1016/j.ijnurstu.2009.08.006

De Winne, S., Marescaux, E., Sels, L., Van Beveren, I., & Vanormelingen, S. (2019). The impact of employee turnover and turnover volatility on labor productivity: A flexible non-linear approach. *International Journal of Human Resource Management, 30*(21), 3049–3079. https://doi.org/10.1080/09585192.2018.1449129

Dieckmann, P., Lippert, A., Glavin, R., & Rall, M. (2010). When things do not go as expected: Scenario life savers. *Simulation in Healthcare, 5*(4), 219–225. https://doi.org/10.1097/SIH.0b013e3181e77f74

Dwyer, T. A., Levett-Jones, T., Flenady, T., Reid-Searl, K., Andersen, P., Guinea, S., Heaton, L., Applegarth, J., & Goodwin, B. C. (2019). Responding to the unexpected: Tag team patient safety simulation. *Clinical Simulation in Nursing, 36,* 8–17. https://doi.org/10.1016/j.ecns.2019.06.007

Ferdous, T., Ali, M., & French, E. (2021). Use of flexible work practices and employee outcomes: The role of work–life balance and employee age. *Journal of Management & Organization,* 1–21. https://doi.org/10.1017/jmo.2020.44

Gaba, D. M. (2021, July 13). *Lesser known uses of simulation in health care.* The Joint Commission. https://www.jointcommission.org/resources/news-and-multimedia/blogs/improvement-insights/2021/07/lesser-known-uses-of-simulation-in-health-care/

Gantt, L. T., & Young, H. M (Eds.). (2016). *Healthcare simulation: A guide for operations specialists.* John Wiley & Son's.

Grenny, J., Patterson, K., & McMillan, R. (2021). *Crucial conversations: Tools for talking when stakes are high* (3rd ed.). McGraw Hill.

Herzberg, F., Mausnes, B., Peter, R. O., & Capwell, D. F. (1957). *Job attitudes: Review of research and opinion.* Psychological Service of Pittsburgh.

Hills, L. (2010). Defusing the angry patient: 25 tips. *The Journal of Medical Practice Management, 26*(3), 158–162.

Hughes, V. (2019). Nurse leader impact. *Nursing Management (Springhouse), 50*(4), 42–49. https://doi.org/10.1097/01.NUMA.0000554338.47637.23

Kramer, M. W., Austin, J. T., & Hansen, G. J. (2021). Toward a model of the influence of motivation and communication on volunteering: Expanding self-determination theory. *Management Communication Quarterly, 35*(4), 572–601. https://doi.org/10.1177/08933189211023993

Langford, J. (n.d). *Moulage recipes.* Collin College Healthcare Simulation. http://www.okhealthcare-workforce.com/Conferences/documents/JackieLangford_ArtofMoulage_Recipes.pdf

Lassche, M., & Scheese, C. (2013). *Effective team work—More than a game of chance* [Poster presentation]. 12th Annual International Nursing Simulation/Learning (INACSL) Resource Centers Conference: Hit the Jackpot with Evidence Based Simulation, Las Vegas, Nevada, United States.

Lee, S. J., Heim, G. R., Sriskandarajah, C., & Zhu, Y. (2018). Outpatient appointment block scheduling under patient heterogeneity and patient no-shows. *Production and Operations Management, 27*(1), 28–48. https://doi.org/10.1111/poms.12791

Marquis, B. L., & Huston, C. J. (2021). *Leadership roles and management function in nursing: Theory and application* (10th ed.). Lippincott Williams & Wilkins.

Massie, R. J. (2019). Repurposing medical equipment. *The Medical Journal of Australia, 211*(11), 527–528. https://doi.org/10.5694/mja2.50410

Muckler, V. C., & Thomas, C. (2019). Exploring suspension of disbelief among graduate and undergraduate nursing students. *Clinical Simulation in Nursing, 35*, 25–32. https://doi.org/10.1016/j.ecns.2019.06.006. ISSN 1876-1399.

Pakroo, P. (2020). E. Gjelten (Ed.), *The small business start-up kit: A step-by-step legal guide* (11th ed.). Nolo.

Passey, D. G., Brown, M. C., Hammerback, K., Harris, J. R., & Hannon, P. A. (2018). Managers' support for employee wellness programs: An integrative review. American Journal of Health Promotion, 32(8), 1789–1799. https://doi.org/10.1177/0890117118764856

Patterson, K., Grenny, J., & McMillan, R. (2004). *Crucial confrontations: Tools for resolving broken promises, violated expectations, and bad behavior*. McGraw Hill.

Porter-O'Grady, T., & Malloch, K. (2018). *Quantum leadership: Sustainable value in health care*. Jones & Bartlett Learning.

Scheese, C. H., & Supiano, K. P. (2013). Learning from grief: Utilizing a simulation center for research. *Nursing Management, 44*(2), 32–37.

Schwalbe, K. (2021). *Healthcare project management, predictive, agile and hybrid approaches* (3rd ed.). Schwalbe Publishing.

Simpson, A., Farr-Wharton, B., & Reddy, P. (2020). Cultivating organizational compassion in healthcare. *Journal of Management & Organization, 26*(3), 340–354. https://doi.org/10.1017/jmo.2019.54

Sinek, S. (2009). *Start with why: How great leaders inspire everyone to take action*. Penguin Books.

Society for Simulation in Healthcare. (2016, August). *Council for accreditation of healthcare simulation programs: Accreditation standards self-study review tool*. https://www.ssih.org/Credentialing/Accreditation/Full-Accreditation

Society for Simulation in Healthcare. (2021). *SSH certified healthcare simulation educatorhandbook*. https://www.ssih.org/Portals/48/Certification/CHSE_Docs/CHSE%20Handbook.pdf

Tian, H., Iqbal, S., Akhtar, S., Qalati, S. A., Anwar, F., & Khan, M. (2020). The impact of transformational leadership on employee retention: Mediation and moderation through organizational citizenship behavior and communication. *Frontiers in Psychology, 11*, 314. https://doi.org/10.3389/fpsyg.2020.00314

# Accreditation of Simulation Laboratories and Simulation Standards

Anthony Battaglia, Fabien Pampaloni, and Beth A. Kuzminsky

*What you get by achieving your goals is not as important as what you become by achieving your goals.*

—Zig Ziglar

This chapter addresses Domain IV: Simulation Resources and Environments (Society for Simulation in Healthcare [SSH], 2021).

## ▶ LEARNING OUTCOMES

- Discuss the importance of simulation laboratory accreditation.
- Describe the accreditation standards of the Society for Simulation in Healthcare (SSH).
- List the 10 standards of best practices in simulation of the International Nursing Association for Clinical Simulation and Learning (INACSL).

## ▶ INTRODUCTION

Globally, simulation education remains at the forefront of learning in the healthcare community and is commonplace in the vast majority of healthcare curricula. Advancements in simulation education are continuous as simulation knowledge, theory, and practice continue to thrive and evolve. This evolution has positioned the healthcare educational community for continued excellence and best outcomes, not only educationally but also excellence that surpasses the classroom and transfers to best patient care. This chapter provides information on the accreditation process of the Society for Simulation in Healthcare (SSH) alongside improvements and updates to the simulation center standards originally developed by the International Nursing Association for Clinical Simulation and Learning (INACSL), which are known today as the Healthcare Simulation Standards of Best Practice™ (HSSOBP™). Both organizations remain committed to excellence in simulation education. These two renowned organizations are international and sponsor journals that contain up-to-date simulation teaching, research, and practice. The SSH supports interprofessional membership, while the INACSL is a nursing-based organization (INACSL, 2014).

## ▶ ACCREDITATION

The Code of Federal Regulations defines *accreditation* as "the status of public recognition that an accrediting agency grants to an educational institution or program that meets the agency's standards and requirements" (National Archives, 1999, p. 1).

Accreditation is a sign to consumers that the recipients have met the highest quality of educational excellence. Accreditation achievement showcases the excellence of the simulation center which resonates with the motivation of students, families, and stakeholders to engage in simulation-based education (SBE). Adherence to accreditation standards and criterion by certified healthcare educators (Certified Healthcare Simulation Educator® [CHSE®], Certified Healthcare

Simulation Operations Specialist® [CHSOS®]), staff, and learners who utilize these accredited centers is an expectation. The duration of accreditation is 5 years (including annual self-study reports), followed by a reaccreditation opportunity.

In addition, accreditation will lead to:

- improved learning processes for the student
- probable ease with budgetary preparedness
- forecasting benefits
- anticipated fixed assets
- improvements in business operations

An understanding of the many benefits of simulation center accreditation can serve as a strong motivator to initiate the process. Improved patient safety is the ultimate outcome of center accreditation, as voiced by many healthcare educators in the simulation industry. One of the major benefits of accreditation is creating stronger opportunities for patient safety efforts that are sustainable through the support of standardized simulation modalities.

Developing a simulation laboratory into one that meets the standards of accreditation places the simulation educators in a mentor capacity. Expect to be the new target of other centers that wish to learn from and with you. This exchange of best practices and effective educational strategies fosters networking and mutual growth. Your center will be considered "a center of excellence" for national and international collaborations that may have never existed.

### Simulation Teaching Tip 23.1

"The value of achieving accreditation should re-energize quality improvement activities that are key to ensuring best practices and improved patient safety efforts that serve the center's mission, vision, and values and should ultimately benefit the care of patients," says John O'Donnell, CRNA, MSN, DrPH, professor and director, University of Pittsburgh School of Nursing Nurse Anesthesia Program, associate director and codirector of Research, Winter Institute for Simulation and Research (personal communication, 2022).

Once program accreditation is achieved, structures and support mechanisms will be in place moving forward that will continue to benefit educators, participants, and support personnel. This infrastructure should further enhance programmatic quality and encourage personnel to seek certification (CHSOS or CHSE), lead to higher quality curriculum and better patient outcomes, and increase confidence and belief in the quality of services and educational opportunities by key stakeholders. In a society that continues to have reservations about the care provided in today's hospitals, your center will be considered a valuable resource for effective learning activities as well as for consultation with clinical partners with a need to engage in broad scale educational initiatives. For example, accredited simulation centers across the United States served as resources for development of just in time training (JIT) in meeting the challenges of the COVID-19 pandemic. Accreditation has the potential to spur faculty and staff achievement and to enhance the value of and satisfaction with educational activities from the perspective of participants. Additionally, accreditation can infuse a sense of pride and accomplishment within the center and engender a growing sense of ownership and enthusiasm that will become contagious.

To ensure success, Dr. O'Donnell also advises the following:

- Embrace a project management process that the center can use to enhance efficiency and organization in curricular development efforts.
- Determine the area(s) in which your institution best qualifies for accreditation and ensure ongoing documentation according to the SSH accreditation standards.

- Maintain an archive of appropriate documentation to validate the category(s) of accreditation you wish to pursue.
- Carefully review the SSH (SSH, 2021) accreditation standards in each category in order to select the domain(s) for which your center is best suited for accreditation.
- Practice strong record keeping and process mapping to prepare for application submission and onsite visits.

Keeping these key principles in mind while reviewing the following standards will open up your pathway to successful accreditation (O'Donnell, 2022).

## ▶ THE SOCIETY FOR SIMULATION IN HEALTHCARE

The SSH was established in January 2004 to represent a rapidly growing group of educators, research scientists, and advocates who use a variety of simulation methodologies for education, testing, and research in healthcare. The SSH accredits simulation programs. The SSH accreditation standards, revised in 2016, now includes the core accreditation standards as well as five areas of concentration:

- assessment
- research
- teaching/education
- systems integration
- fellowship

*Note:* The completion of core accreditation standards and at least one of assessment, research, or teaching/education is mandatory for accreditation consideration (SSH, 2021).

Due to the complexity of the accreditation process, all guidelines, documentations, and forms are available on the SSH home page (www.ssih.org) using the "Full Accreditation" option under the "Accreditation" tab.

## ▶ STANDARDS

The HSSOBP are created and constantly revised to enhance simulation science, promote best practices, and build a solid foundation for evidence-based methodologies.

These standards provide road maps for simulation science operations. Their existence promotes a continuous improvement of both quality and safety within simulation laboratories. Adherence to standards demonstrates a seal of commitment to excellence in evidence-based sciences, ultimately improving patient care.

### Evidence-Based Simulation Practice 23.1

"Health professions education without quality simulation experiences is an ancient and outdated method. I am proud of our simulation center, where students at the undergraduate level start simulation before entering clinicals and continue simulation throughout their curriculum. All of our clinical courses at the undergraduate and graduate level have quality simulation experiences attached, and we continue to focus on students defining clinical judgement for their nursing practice. Students need to understand what clinical judgment is and simulation allows us to foster their development of technical skills and non-technical skills that these young professionals need in order to mature into their own professional identities. It is through the magic of simulation, coaching, and skilled debriefing models guided by INACSL best practices that we are able to succeed."

—Nicole Szalla, DNP, RN, CHSE, CMSRN, Director, RISE Center at Robert Morris University

# ▶ THE INTERNATIONAL NURSING ACCREDITATION FOR CLINICAL SIMULATION AND LEARNING

The standards of INACSL accreditation were created based on a detailed survey geared toward the needs and importance of maintaining an educational homogeneity among clinical practices. The initial standards were published in August of 2011 and the first revisions were completed in 2016. In 2021, the INACSL rereleased the INACSL Standards of Best Practice: Simulation$^{SM}$ as the HSSOBP to reflect better positioning within the field of simulation. Two additional areas of expertise were added: Prebriefing and Professional Development.

The newly revised HSSOBP are as follows (INACSL, 2021l):

- Professional Development
- Prebriefing: Preparation and Briefing
- Simulation Design
- Facilitation
- The Debriefing Process
- Operations
- Outcomes and Objectives)
- Professional Integrity
- Simulation-enhanced Interprofessional Education (Sim-IPE)
- Evaluation of Learning and Performance (INACSL, 2021e)

# ▶ STANDARDS OVERVIEW

## PROFESSIONAL DEVELOPMENT

This new standard targets the initial and ongoing professional development supporting the simulationist across their career. As the practice of simulation-based education grows, professional development allows the simulationist to stay current with new knowledge, provide high-quality simulation experiences, and meet the educational needs of the learners.

There are three criteria necessary to meet this standard:

- Perform an educational needs assessment that includes a gap analysis to provide the foundational evidence for a well-designed professional development plan.
- Participate in professional development activities that address desired learning outcomes and align with an individual's role and the priorities of the institution.
- Reevaluate the professional development plan on a regular basis using formative and summative methods by both the individual and the organization (INACSL, 2021d).

## PREBRIEFING: PREPARATION AND BRIEFING

This new standard defines prebriefing as a process which involves preparation and briefing. Prebriefing ensures that simulation learners are prepared for the educational content and are aware of the ground rules for the simulation-based experience. Prior to the development of this standard, the preparation phase of prebriefing was part of the INACSL Standards of Best Practice$^{SM}$: Simulation Design and remains a crucial component of simulation design. According to the most current literature review, prebriefing is referred to as both preparation activities and briefing activities. For the purposes of this prebriefing standard, prebriefing will refer to the activities *prior* to the start of the simulation, including the preparation and briefing aspects of the simulation-based experience. Guidelines for this standard will be provided that apply to both preparation and briefing, and then each of these components will have its own guidelines to ensure they are met.

There are three criteria necessary to meet this standard:

1. The simulationist should be knowledgeable about the scenario and competent in concepts related to prebriefing.
2. Prebriefing should be developed according to the purpose and learning objectives of the simulation-based experience.
3. The experience and knowledge level of the simulation learner should be considered when planning the prebriefing (INACSL, 2021c).

## SIMULATION DESIGN

This standard targets the creation of simulation-based experiences that are constructed to meet objectives and ensure achievement of expected outcomes. It outlines the framework for developing effective simulation-based experiences. Its design reflects best practices from adult learning, education, instructional design, clinical standards of care, evaluation, and simulation pedagogy (Rogers et al., 2023).

There are 11 criteria necessary to meet this standard:

1. Simulation-based experiences (SBE) should be designed in consultation with content experts and simulationists knowledgeable in best practices in simulation education, pedagogy, and practice.
2. Perform a needs assessment to provide the foundational evidence of the need for a well-designed simulation-based experience.
3. Construct measurable objectives that build upon learners' foundational knowledge.
4. Build the simulation-based experience to align the modality with the objectives.
5. Design a scenario, case, or activity to provide the context for the simulation-based experience.
6. Use various types of fidelity to create the required perception of realism.
7. Plan a learner-centered facilitative approach driven by the objectives, learners' knowledge and level of experience, and the expected outcomes.
8. Create a prebriefing plan that includes preparation materials and briefing to guide participant success in the simulation-based experience.
9. Create a debriefing or feedback session and/or a guided reflection exercise to follow the simulation-based experience.
10. Develop a plan for evaluation of the learner and of the simulation-based experience.
11. Pilot-test simulation-based experiences before full implementation (INACSL, 2021j).

## FACILITATION

This standard describes facilitation methods and presents the key qualities of an effective facilitator. Facilitation methods vary and are dependent on the learning needs of participants and the expected outcomes. Facilitators assume responsibility and oversight for managing the entire simulation-based experience. Facilitators must be qualified, educated, and skilled, and possess the ability to guide, support, and seek out ways to assist learners in successful completion of desired outcomes.

"Through the use of facilitation methods, the facilitator's role is to help participants in their skill development and explore their thought processes in critical thinking, problem solving, clinical reasoning, clinical judgment, and apply their theoretical knowledge to patient care in a range of health care settings." (INACSL, 2021h, p. 1)

For these reasons, facilitator continuing education is essential to maintain the skills of the individual and for them to remain current and effective. There are five necessary criteria to meet this standard:

1. Effective facilitation requires a facilitator who has specific skills and knowledge in simulation pedagogy.
2. The facilitative approach is appropriate to the level of learning, experience, and competency of the participants.
3. Facilitation methods before the simulation-based experience include preparatory activities and a prebriefing to prepare participants for the simulation-based experience (follow the HSSOBP Prebriefing: Preparation and Briefing).
4. Facilitation methods during a simulation-based experience involve the delivery of cues (predetermined and/or unplanned) aimed to assist participants in achieving expected outcomes.
5. Facilitation after and beyond the simulation-based experience aims to support participants in achieving expected outcomes (INACSL, 2021h).

## ▶ THE DEBRIEFING PROCESS

The literature supports that essential learning occurs in the debriefing phase of the simulation-based experience. Moreover, the skills of the debriefer are critical to ensure the best possible learning outcomes. This standard describes the significance and background of the debriefing process in simulation-based experiences and supporting criteria with required elements for successful debriefing. It advises that all simulation-based experiences include a planned debriefing session aimed at promoting reflective learning for improvement in future participant performance. There are five necessary criteria to meet this standard. Failure to follow this standard may lead to poor educational consequences to including unsuccessful debriefing sessions and potential uncomfortable experiences for participants (INACSL, 2021k).

### OPERATIONS

This standard emphasizes that all simulation-based education programs require systems and infrastructure to support and maintain operations. It also encompasses all components necessary to efficiently and effectively implement simulation-based education (SBE). These components include infrastructure, people, and processes. The effective application of this standard will guarantee cohesive simulation operations and improve interprofessional collaboration.

There are six necessary criteria to meet this standard:

1. Implement a strategic plan that coordinates and aligns the resources of the SBE program to achieve its goals.
2. Provide personnel with appropriate expertise to support and sustain the SBE program.
3. Use a system to manage space, equipment, and personnel resources.
4. Secure and manage the financial resources to support stability, sustainability, and growth of the SBE program's goals and outcomes.

5. Use a formal process for effective systems integration.
6. Create policies and procedures to support, sustain, and/or grow the SBE program (INACSL, 2021b).

## OUTCOMES AND OBJECTIVES

This standard states that all simulation-based experiences originate with the development of measurable objectives designed to achieve expected behaviors and outcomes. *Simulation-based experience* is defined as "[a]n array of structured activities that represent actual or potential situations in education and practice. These activities allow learners to develop or enhance their knowledge, skills, and attitudes, or to analyze and respond to realistic situations in a simulated environment" (INACSL, 2021g, p. 1). Current literature demonstrates the use of simulation in educational settings to facilitate achievement of cognitive, psychomotor, and affective skills.

There are five necessary criteria to meet this standard:

1. Establish learning outcomes influenced by accreditation, program, curriculum, and/ or patient care needs that are measurable and appropriately scaffolded to learners' knowledge, skills, and attitudes.
2. Create objectives for the simulation-based experience to meet the defined outcomes based on formative or summative evaluation.
3. Identify appropriate simulation modality to meet the learning objectives/outcomes.
4. Identify appropriate fidelity to meet the learning objectives/outcomes.
5. Establish guidelines for facilitation of SBE to meet the objectives (INACSL, 2021g).

## PROFESSIONAL INTEGRITY

This standard emphasizes the importance of ethical behavior for all individuals involved in simulation-based experiences. Regardless of one's role or responsibilities, it is important to encourage communication among team members in order to strengthen professional integrity during the somewhat unpredictable simulation-based experiences. The inability to maintain a professional and ethical balance during experiences may cause participants to present altered and biased performance, as well as develop a sense of distrust in professional relationships.

There are five necessary criteria to meet this standard:

1. Honor and uphold the Healthcare Simulationist Code of Ethics.
2. Follow the standards of practice, guidelines, principles, and ethics of one's profession.
3. Create and maintain a safe learning environment (follow HSSOBP Facilitation).
4. Practice inclusion by respecting equity, diversity, and inclusivity among all involved and in all aspects of SBE.
5. Require confidentiality of the performances and scenario content based on institution policy and procedures (INACSL, 2021a).

## SIMULATION-ENHANCED INTERPROFESSIONAL EDUCATION

This standard's sole purpose is to obtain ultimate learning outcomes while performing interprofessional simulation experiences. Nowadays, healthcare providers from all specialties often collaborate in order to reach a mutual outcome. It is of critical importance that communication, cooperation, and skill sharing are mastered during such collaborations. The

Sim-IPE effectively creates learning objectives, giving individuals the ability to "learn about, from, and with each other to enable effective collaboration and improve health outcome" (Xavier et al., 2022, p. 31).

There are four necessary criteria to meet this standard:

1. Conduct Sim-IPE based on a theoretical or a conceptual framework.
2. Utilize best practices in the design and development of Sim-IPE.
3. Recognize and address potential barriers to Sim-IPE.
4. Devise an appropriate evaluation plan for Sim-IPE (INACSL, 2021i).

## EVALUATION OF LEARNING AND PERFORMANCE

This standard advises that all simulation-based experiences require participant evaluation. Formative, summative, high-stakes, and authentic evaluations are types of assessment used to determine the participant's skill level, competency, and overall performance.

There are four necessary criteria to meet this standard:

1. Determine the method of learner evaluation before the SBE.
2. SBEs may be selected for formative evaluation.
3. SBEs may be selected for summative evaluation.
4. SBEs may be selected for high-stakes evaluation (INACSL, 2021f).

## ▶ SUMMARY

The prestigious recognition of accreditation brings a sense of accomplishment to the faculty and staff as participants reap the benefits of learning in a simulation center that has gone the distance and has reached this remarkable benchmark. It is the hope of the authors that this chapter has equipped you with enough references to pursue accreditation and receive global acknowledgment for your accomplishment. Recruitment, retention, grant funding, and publications are only examples of the many opportunities that will follow such an achievement. This is an ideal time to be a member of the simulation community and contribute to its success, development, and evolution.

 CASE STUDY 23.1

A newly certified healthcare simulation educator is developing a strategic plan for their interdisciplinary laboratory. The laboratory is a converted skills laboratory in a school of physical therapy. The laboratory has been functioning for a year and has one laboratory technician. How would you advise the simulation educator to go about starting the process for Society for Simulation in Healthcare (SSH) accreditation or meeting the International Nursing Association for Clinical Simulation and Learning (INACSL) standards? What resources would you recommend to the simulation educator? How long do you think either process should take?

1.  Which statement is TRUE about the standard "Prebriefing: Preparation and Briefing"?

    A. "This standard's sole purpose is to obtain ultimate learning outcomes while performing interprofessional simulation experiences."
    B. "This standard describes facilitation methods and presents the key qualities of an effective facilitator."
    C. "This standard emphasizes that all simulation-based education programs require systems and infrastructure to support and maintain operations."
    D. "This standard should be developed according to the purpose and learning objectives of the simulation-based experience."

2.  The _____ prepares activities and prebriefings prior to simulation-based experiences and also delivers cues aimed to assist participants in achieving expected outcomes.

    A. Project manager
    B. Director of simulation operations
    C. Facilitator
    D. Information technologist

3.  A simulation educator is developing a self-study report for an accreditation process and is describing a simulation about the goals and responsibilities of a rapid-response team. This should be integrated in which of the following standards?

    A. Evaluation of Learning and Performance
    B. The Debriefing Process
    C. Facilitation
    D. Outcomes and Objectives

4.  End-of-semester competency checkoffs using a standardized patient (SP) is an example of what type of assessment?

    A. Formative
    B. Summative
    C. Self
    D. Midterm

5.  Which standard emphasizes the need for gap analysis assessment as well as encourages the continuous learning development of the simulationist?

    A. Outcomes and Objectives
    B. The Debriefing Process
    C. Professional Development
    D. Facilitation

**1. D) "This standard should be developed according to the purpose and learning objectives of the simulation-based experience."**

Prebriefing should be developed according to the learning outcomes, the simulation educator should have competency in prebriefing, and the prebrief should be at the correct level. Learning outcomes are not the "sole purpose" of prebriefing and the facilitator's effectiveness is not being judged. Prebriefing does not include infrastructure.

## 2. C) Facilitator

The facilitator is the person that prepares activities and prebriefing to assist students in achieving the learning outcomes. Project managers or directors have a larger role and oversee simulation laboratories, while information technologists assist with the computerization of the simulation laboratories.

## 3. D) Outcomes and Objectives

Outcomes and objectives include defining the goals and outcomes of simulation scenarios as they are being planned. Evaluation of learners is formative and summative evaluation methods. Debriefing is the reflective learning that takes place after the simulation experience, while facilitation has to do with program outcomes.

## 4. B) Summative

Summative evaluation is the final grade of an experience or a course. Formative evaluation is done as a learning experience so competencies can improve; this is also true for a midterm or midpoint assessment. Self-assessment is a reflective process that promotes self-improvement.

## 5. C) Professional Development

Simulation educators need continuous professional development to keep up to date on methodologies and theories. Professional development also includes gap analysis in order to enact process improvement. The simulationist should already understand how to develop outcomes and objectives and how to debrief after a scenario. Facilitation is the type of teaching that is promoted in the simulation laboratory and is also part of the simulationist's job description.

6. A key ingredient for a successful accreditation process is to have a:

   A. Simulation educator
   B. Accreditations liaison
   C. Consultant
   D. Project manager

7. A simulation educator is developing a self-study report for accreditation and includes a section on personnel qualification; this information should be included in:

   A. Professional Integrity
   B. The Debriefing Process
   C. Simulation Design
   D. Facilitation

8. During the accreditation application process, the applicant needs consultation about learning domains. The MOST appropriate organization to contact is the:

   A. Society for Simulation in Healthcare (SSH)
   B. International Nursing Association for Clinical Simulation and Learning
   C. National Board of Nursing
   D. National League for Nursing

9. Best practice is a method that has been generally accepted as superior to any alternatives because it produces results that are supported by research. Which standard incorporates best practice for adult learning?

   A. The Debriefing Process
   B. Outcomes and Objectives
   C. Facilitation
   D. Simulation Design

10. The duration of a simulation center accreditation is:

   A. 1 year
   B. 3 years
   C. 5 years
   D. 8 years

### 6. A) Simulation educator

A simulation educator who is certified in simulation and understands the accreditation process and expectations is needed. A consultant, liaison, or manager is not necessary to ensure good accreditation outcome. The simulation educator is the key person needed.

### 7. D) Facilitation

Facilitation includes professional qualifications and continuous professional improvement. Professional integrity has to do with ethical practices. The debriefing process and simulation design have to do with the development of simulation scenario and reflective learning. All simulation specialists should be educating students with a facilitation methodology.

### 8. A) Society for Simulation in Healthcare (SSH)

The SSH is the appropriate organization that accredits simulation programs. The International Nursing Association for Clinical Simulation and Learning, the National Board of Nursing, and the National League for Nursing are not accrediting bodies.

### 9. C) Facilitation

Facilitation is the best simulation teaching practice and makes the learning experience as rich as possible and meet the student learning outcomes. The debriefing process is important, but facilitation is also used in debriefing. Outcomes and objectives are made prior to the teaching process as is the simulation design.

### 10. C) 5 years

The accreditation process is every 5 years with annual reports. Accreditation does not last 1, 3, or 8 years in simulation.

# REFERENCES

International Nursing Association for Clinical Simulation and Learning Standards Committee, Bowler, F., Klein, M., & Wilford, A. (2021a, September). Healthcare simulation standards of best practice™: Professional integrity. *Clinical Simulation in Nursing, 58*, 45–48. https://doi.org/10.1016/j.ecns.2021.08.014

International Nursing Association for Clinical Simulation and Learning Standards Committee, Charnetski, M., & Jarvill, M. (2021b, September). Healthcare simulation standards of best practice™: Operations. *Clinical Simulation in Nursing, 58*, 33–39. https://doi.org/10.1016/j.ecns.2021.08.012

International Nursing Association for Clinical Simulation and Learning Standards Committee, Decker, S., Alinier, G., Crawford, S. B., Gordon, R. M., & Wilson, C. (2021c, September). Healthcare simulation standards of best practice™: The debriefing process. *Clinical Simulation in Nursing, 58*, 27–32. https://doi.org/10.1016/j.ecns.2021.08.011

International Nursing Association for Clinical Simulation and Learning Standards Committee, Hallmark, B., Brown, M., Peterson, D. T., Fey, M., & Morse, C. (2021d, September). Healthcare simulation standards of best practice™: Professional development. *Clinical Simulation in Nursing, 58*, 5–8. https://doi.org/10.1016/j.ecns.2021.08.007

International Nursing Association for Clinical Simulation and Learning Standards Committee, McDermott, D. S., Ludlow, J., Horsley, E., & Meakim, C. (2021e, September). Healthcare simulation standards of best practice™ prebriefing: Preparation and briefing. *Clinical Simulation in Nursing, 58*, 9–13. https://doi.org/10.1016/j.ecns.2021.08.008

International Nursing Association for Clinical Simulation and Learning Standards Committee, McMahon, E., Jimenez, F. A., Lawrence, K., & Victor, J. (2021f, September). Healthcare simulation standards of best practice™: Evaluation of learning and performance. *Clinical Simulation in Nursing, 58*, 54–56. https://doi.org/10.1016/j.ecns.2021.08.016

International Nursing Association for Clinical Simulation and Learning Standards Committee, Miller, C., Deckers, C., Jones, M., Wells-Beede, E., & McGee, E. (2021g, September). Healthcare simulation standards of best practice™: Outcomes and objectives. *Clinical Simulation in Nursing, 58*, 40–44. https://doi.org/10.1016/j.ecns.2021.08.013

International Nursing Association for Clinical Simulation and Learning Standards Committee, Persico, L., Belle, A., DiGregorio, H., Wilson-Keates, B., & Shelton, C. (2021h, September). Healthcare simulation standards of best practice™: Facilitation. *Clinical Simulation in Nursing, 58*, 22–26. https://doi.org/10.1016/j.ecns.2021.08.010

International Nursing Association for Clinical Simulation and Learning Standards Committee, Rossler, K., Molloy, M. A., Pastva, A. M., Brown, M., & Xavier, N. (2021i, September). Healthcare simulation standards of best practice™: Simulation-enhanced interprofessional education. *Clinical Simulation in Nursing, 58*, 49–53. https://doi.org/10.1016/j.ecns.2021.08.015

International Nursing Association for Clinical Simulation and Learning Standards Committee, Watts, P., I., McDermott, D. S., Alinier, G., Charnetski, M., & Nawathe, P. A. (2021j, September). Healthcare simulation standards of best practice™: Simulation design. *Clinical Simulation in Nursing, 58*, 14–21. https://doi.org/10.1016/j.ecns.2021.08.009

International Nursing Association for Clinical and Simulation Learning. (2021l). Healthcare standards of best practice.https://www.inacsl.org/healthcare-simulation-standards-ql

INACSLk, 2021) International Nursing Association for Clinical Simulation and Learning Standards Committee, Decker, S., Alinier, G., Crawford, S. B, Gordon, R. M., Jenkins, D., & Wilson, C. (2021k) Healthcare simulation standards of best practice™: The debriefing process. *Clinical Simulation in Nursing, 58*, 27–32. https://doi.org/10.1016/j.ecns.2021.08.

National Archives. (1999). The code of federal regulations. https://www.ecfr.gov/

O'Donnell, L., Ambrose, H., Barreca, R., Brooks, K., Hayden, M., Henry, C., Nelson, K., Stark, S., Watters, S., & Wolff, L. (2022). Leading nursing excellence through a system Magnet ® program director council. *The Journal of Nursing Administration, 52*(7/8), 389–391. https://doi.org/10.1097/NNA.0000000000001170

Rogers, B. A., & Franklin, A. E. (2023). Lasater clinical judgment rubric reliability for scoring clinical judgment after observing asynchronous simulation and feasibility/usability with learners. *Nurse Education Today, 125.* https://doi.org/10.1016/j.nedt.2023.105769

Society for Simulation in Healthcare. (2021). *Core accreditation standards—2021 standards revision.* https://www.ssih.org/Portals/48/2021%20SSH%20ACCREDITATION%20STANDARDS.pdf

Xavier, N. A., & Brown, M. R. (2022). *Interprofessional education in a simultion setting.* National Library of Medicine. https://www.ncbi.nlm.nih.gov/books/NBK557471/#:~:text=Simulation-enhanced%20interprofessional%20education%20%28Sim-IPE%29%20is%20%E2%80%9Cwhen%20participants%20and,experience%20to%20achieve%20shared%20learning%20outcomes%20or%20goals

# Practice Test

Linda Wilson and Ruth A. Wittmann-Price

1. What is the BEST simulation modality to promote changes in learner behavior in the affective domain?

    **A.** Simulated participants

    **B.** Part-task trainers

    **C.** High-fidelity manikins

    **D.** Virtual reality

2. When considering psychological fidelity, what is MOST important to consider?

    **A.** Certified simulation educators

    **B.** Learner-centric approaches

    **C.** Learning outcomes to guide the simulation

    **D.** High-fidelity simulators

3. Which simulated participant attributes need to be considered for realism?

    **A.** Hair and skin color

    **B.** Ethnicity and education level

    **C.** Race and articulation

    **D.** Age and gender

4. The new simulation educator needs a better understanding of simulation techniques when they state that according to the National League for Nursing (NLN) Jeffries Simulation Theory the following component of simulation is important:

    **A.** Educational strategies

    **B.** Participants

    **C.** Simulation experiences

    **D.** Specific prebrief times

5. A simulation researcher would like to investigate Kirkpatrick's levels of evaluation and would like to focus on the levels that need more evidence. Therefore, the simulation researcher should choose to study:

    **A.** Level 1 (reaction) and level 2 (learning)

    **B.** Level 2 (learning) and level 3 (behavior)

    **C.** Level 3 (behavior) and level 4 (results)

    **D.** Level 4 (results) and level 1 (reaction)

6. The simulation educator understands education and learning in simulation when they state using a simulation video in what manner?

   A. Show the entire video without comments
   B. Bookmark while videotaping and show critical points
   C. Bookmark while videotaping and just show negative points
   D. Send the video to participants to watch on their own time

7. The novice simulation educator needs a better understanding of simulation research efforts when they state:

   A. "A gold standard for debriefing processes is needed."
   B. "Learner satisfaction with simulation pedagogy is understudied."
   C. "The impact of participant's race on simulation outcomes is under studied."
   D. "We need to know more about the effectiveness of virtual and screen-based learning."

8. From the national survey, what is the ratio of clinical to simulation time?

   A. 2:1
   B. 2:2
   C. 1:2
   D. No evidence supports a particular ratio

9. The simulation educator did a literature search and found that most published data pertain to which of the following levels of Kirkpatrick's evaluation process?

   A. Level 1 (reaction)
   B. Level 2 (learning)
   C. Level 3 (behavior)
   D. Level 4 (results)

10. A novice simulation educator needs better understanding of simulation learning when they indicate that they plan to use which of the following modalities for mental health simulation?

    A. Virtual game
    B. High-fidelity simulator
    C. Part-task trainer
    D. A simulated participant

11. The novice simulation educator needs further education when they state a debriefing framework is:

    A. "Debriefing with good judgment."
    B. "Preview advocacy inquiry."
    C. "Debriefing for meaningful learning."
    D. "Plus delta."

12. The organization that maintains healthcare simulation standards of best practice is the:

    A. National League for Nursing
    B. Society for Simulation in Healthcare
    C. International Nursing Association for Clinical Simulation and Learning
    D. Association of Standardized Patient Educators

13. A simulation educator receives an accommodation letter from the university's disabilities office that states the student has an accommodation, which is a special stethoscope for people with hearing impairment. The simulation educator should:

    A. Develop a scenario in which a stethoscope is not needed
    B. Assign the student to be an observer or a participant
    C. Ask the student in prebriefing if it works well for them
    D. Allow the student to use the stethoscope

14. The simulation educator needs to set up the laboratory for advanced healthcare learners to practice central line insertion. The BEST modality to practice this skill would be:

    A. Simulated participant
    B. High-fidelity manikin
    C. Part-task trainer
    D. Virtual reality

15. A simulation educator is debriefing a group of junior learners and properly focuses the discussion by stating:

    A. "I think the best start is to review the entire scenario."
    B. "You worked well as a team."
    C. "Let's take a vote to see what the best part of the experience was."
    D. "We can discuss how we would do that the next time."

16. A simulation consultant was hired by a healthcare academic unit to assist with developing a simulation program. The BEST advice would include:

    A. Scheduling simulation at a specific time during each semester
    B. Having the students sign up on their own for simulation experiences
    C. Using simulation as a remediation tool to enhance understanding
    D. Integrating simulation throughout the curriculum

17. A novice simulation educator has new video equipment capabilities and would like to use the video equipment. The seasoned simulation educator looks at the upcoming laboratory schedule and suggests:

    A. Interviewing a patient (standardized patient [SP])
    B. Megacode in advanced cardiac life support (ACLS)
    C. Medication administration
    D. Intraosseous vascular insertion

18. A simulation consultant is using Kern et al.'s (2009) method of curriculum integration and is therefore expected to begin the curriculum change by:

    A. Performing a needs assessment
    B. Undertaking a learner assessment
    C. Choosing the appropriate environment
    D. Establishing learning objectives

19. The novice simulation educator needs additional understanding when they state the following is a protection of students' ethical, legal, and regulatory rights in a simulation laboratory:

    A. Having codes of conduct accessible to students
    B. Maintaining fair evaluation processes throughout the learning activities
    C. Implied consent to record when tapes will be destroyed after debriefing
    D. Consent for picture taking for any use

20. Which assessment method should the simulation educator use to measure competency attainment?

    A. Validated checklists
    B. Multiple-choice test
    C. Peer critique
    D. Focus group

21. Studies have consistently demonstrated that simulation is a good learning experience to improve:

    A. Clinical outcomes
    B. Teamwork
    C. Patient outcomes
    D. Knowledge

22. Interprofessional education (IPE) is used in simulation as a modality consistent with:

    A. Experiential learning
    B. Behavioralism
    C. Deliberate practice
    D. Self-directed learning

23. A simulation educator wants to improve healthcare learners' skill in central venous catheter placement. The BEST teaching method to accomplish this is:

    A Deliberate practice
    B. High-fidelity scenario
    C. Case studies
    D. Standardized patient encounter

24. A simulation educator is providing a healthcare learner with a documented formative feedback on interpersonal communication skills. The purpose of this is to:

    A. Assign a grade for the activity
    B. Provide information for prebriefing
    C. Give constructive feedback
    D. Add to a pass/fail in clinical skills

25. During a scenario, the simulation educator programs the manikin to cough in order to have the learners listen to lung sounds that they did not complete on a head-to-toe patient assessment. This technique is which activity element/modality?

    A. Passive element
    B. Active element
    C. Interactive element
    D. Transference

26. A standardized patient is providing the learner with feedback after the encounter in order to:

    A. Provide a grade for the student
    B. Identify remediation needs
    C. Have students self-reflect
    D. Promote student development

27. A simulation manager is interviewing actors for a standardized patient (SP) role and is assessing which important attribute?

    A. Articulation skills
    B. Disease manifestations
    C. Emotional intelligence
    D. Honesty

28. A simulation educator has developed a simulation scenario for the critical care course. After the scenario, the educator should undertake which of the following activities first?

    A. Write another simulation scenario on a topic of interest
    B. Evaluate the students' feedback about the scenario
    C. Determine the methods of evaluation to be used
    D. Make process improvements based on observation by the educator

29. A simulation manager is making an anticipated budget for the next fiscal year and allocates money for part-task trainers because they are:

    A. Lightweight
    B. Disposable
    C. Small and store easily
    D. Cost-effective

30. A simulation educator is planning a learning event and understands that:

    A. Student skills should all be at an acceptable level
    B. Scenarios that are challenging will enhance learning
    C. Topic areas should include common clinical issues
    D. Activities should meet student learning outcomes

**31.** A simulation educator is developing goals for a simulation activity. A goal written in the affective domain is to:

   **A.** Demonstrate the correct technique for inserting an intravenous catheter
   **B.** Understand the technique for administering intramuscular medications
   **C.** Empathize with the chronically ill patient and family members
   **D.** List the steps of checking tube feeding residuals

**32.** Which of the following would be an example of a summative evaluation?

   **A.** Performing an end-of-course objective structured clinical examination (OSCE)
   **B.** Completing one of four didactic tests given throughout the semester
   **C.** Deliberate practice of Foley catheter insertion in open laboratory hours
   **D.** A simulation scenario about a cardiac infarction that is recorded for review

**33.** The simulation educator needs additional understanding of an integrated curriculum development when they state:

   **A.** "I need to identify every place where I can get resources for simulation."
   **B.** "This simulation curriculum needs to be evaluated after a year."
   **C.** "I am positive that we have political support for this simulation curriculum."
   **D.** "We can address simulation implementation barriers as they arise."

**34.** In order to ensure interprofessional collaboration, the simulation educator must promote the four main interprofessional concepts, including:

   **A.** Leadership
   **B.** Evidence-based practice
   **C.** Reflection
   **D.** Communication

**35.** During an advocacy-inquiry debriefing session, the simulation educator addresses a need for process improvement by stating:

   **A.** "I am concerned because I noticed the team took 4 minutes to organize themselves."
   **B.** "The team took too long to organize themselves but met the goal."
   **C.** "Let's list what went well and what needs improvement for next time."
   **D.** "Can you all tell me as a group what took you so long and how to improve?"

**36.** During a formative evaluation with a student after a simulation scenario about patient safety, which of the following is the BEST response to promote learning?

   **A.** "Not identifying the patient could result in you eventually losing your license."
   **B.** "You will fail the course if you do not identify patients correctly."
   **C.** "Understanding patient safety is priority of every nurse."
   **D.** "Can you think of how to increase patient safety in the next scenario?"

37. The simulation educator would like to meet the following competency with students: demonstrate and explain IV insertion on an adult patient. The BEST method to meet this student learning outcome is:

    A. Using a standardized patient and virtual simulation
    B. Using a part-task trainer with a standardized patient
    C. Using a high-fidelity manikin with part-task trainer
    D. Using a peer who is role-playing and a part-task trainer

38. The simulation educator notices that during a scenario a learner stops and begins to cry uncontrollably. The BEST action for the simulation educator to take is to:

    A. Stop the scenario and ask the student to come out then continue with the other learners
    B. Continue the scenario and provide feedback to the student individually immediately after
    C. Give the other students a "lifesaver" to focus their attention on the student having the issue
    D. Stop the scenario and debrief the group in situ to better understand the reaction

39. A simulation educator has developed and used an evaluation tool for six different groups and the scores are consistent. The simulation educator concludes the tool is:

    A. Valid
    B. Realistic
    C. Reliable
    D. Feasible

40. One of the primary reasons healthcare education programs integrate simulation throughout a curriculum is to:

    A. Promote skill attainment
    B. Practice missing procedures
    C. Close knowledge gaps
    D. Assist at-risk students

41. The simulation educator is using moulage to make a wound on a part-task trainer in order to promote realism and increase:

    A. Physical fidelity
    B. Psychological fidelity
    C. Environmental fidelity
    D. Equipment fidelity

42. The simulation educator is providing standardized patient (SP) orientation and an actor asks if there are any instances that would warrant "coming out of character." The simulation educator correctly answers the question from the SP when they say: "Yes, when the student . . .":

    A. Makes an error
    B. Requests further information
    C. Is finished
    D. Requests the SP to come out of character

43. The novice simulation educator states which of the following about the concept of realism and the seasoned simulation educator corrects them?

    **A.** "Increased realism will ensure the learning outcomes are met."
    **B.** "Realism should be created within a safe environment."
    **C.** "Realism increases the fidelity of the simulation scenario."
    **D.** "Realism may assist the students to better understand the situation."

44. Deliberate practice is a teaching methodology in simulation education with the intent that it will:

    **A.** Keep learners motivated
    **B.** Lead to intervention perfection
    **C.** Lead to skills becoming automatic habits
    **D.** Provide new understanding about practice

45. The simulation educator is teaching learners about interprofessional collaboration and should include which essential core competency?

    **A.** Leadership
    **B.** Responsibility
    **C.** Reflection
    **D.** Demonstration

46. The novice simulation educator needs a better understanding of the role of standardized patients when they state, "Standardized patients can . . .":

    **A.** Provide a score for the experience
    **B.** Provide individual feedback
    **C.** Use a script and also ad lib if needed
    **D.** Display healthcare knowledge and emotions

47. Microethical situations can be simulated and used as learning activities and can include all of the following EXCEPT:

    **A.** Work around medication administration practices
    **B.** Poor handwashing techniques
    **C.** Breaches in confidentiality about laboratory performance
    **D.** Inappropriately touching another person

48. The simulation educator encourages a prebriefing that promotes students to touch the manikins. This activity assist in promoting:

    **A.** Physical fidelity
    **B.** Psychological fidelity
    **C.** Environmental fidelity
    **D.** Equipment fidelity

49. Four simulation educators provided feedback after reviewing a video activity. Which simulation educator provided feedback in a "sandwich format"?

    A. "You did a good patient assessment and need to improve on both heart sounds and lung sound stethoscope placement."

    B. "The heart sound stethoscope placement was incorrect so let us review, but the lung sound stethoscope placement on the standardized patient was correct."

    C. "You did an overall thorough patient head-to-toe assessment but need practice in lung sound stethoscope placement, but your heart stethoscope placement was fine."

    D. "Let us consider going over the placement of your stethoscope for the heart sounds one more time."

50. A simulation educator consults the literature to ensure they are developing an "as if" scenario and finds the BEST element to include is:

    A. Higher fidelity
    B. Moulage
    C. Believable information
    D. Complex cases

51. During a debriefing session, a student states they felt as if there was an ethical issue when the feeding tube was inserted in the patient who was not likely to survive. The domain that is reflected in this student's learning regarding ethical thinking is:

    A. Cognitive
    B. Psychomotor
    C. Internalization
    D. Affective

52. A learning outcome for a simulation activity states: "At the end of this scenario the students will demonstrate correct sterile technique." This student learning outcome is written in which domain?

    A. Cognitive
    B. Psychomotor
    C. Somatic
    D. Affective

53. The important principles used by the TeamSTEPPS approach include:

    A. Concerned, uncommunicated, strategies
    B. Cognitive, uncomfortable, safety
    C. Cognitive, uncommunicated, scenario
    D. Concerned, uncomfortable, safety

54. "At the end of this simulation session the student will describe correct sterile technique." This is a student learning outcome written in which learning domain?

    A. Cognition
    B. Psychomotor
    C. Internalization
    D. Affective

55. A dean would like to provide healthcare faculty with a professional development opportunity due to a growing simulation program. The MOST beneficial professional development workshop would include:

   **A.** Working the manikins
   **B.** Developing scenarios
   **C.** Understanding debriefing
   **D.** Learning how to troubleshoot

56. A simulationist is developing a rubric for a team simulation activity and understands that the following attribute is not necessarily displayed in all team simulation activities and may not be needed on the rubric?

   **A.** Role understanding
   **B.** A plan to correct mistakes
   **C.** An evaluation for the team effort
   **D.** An identified leader

57. The simulation educator is creating a rubric for a team activity that includes the core components of interprofessional collaboration. The rubric should include:

   **A.** Leadership
   **B.** Delegation
   **C.** Values
   **D.** Demonstration

58. The simulation educator debriefs a learner who got upset during a team-based simulation scenario and used a raised voice. The central theme of the debriefing is to address:

   **A.** Receiving
   **B.** Valuing
   **C.** Internalizing
   **D.** Organizing

59. The first priority the simulationist should have when recruiting and working with standardized patients is:

   **A.** Provide orientation and training for the people involved
   **B.** Recruit only trained actors to serve as standardized patients
   **C.** Ensure that the actors are paid prior to the simulation day
   **D.** Provide an exact script for the actors to follow

60. A good planning activity for new simulation scenarios is:

   **A.** Seek the input of students who will be participating
   **B.** Ask other faculty whether they can foresee any issues
   **C.** Conduct a run-through or field test of the new simulation
   **D.** Ask for real-life patient situations from practice partners

61. A simulation laboratory manager is placing an ad on the university website for standardized patients. The priority item that the ad should request is:

    **A.** A reference
    **B.** A curriculum vitae (CV)
    **C.** Application
    **D.** Video of acting skills

62. A simulation educator is critiquing four debriefing videos. A statement or question from each video is below. Which statement or question warrants immediate attention?

    **A.** "Help me to understand why you did this."
    **B.** "How do you think the group did overall?"
    **C.** "You know this is the wrong way to do this."
    **D.** "Can you tell me what you were thinking at the time?"

63. The simulationist is using a computer-generated, three-dimensional (3D) IV program to allow learners to practice the skill. This is an example of what type of simulation modality?

    **A.** High-fidelity
    **B.** Virtual reality
    **C.** Task trainer
    **D.** Standardized patient

64. The novice simulation educator needs a better understanding of the purpose and goal of simulation education when they state:

    **A.** "Simulation can substitute for some clinical hours in difficult-to-find specialty areas."
    **B.** "Simulation is useful in helping students to experience uncommon clinical situations."
    **C.** "Simulation can help students to develop confidence before entering the hospital setting."
    **D.** "Simulation is something that can be done at the last minute if needed for makeup days."

65. A simulation educator has developed a simulation experience involving physicians, registered nurses, emergency medical technicians, and licensed practical nurses. Which standard's guidelines would the educator have to follow in order to reach learning outcomes shared by all specialties?

    **A.** Simulation$^{SM}$ Simulation Design
    **B.** Simulation$^{SM}$ Outcomes and Objectives
    **C.** Simulation$^{SM}$ Professional Integrity
    **D.** Simulation$^{SM}$ Simulation-Enhanced Interprofessional Education

66. The simulation educator needs to review the Simulation[SM] Debriefing standard when they state that the standard facilitates:

   A. "Reflection on individual and team performance to achieve targeted performance improvement."
   B. "Critical thinking, clinical judgment, reasoning, reflection, and reflective thinking."
   C. "Recognition and curtailment of unprofessional and unethical behavior during simulation."
   D. "Modification based on assessed participant needs and the impact of the experience."

67. In a team training simulation activity, the simulation educator would expect to see which leadership element demonstrated by learners?

   A. A shared understanding
   B. Delegation
   C. Balance of work
   D. Mutual trust

68. Interprofessional collaborative practice includes which element?

   A. Teamwork
   B. Delegation
   C. Prioritization
   D. Demonstration

69. When simulation is used as an evaluative activity rather than a learning activity, there must be:

   A. Effective evaluation tools that are valid and reliable
   B. Videotaping of learners' performance in case of review
   C. Learners who are aware of the grading criteria
   D. Content in the scenario that has been taught and objectively tested in class

70. A simulationist is doing a simulation project and would like to collect data about students' perceptions of using simulation as a learning modality. The BEST method to collect this data would be:

   A. Objective structured clinical exams (OSCEs)
   B. Self-reporting surveys
   C. Skills checklists
   D. Direct questioning

71. Which statement demonstrates poor simulation management on the part of the novice simulationist?

   A. "I will have students arrive at 7:00 a.m., and we will see how long the simulation takes."
   B. "I will schedule small groups of learners for each simulation activity."
   C. "I will have the course faculty help develop objectives for the simulation activity."
   D. "I will bring each group of students in for prebriefing and keep them together for debriefing."

72. A new simulation educator demonstrates lack of knowledge about simulation modalities when they state:

    **A.** "IV arms are a great use of low-fidelity simulation."
    **B.** "High-fidelity manikins can be used effectively with new nursing students."
    **C.** "A task trainer can be effective in teaching new skills."
    **D.** "Debriefing is an effective method for evaluating skill acquisition with task trainers."

73. Continuous professional development (CPD) in simulation has been demonstrated to increase:

    **A.** Learner knowledge
    **B.** Professional career attainment
    **C.** Higher fidelity
    **D.** Critical analysis

74. The simulation educator gets the same results with six different groups of students using a newly made skills checkoff list for skill attainment of second-year physical therapy students. The simulation educator understands this supports:

    **A.** Credibility
    **B.** Validity
    **C.** Reliability
    **D.** Content

75. The BEST description about a simulation educator who demonstrates transformational leadership is:

    **A.** "The simulation educator moves people toward the future by providing us with what simulation can do for learners."
    **B.** "The simulation educator organizes the simulation laboratory so it is easy for students to learn."
    **C.** "The simulation educator supports faculty by developing scenarios that depict hard-to-get student clinical experiences."
    **D.** "The simulation educator is excellent at scheduling the simulation experiences needed for learners throughout the semester."

76. The simulation educator promotes interprofessionality by:

    **A.** Sharing knowledge
    **B.** Demonstrating leadership
    **C.** Delegating tasks
    **D.** Prioritizing interventions

77. Debriefing should create an overall climate of:

    **A.** Mutual respect
    **B.** Straightforwardness
    **C.** Shared perspectives
    **D.** Psychological safety

78. The simulation educator writes the following student learning outcomes: "Demonstrate interprofessional communication skills." This student learning outcome is at what level of Bloom's taxonomy?

    **A.** Understanding
    **B.** Applying
    **C.** Comprehending
    **D.** Analyzing

79. The certification for simulation healthcare education is a certification that:

    **A.** Travels with nurses through their careers
    **B.** Can be revoked if wrongdoing is noted in a career
    **C.** Has to be renewed every 3 years
    **D.** Demonstrates to others a level of proficiency

80. A transactional simulation leader may perform which of the following activities?

    **A.** Describe the new and upcoming simulation technologies being developed
    **B.** Organize the simulation laboratory so it is easy for students to learn
    **C.** Provide the resources needed so simulation educators can be creative
    **D.** Maintain the mission of the simulation laboratory learning environment in focus

81. The simulation educator uses a lifesaver to assist students in staying on track when there is an indication that there will be a deviation from the student learning outcomes at which level?

    **A.** Advanced beginner
    **B.** Competent
    **C.** Proficient
    **D.** Expert

82. A learner presents the simulation educator with an accommodation letter stating they need instructions read to them. The simulation educator is obligated by law to provide:

    **A.** Special equipment
    **B.** More time for debriefing
    **C.** Reasonable accommodations
    **D.** One on one instruction

83. Evidence-based simulation education has demonstrated that student learning outcomes in healthcare programs are:

    **A.** Negatively impacted by the overuse of simulation
    **B.** Positively impacted by the use of simulation
    **C.** Not significantly affected by simulation
    **D.** Obscured by simulation learning experiences

84. Simulation laboratories can promote diversity and interprofessional training due to:

   A. Standardized patients (SPs) who can pretend to be of any ethnicity or race and provide feedback
   B. Manikins that can be altered with moulage to depict a marginalized patient
   C. Learners checking their social determinants at the door to start learning without bias
   D. Learning which can take place for all under the guidance of experienced simulation educators

85. The first steps learners assume when developing their professional identity is:

   A. Feeling like an imposter
   B. Using trial-and-error methods to learn
   C. Understanding the seriousness of the role
   D. Gaining confidence in the role

86. The simulation educator observes a healthcare learner stopping and looking around the simulation laboratory before an activity starts. The simulation educator understands that the learner is:

   A. Gaining understanding of their role
   B. Requesting more unstructured time
   C. Socializing to a modulation frame
   D. Acclimating to the primary frame

87. A wrong assumption by a simulation educator about the learning needs of minority students includes which of the following beliefs?

   A. Minority students may do just as well in simulation because they will join in
   B. Minority students may feel marginalized in the learning environment
   C. Minority students may not feel they belong in the scenario with everyone else
   D. Minority students may need additional resources due to social determinants

88. A student receives time and a half during classroom testing. During an evaluative scenario in the simulation laboratory, students have to read the patient's case history and the student requests extra time. The simulation educator should:

   A. Refer the student to the university's Americans With Disabilities Act (ADA) officer
   B. Provide time and half to the student to read the case
   C. Explain to the student that the request is not reasonable
   D. Provide a private place for the student to read the case history

89. The simulation educator arranges an interprofessional education (IPE) activity. The goal of IPE is to:

   A. Understand each other's role
   B. Make environments more congenial
   C. Provide different perspectives
   D. Provide safe patient care

90. A simulation educator is orientating a group of standardized patients and discussing how students store and recall information. This is specifically referring to:

    **A.** Worldviews
    **B.** Philosophies
    **C.** Teaching theories
    **D.** Learning theories

91. What educational theory is the simulation educator using when they write the following student learning outcome: "At the end of this simulation experience the learner will correctly demonstrate IV insertion"?

    **A.** Constructivism
    **B.** Behaviorism
    **C.** Idealism
    **D.** Realism

92. The simulation educator is conducting a simulation using both a high-fidelity simulator as the patient and a standardized participant who is acting as a concerned and agitated family member who needs deescalating assistance. Which method of simulation is being used?

    **A.** Task trainer
    **B.** Human patient simulators
    **C.** Hybrid simulation
    **D.** Mixed simulation

93. During a simulation activity, the simulation educator orients learners to the environment and provides information about the scenario. The simulation educator is enacting which stage of simulation development?

    **A.** Designing
    **B.** Planning
    **C.** Implementation
    **D.** Debriefing

94. A simulation educator begins a prebriefing session by asking the learners to recall information from a previous session before providing them with information for the upcoming simulation activity. The simulation educator is enacting which educational theory?

    **A.** Constructivism
    **B.** Behaviorism
    **C.** Scaffolding
    **D.** Realism

95. The novice simulation educator needs better understanding of the adult learning theory when they state: "Adult learners . . .":

    **A.** Prefer self-directed instruction
    **B.** Are motivated to learn
    **C.** Demonstrate independence in decision-making
    **D.** Seek out theoretical knowledge

96. When a healthcare learner enters a simulation scenario and reflects on a past simulation experience, the socialization is in the form of a(n):

    A. Reflection frame
    B. Expert frame
    C. Modulation frame
    D. Primary frame

97. The novice simulation educator needs a better understanding of the purposes of simulation education when they state:

    A. "Simulation can be used for pharmacology practice."
    B. "Using simulation for basic science is difficult."
    C. "Practicing skills is done well using part-task trainers."
    D. "Crisis management can be taught effectively with simulation."

98. A learner is trying over and over to gain skill in placing a nasogastric tube on a part-task trainer. The student is displaying which concept in Kolb's experiential learning theory?

    A. Concrete experience
    B. Abstract conceptualization
    C. Reflective observation
    D. Active experimentation

99. A simulation educator is asking the standardized patients (SPs) for feedback about the learner's performance and skills. The simulation educator is using which educational philosophy?

    A. Constructivism
    B. Behaviorism
    C. Scaffolding
    D. Realism

100. Which of the following is an example of closed-loop communication?

    A. "Did you get a regular heart rhythm, if so how did it sound?"
    B. "Please provide the patient with a shock when I motion with my hand."
    C. "Please let me know what you heard me say about the treatment plan."
    D. "Are you going to tell me what you would like first?"

101. The goal of simulation education is to:

    A. Make up clinical hours
    B. Understand didactic content
    C. Create innovative therapies
    D. Promote positive patient outcomes

102. A learner is watching the scenario of cardiac arrest on a patient and a resuscitation effort and chooses to be the "recorder" for the event. The student is displaying which concept in Kolb's experiential learning theory?

    A. Concrete experience
    B. Abstract conceptualization
    C. Reflective observation
    D. Active experimentation

103. The simulation educator develops an evaluative instrument that demonstrates validity between the responses and the expectations. This type of validity is considered:

    A. Content
    B. Construct
    C. Face
    D. Predictive

104. The simulation educator is in the process of developing a scenario for a simulation experience. The simulation educator now needs to decide on an appropriate assessment tool to be used to evaluate the learners. This describes which simulation stage?

    A. Designing
    B. Planning
    C. Implementation
    D. Evaluation

105. Certification for Advanced Healthcare Simulation Educators considers expertise in which area of simulation education?

    A. Displaying professional values related to simulation
    B. Using several debriefing methods
    C. Maintaining the technical facilities
    D. Providing staff professional development

106. A learner approaches the simulation educator the day following a scenario and tells the simulation educator that after some thoughts they were capable of better communication about a controversial issue. The student is displaying which concept in Kolb's experiential learning theory?

    A. Concrete experience
    B. Abstract conceptualization
    C. Reflective observation
    D. Active experimentation

107. The novice simulation educator needs a better understanding of simulation learning when they state:

    A. "Simulation is safe space for learning."
    B. "Simulation can be less anxiety-provoking."
    C. "Simulation is spontaneous learning."
    D. "Simulation teaches safe patient care."

108. During a simulation scenario, a student performs skills on the manikin and reacts and changes directions appropriately when the cardiac monitor strip changes. The student is displaying which concept in Kolb's experiential learning theory?

    A. Concrete experience
    B. Abstract conceptualization
    C. Reflective observation
    D. Active experimentation

109. A simulation educator is debriefing learners and provides them with internet resources and poses questions that stretch their current knowledge base to consider different approaches. The simulation educator is using which learning?

    A. Constructivism
    B. Behaviorism
    C. Scaffolding
    D. Realism

110. The novice simulation educator needs a better understanding of Kneebone's essential elements for successful simulation when they state simulation should:

    A. "Allow for deliberate practice."
    B. "Can include experiences as close to real life as possible."
    C. "Be learner-centered."
    D. "Encourage students to learn skills using peer tutoring."

111. The standardized patient is using a reflective debriefing technique to better understand the learner's:

    A. Frame of reference
    B. Social determinants
    C. Prior learning
    D. Role and responsibilities

112. The Simulation[SM] Simulation Operations standard focuses on which of the following simulation education attributes?

    A. Reducing nonessential members of the simulation team
    B. Accepting variable student performance in the simulation lab
    C. Successfully advancing the simulation program
    D. Improving interprofessional collaboration

113. An effective method of studying for the Certified Simulation Healthcare Educator (CHSE) examination is:

    A. Reviewing the Society for Simulation in Healthcare (SSH) website
    B. Reading the examination handbook
    C. Establishing a peer study group
    D. Asking others about test specifics

**114.** During a simulation activity using a part-task trainer haptic body part and a computer to insert a central line, students ask why they need the leg and torso when they can see them on the computer. The simulation educator's BEST answer is:

**A.** "To visualize the anatomy in three dimensions (3D)."

**B.** "To better understand where to place the line."

**C.** "To get the real feel of the puncture site."

**D.** "To further demonstrate the invasive technique."

**115.** The novice simulation educator states that they intent to become certified in simulation education; however, they do not really understand the rationale for certification when they state:

**A.** "It is for personal accomplishment and professional competence."

**B.** "It provides the ability to develop well-designed interdisciplinary scenarios."

**C.** "I will be able to publish about effective uses of simulation."

**D.** "It is mandated in order to conduct any simulation activity."

**116.** A simulation educator requests equipment for a new simulation scenario, which requires an IV pump for medications. Programming and setting up the pump is a student learning outcomes. At $1,200 each, the simulation budget does not have sufficient funds in the equipment budget to purchase the new IV pump. What is the BEST response for trying to meet this educational equipment request?

**A.** Examine the budget and note that there is exactly $1,200 left over in the research grant funds and reallocate this money to purchase the IV pump

**B.** Identify alternatives including renting or borrowing an IV pump from another simulation center or purchasing a refurbished pump

**C.** Ask your artistically gifted simulation technology specialist (STS) to design a look-alike pump, including a complete remake of the display

**D.** Contact the educator and let them know that there is no money in the budget, and they will have to wait until next year to run this new simulation scenario

**117.** The simulation educator provides the standardized patient with proper instructions when they instruct them to:

**A.** Be flexible and tell the student how they feel during the simulation activity

**B.** Share personal experiences with the student

**C.** Answer the questions asked by the student

**D.** Go off script if it provides more situation complexity

**118.** An older and poorly funded simulation center has an increasing probability of replacing several expensive items. Administration leaders and stakeholders are enthusiastic about the center, but it lacks resources. A new donor has recently been identified who wants to fund areas that will make the greatest simulation impact. The donor requests that the simulation educator identify the center's needs and rank them in order of importance. What process can the simulation educator use to help gather data and synthesize this information?

**A.** Complete a probability impact risk matrix and risk register

**B.** Conduct a process audit and update the business plan accordingly

**C.** Review and revise the annual report and strategic plan

**D.** Start an issues log to track the items that are most troublesome

119. The simulation educator understands that using moulage:

    A. Promotes reactive learning
    B. Meets objectives
    C. Increases realism
    D. Decreases student anxiety

120. The simulation educator has been asked to create a schedule for an objective standardized clinical exam (OSCE). The faculty want to start at 3:00 p.m. and run several 15-minute OSCEs using nine rooms, nine graders, and nine standardized patients (SPs), with nine students per time slot and 5 minutes in between each round. There are 45 students. The simulation educator will need 60 minutes prior to the start of the OSCE to set up and train the SPs and 30 minutes after the last round to clean up. How much total time is needed to schedule and plan for this event?

    A. 1 hour 15 minutes
    B. 2 hours 45 minutes
    C. 3 hours 5 minutes
    D. 4 hours 35 minutes

121. The learner in a simulation activity uses closed-loop communication appropriately when they:

    A. Make eye contact with the listener
    B. Address each team member of different disciplines
    C. Record the prescription in the computer
    D. Repeat what was said out loud

122. A major goal of expanding simulation research is to:

    A. Provide standardization for student evaluations
    B. Have participants reflect on their thoughts and feelings
    C. Close the gap between theory and practice
    D. Discover learning through innovative teaching

123. The simulation educator has just joined the operations team of a simulation center that opened 18 months ago. After a simulation event, one of the users sits down with the simulation educator and expresses their frustration with the inconsistency between events and between working with various personnel. Sometimes the services are excellent and all the requested items for the scenario are there, and other times many items are missing. What recommendation can you make that will have the biggest impact on resolving this issue?

    A. Implement a timeline and checklist for each simulation
    B. Review the center's past 18 months for user complaints
    C. Assess the center's scheduling practices
    D. Plan a staff retreat that emphasizes good customer service

124. A team of simulation educators are developing a checklist for senior healthcare students. The checklist has some affective attributes such as professionalism and advocacy that need to be demonstrated. In order to score students in a like manner with many graders, it is advisable to:

    A. Use one evaluator for all learners
    B. Add descriptions
    C. Ask for student input
    D. Ask the standardized patient's input

125. A key concept of debriefing is to:

    A. Critique the event
    B. Identify peer interaction
    C. Build consensus
    D. Develop improvement strategies

126. A healthcare simulation educator is developing a scenario for a student to learn pediatric care on a manikin and would like to use the constructivist theory as the foundation. The BEST method would be to:

    A. Have the student repeat a pediatric assessment several times to get the procedures correct
    B. Have the student approach the assessment using what they have learned and discuss later
    C. Develop a scenario that changes the child's status if an assessment is performed incorrectly
    D. Change the newborn's status to mimic a healthy child if the assessment is done correctly

127. During a scenario, the simulation technology specialist (STS) leaves the center, returning 30 minutes later. The simulation educator is left with equipment that malfunctioned and supplies that were missing. The simulation educator has only 5 minutes before the scenario begins. What is the BEST initial course of action?

    A. Report this incident to the director and have them deal with the incident
    B. Confront the STS, letting them know leaving was inappropriate and what happened
    C. Ignore the situation and do not address it since it was a one-time incident
    D. Schedule a time in the near future to meet with the STS to discuss the incident

128. The simulation educator needs additional understanding when they state to students: "A constructivist approach to this scenario includes . . .":

    A. Using the material we learned yesterday and applying it today
    B. Starting with what we know about this situation and then assessing the patient
    C. Approaching the patient as if we have no information
    D. Relating what is similar in this case to other cases we have worked through

129. The individual who schedules events (the scheduler) in the simulation center cancels a high-priority user and in that place schedules one of their friend's groups (a mid-priority user) in the center. As the director of the center, an email complaint from your high-priority user is received. What is the MOST appropriate immediate action?

    A. Speak with the scheduler to find out why this action was taken
    B. Reschedule the event for the high-priority user and cancel the second group
    C. Do a resource assessment, and if able, negotiate so that both groups can use the center
    D. Remove scheduling privileges until the scheduler undergoes retraining on policies

130. During a team-based simulation scenario, a student takes the lead and approaches the patient first and takes the patient's blood pressure when the manikin tells the group that they feel lightheaded. The student who takes the blood pressure is displaying which learning style?

    A. Concrete experience (CE)
    B. Abstract conceptualization (AC)
    C. Reflective observation (RO)
    D. Active experimentation (AE)

131. One of the goals of the simulation educator is to apply for simulation accreditation. Which activity will BEST help the simulation educator identify areas where the program meets the criteria?

    A. Download the accreditation application
    B. Hold a stakeholder meeting to discuss the accreditation process
    C. Submit your application for accreditation
    D. Perform a gap analysis on the accreditation standards

132. The simulation educator has developed a simulation scenario based on the scaffolding learning theory and presents it to a group of students. The students are provided with an explanation of the case that becomes increasingly difficult. The group was unable to formulate a cohesive plan for the patient. One learning element that is most likely missing may have been:

    A. Instructor presence
    B. Realism
    C. Constructive feedback
    D. Knowledge

133. The simulation educator has been asked to create a schedule for an objective standardized clinical exam (OSCE) where the college of pharmacy wants to run several 15-minute OSCE events using nine rooms, nine graders, and nine standardized patients (SPs), for nine students per time slot and with 5 minutes in between each event. There are 45 students in total. How many total rounds will you need to plan for this event?

    A. Four rounds
    B. Five rounds
    C. Six rounds
    D. Nine rounds

**134.** Guided by the social learning theory, the simulation educator demonstrates to a student who has low self-efficacy how to insert IV lines correctly. The principle that the healthcare simulation educator is using is:

**A.** Mastering experience learning

**B.** Vicarious experience learning

**C.** Verbal persuasion

**D.** Physiologic state

**135.** A simulation center is experiencing a high turnover in simulation technicians and support staff. Staff are unhappy and complain that they are exhausted and burned out. Which of the following leadership styles will MOST likely result in improved employee retention and satisfaction?

**A.** Transformational

**B.** Democratic

**C.** Laissez-faire

**D.** Authoritarian

**136.** One of the healthcare students was previously an emergency medical technician (EMT), and during a simulation prebriefing the student states that they would like to advance their splinting skills. The student is demonstrating which type of educational concept?

**A.** Pedagogy

**B.** Realism

**C.** Behaviorism

**D.** Andragogy

**137.** An important tour is scheduled after normal working hours in 2 months. Staffing this event has become a challenge because one of the employees in a leadership position has openly refused to modify their schedule to support this event and has encouraged other employees to refuse as well. Alternate time-off and compensation have been offered; their schedules are seldom modified. What resource can BEST help with this problem?

**A.** Human resources personnel

**B.** Resource allocation

**C.** Benefits specialist

**D.** Policies and procedures

**138.** The novice simulation educator needs additional information when they provide a list of Kneebone's (2005) simulation learning principles as:

**A.** Occurring in a safe environment

**B.** Tutors being available to learners

**C.** Teacher-centered

**D.** Mimicking real life

**139.** Kirkpatrick's (1998) simulation learning principles are orderly, and once learning is achieved the simulation educator should expect the students to:

A. React to the debriefing questions positively

B. Apply the learning to patient care with positive outcomes

C. Learn through a premodule requirement and quiz

D. Demonstrate a change in behavior during simulation

**140.** The last step of Doerr and Murray's (2008) simulation teaching–learning process is:

A. Debriefing

B. Transference

C. Developing learning outcomes

D. Creating the situation

**141.** A simulation educator is developing student objectives/learning outcomes and would like learners to reach a level of application. Which objective/learning outcome would BEST fit the application level?

A. Defining the hybrid simulation procedure

B. Discussing the clinical decision for starting CPR

C. Prioritizing the intervention

D. Evaluating the intervention's effect

**142.** A simulation educator completes an educational style scenario with learners and enters the room to debrief. The simulation educator informs the students that their performance was terrible and that they failed the scenario. This action would be considered:

A. Appropriate because the learners did not perform well

B. Appropriate because students should know when they underperform

C. Inappropriate because the scenario's purpose was for learning

D. Inappropriate because learners should never be failed in simulation

**143.** The simulation educator is completing a scenario during which a patient dies. Prebriefing is essential in a scenario that can be poignant because:

A. The simulation educator can determine what the students know before starting

B. The simulation educator sets the stage to help learners deal with their emotions

C. Demonstrative scenarios of this nature are not ideal but needed

D. Learners may cry during the scenario and disrupt the learning

**144.** During a scenario, an interprofessional healthcare provider enters the room and does not wash or gel their hands. This would be discussed in debriefing and would be:

A. A microethical situation or dilemma

B. An appropriate action since their hands may have just been washed

C. Something to be addressed by the simulation educator during the scenario

D. A scenario that is too difficult for the learners to manage

145. Learners and the simulation educator are about to begin a simulation scenario and the learners will be recorded. When using video recording during simulation experiences, it is important for:

    A. Simulation educators to learn how to use the equipment
    B. Technical support to be available in case of technical issues
    C. Learners to have signed a consent agreement to be recorded
    D. All participants to work companionably to enhance the recording

146. Certified Simulation Healthcare Educator (CHSE) recertification for initial or advanced recertification should be completed:

    A. Every 5 years
    B. Every 4 years
    C. Every 3 years
    D. Every 2 years

147. A simulation educator receives the following question from an academic colleague: "Why bother recertifying since you are already a simulation expert?" The BEST response would be:

    A. "I do not want to take the examination again."
    B. "The initials after my name increase my job prospects."
    C. "It is an expectation of administrators in academia."
    D. "It demonstrates that my expertise is ongoing."

148. Participants are experiencing a simulation activity for the purpose of learning crutch walking. What type of experience would this be considered?

    A. Formative
    B. Summative
    C. Cumulative
    D. Additive

149. Certification as a simulation healthcare educator provides societal reassurance that the educator:

    A. Has met the maximum standards in the field of certification
    B. Has completed an intense course of study about simulation learning
    C. Can develop simulation scenarios that promote clinical judgment
    D. Has met the minimum standards in the discipline of simulation learning

150. Equivalency to the expected academic degree needed for certification includes:

    A. Developing a simulation program that is fully functioning
    B. Promoting simulation as a needed learning strategy
    C. Being an expert in the field through practice initiatives
    D. Speaking at simulation conferences about best practices

# Practice Test Answers and Rationales

Linda Wilson and Ruth A. Wittmann-Price

1. **A) Simulated participants**
   Simulated participants will provide the learner with a human that can assist them with reflecting on how they made a patient feel during their interaction. Part-task trainers, high-fidelity manikins, and virtual reality cannot replace the humanness for affective learning.

2. **C) Learning outcomes to guide the simulation**
   Having a planned simulation learning experience with learning outcomes to guide the simulation is important and maintains psychological fidelity. Learner-centric approaches are also important but do not guarantee that the scenario or the learning activity will be psychologically sound for all learners. Neither does having a certified simulation educator or a high-fidelity simulator.

3. **D) Age and gender**
   Learners are assisted if age and person-identified gender are congruent with the simulation scenario. This will increase realism more than hair or skin color, ethnicity, race, articulation, and education level.

4. **D) Specific prebrief times**
   The prebrief and debrief should not have specific or strict times to be completed. Each group of participants may have different learning needs. There needs to be an experience, educational strategies, and participants or learners.

5. **C) Level 3 (behavior) and level 4 (results)**
   How simulation changes behavior and produces results that benefit quality patient care are areas still in need of additional evidence. There are studies about learning and reaction in the literature.

6. **B) Bookmark while videotaping and show critical points**
   Showing the video's important or critical points, both positive and negative, is more effective than showing the entire video, just showing negative implementations, or letting learners watch the video on their own.

7. **B) "Learner satisfaction with simulation pedagogy is understudied."**
   Learners' perceptions of simulation is one area that has been studied. Debriefing processes, learner satisfaction with simulation pedagogy, and the impact of a participant's race are in need of further investigation and data to determine best practice.

8. **C) 1:2**
   One hour of simulation is comparable to 2 hours of direct patient clinical learning experiences due to the intenseness, reflection, and clinical decision-making components. Research does not support 2:1 or 2:2 ratios, while there is evidence for the 1:2 ratio.

9.  **A) Level 1 (reaction)**
    The most researched level is reaction, which has to do with learners' perceptions of the simulation experience. The second most researched areas are learning and behavior changes. More research is needed about long-term outcomes or results.

10. **C) Part-task trainer**
    A part-task trainer is probably the least effective modality to use for affective simulation learning. A better choice may be a simulated patient so they could display the mental health issue. High-fidelity may be used if the controller can use audio, but it is still not as effective as a live person who can demonstrate emotion. Virtual gaming will also lack the emotion needed.

11. **C) "Debriefing for meaningful learning."**
    Debriefing for meaningful learning is not actually a debriefing framework. Debriefing with good judgment, preview advocacy inquiry, and plus delta are techniques used to debrief.

12. **B) Society for Simulation in Healthcare**
    The Society for Simulation in Healthcare establishes standards of best practice and certifications for simulation healthcare educators. The National League for Nursing is a nursing faculty organization that promotes best practice in nursing education The International Nursing Association for Clinical Simulation and Learning promotes best practices for simulation learning but does not offer certifications. The Association of Standardized Patient Educators promotes best practice for standardized patients used in simulation scenarios.

13. **D) Allow the student to use the stethoscope**
    An amplified stethoscope is a reasonable accommodation and the simulation educator should not interfere with the student using it or bring attention to it. Developing a scenario in which a stethoscope is not needed is not necessary. The student should not be assigned another role since they are a learner, and calling out the student in prebriefing is not appropriate.

14. **C) Part-task trainer**
    A part-task trainer is the best modality because it can elicit the skill and is durable, so students can practice over and over without the wear and tear of a more expensive manikin or high-fidelity manikin. Virtual reality does not provide hands-on experience, and a simulated participant is not used for invasive procedures.

15. **D) "We can discuss how we would do that the next time."**
    The purpose of debriefing is process improvement. There is only a need to review important parts, not review the entire scenario. The learners should reflect on their team effort, and the best part of the experience may be different for different learners.

16. **D) Integrating simulation throughout the curriculum**
    Simulation experiences should be integrated throughout the curriculum to effectively enhance knowledge acquisition. It does not have to be a specific time, and all students should have the experience as a learning tool rather than just a remediation methodology.

17. **A) Interviewing a patient (standardized patient [SP])**
    Interviewing a patient is an ideal situation to videotape and have the learner rewatch and reflect. Megacode in ACLS, medication administration, and intraosseous vascular insertion concentrate on skills and actions that can be recorded by other methods. Interpersonal interactions are captured well on video.

18. **A) Performing a needs assessment**
   A needs assessment is the first step to identify if the change is needed and the gaps in the curriculum that must be addressed. Learner assessments can be added to the needs assessment once gaps have been established. The environment is the entire learning organization or unit, and the learning objectives should be established when a new curriculum model is decided upon by the faculty.

19. **C) Implied consent to record when tapes will be destroyed after debriefing**
   Even if a tape is going to be destroyed, there still should be permission before its taped. Having codes of conduct accessible to students, maintaining fair evaluation processes throughout the learning activities, and consent for picture taking for any use are correct to do.

20. **A) Validated checklists**
   A checklist that is validated is a good objective method to measure competency. Multiple-choice testing is better suited for cognitive evaluation; peer critique is good for feedback but the learners are not experts; and a focus group is good for understanding perceptions.

21. **B) Teamwork**
   There are studies that support simulation as a learning methodology that positively affects teamwork. More studies are needed long term to understand simulation's effect on knowledge retention and clinical and patient outcomes.

22. **A) Experiential learning**
   IPE is a form of experiential learning because it encompasses in-person, hands-on learning. Behaviorism is a learning theory that uses a reward system, deliberate practice does not have to encompass interprofessional students, and IPE is not usually self-directed learning.

23. **A) Deliberate practice**
   Deliberate practice is a modality that assists mastery in psychomotor competency. High-fidelity manikins are not needed for tasks, case studies do not provide the psychomotor skills, and standardized patients cannot be used for invasive procedures.

24. **C) Give constructive feedback**
   Formative evaluation is used for improvement and therefore it is constructive feedback. Assigning a grade or a pass/fail score is summative. Providing information is not an assessment; it is learning.

25. **C) Interactive element**
   Inserting a clue during a scenario to assist learners is "an interactive element." This is not passive or active learning and there is no transference into practice because the students are practicing.

26. **D) Promote student development**
   Feedback is providing for formative process improvement. Standardized patients cannot recommend remediation or provide a grade. Students may self-reflect, but the main point is to promote professional development by listening to how they made the patient (standardized patient) feel during the encounter.

27. **C) Emotional intelligence**
    SPs need emotional intellect in order to assess students' actions and provide appropriate feedback. SPs do not need to have the disease, but symptomatic SPs are used in some cases and are a helpful teaching tool. Honesty is good, but providing honest assessments takes emotional intelligence. Articulation skills are helpful but not critical.

28. **B) Evaluate the students' feedback about the scenario**
    Student feedback is a priority when assessing if a scenario worked well and met the student learning objectives. Knowing students' perceptions, before including observations and staff feedback, is important in revising scenarios. Determining the valuation should be done in the planning stage, and moving forward to write another scenario is not the priority.

29. **D) Cost-effective**
    Part-task trainers (PTTs) are cost-effective. PTTs are not always small and lightweight. PTTs are not disposable; they are durable.

30. **D) Activities should meet student learning outcomes**
    The learning activities planned in any simulation event should directly relate back to the student learning outcomes. Meeting the student learning outcomes should place the activity at the correct level for the students' skills. Challenging scenarios may or may not meet the leveled student learning outcomes. The learning event does not have to be common clinical scenarios.

31. **C) Empathize with the chronically ill patient and family members**
    Empathy is an affective attribute of healthcare professionals. Demonstrating is in the psychomotor domain, while listing and understanding are in the cognitive domain.

32. **A) Performing an end-of-course objective structured clinical examination (OSCE)**
    The OSCE at the end is summative. One didactic test is not summative; it is a score that leads to the end grade. Deliberate practice is formative to increase skills, and a reviewed scenario would be formative.

33. **D) "We can address simulation implementation barriers as they arise."**
    Barriers need to be anticipated and worked through to fully integrate simulation into a curriculum. The curriculum needs to be evaluated in an ongoing fashion and resources need to be established before implementation. Political support for a simulation program needs to be established in the planning stage.

34. **D) Communication**
    Communication is one of the four interprofessional education (IPE) principles. Leadership, evidence-based practice, and reflection are not included in the four essential principles but are important attributes of healthcare professionals. Other IPE elements include responsibility, accountability, coordination, communication, cooperation, assertiveness, autonomy, and mutual trust and respect.

35. **A) "I am concerned because I noticed the team took 4 minutes to organize themselves."**
"I am concerned because I noticed the team took 4 minutes to organize themselves" is in the format of an advocacy-inquiry debriefing. "The team took too long to organize themselves but met the goal" would not be used to start a debriefing. "Let's list what went well and what needs improvement for next time" is a plus-delta technique. "Can you all tell me as a group what took you so long and how to improve?" is not a debriefing technique because it is placing the learners on the spot.

36. **D) "Can you think of how to increase patient safety in the next scenario?"**
The last option asks the student to reflect, which is a method for them to learn from their mistakes. "Not identifying the patient could result in you eventually losing your license" and "You will fail the course if you do not identify patients correctly" are threatening, while "Understanding patient safety is priority of every nurse" is general and condescending.

37. **B) Using a part-task trainer with a standardized patient**
Using a part-task trainer and a standardized patient is the best method to educate and practice. Virtual simulation is also acceptable, but actually practicing the procedure using the equipment may increase competency. Peers are not as objective as standardized patients, while high-fidelity manikins cannot provide feedback.

38. **A) Stop the scenario and ask the student to come out then continue with the other learners**
Stopping the scenario and removing the student who is upset and then continuing the learning with the rest of the students is the best thing to do. The student who is having an issue should be dealt with individually and confidentially. Continuing the scenario is not recognizing the human reaction taking place. Focusing on the upset student is not appropriate.

39. **C) Reliable**
Reliability is eliciting the same results group after group on an evaluation tool or instrument. Validity is having the tool look at the appropriate constructs. Realism is a theory, while feasibility has to do with how easy a tool is to administer.

40. **C) Close knowledge gaps**
Simulation programs can close knowledge gaps through well-integrated and constructed simulation activities. They are more than a learning procedure and they are not just for assisting at-risk students. Simulation learning is not just to practice psychomotor skills because it includes affective and cognitive learning. Practicing missing procedures is one asset but not the primary reason.

41. **A) Physical fidelity**
Making the wound look as real as possible increases the physical fidelity of simulation learning. Psychological fidelity is an affective issue addressed in simulation, while environmental fidelity is increasing the realism of the setting. Equipment is not specifically addressed as fidelity.

42. **C) Is finished**

The SP should stay in character until the scenario is finished, then come out of character to provide the learners feedback. If an error is made that is not life-threatening, it should be discussed and reflected upon during debriefing. The student should not request information from the SP that they should know prior to the simulation learning activity and should not request the SP to come out of character.

43. **A) "Increased realism will ensure the learning outcomes are met."**

Realism in itself does not ensure that student learning outcomes are met; realism should be created as all simulation activities, in a safe environment. Realism can increase the fidelity and assist students with better grasping the situation.

44. **C) Become automatic habits**

Deliberate practice is done to repeat procedures that will become automatic when needed in the clinical area. It may or may not motivate learners and is usually not done for understanding. Practice is never done for perfection.

45. **B) Responsibility**

Responsibility is a competency for interprofessional education. Leadership, reflection, and demonstration are not identified as core leadership competencies. Other leadership competencies include accountability, coordination, communication, cooperation, assertiveness, autonomy, and mutual trust and respect.

46. **A) Provide a score for the experience**

Only the faculty can provide a score or final grade for the experience. The standardized patient can provide feedback, use knowledge and emotions, and ad lib if needed, but they cannot grade.

47. **D) Inappropriately touching another person**

Any sexual harassment is a larger issue than a microethical issue and needs to be reported immediately. Work around medication administration practices, poor handwashing techniques, and breaches in confidentiality about laboratory performance can be dealt with and discussed in a simulation activity to increase learner awareness.

48. **B) Psychological fidelity**

Having learners become familiar with the equipment and environment promotes psychological fidelity. Promoting psychological fidelity will enhance students' performance during the simulation activity. Physical fidelity has to do with the equipment being used, while environmental fidelity is the scenario setup. There is no equipment fidelity recognized in simulation.

49. **C) "You did an overall thorough patient head-to-toe assessment but need practice in lung sound stethoscope placement, but your heart stethoscope placement was fine."**

"You did an overall thorough patient head-to-toe assessment but need practice in lung sound stethoscope placement, but your heart stethoscope placement was fine" provided a positive, a needs improvement, and then a positive, which is a "sandwich feedback" technique. The other simulation educators did not provide all three components in their feedback statement.

50. **C) Believable information**

    Fiction contracts that treat the simulation activity as "as if" are easier if the case and the setup are as believable as possible. The case does not have to be complex, high fidelity, or contain moulage to make it believable.

51. **D) Affective**

    Ethical considerations in a patient scenario involve values and judgment, which is affective learning. Cognitive is reasoning and knowledge, psychomotor is skill-based, and internalization is taking on another's values.

52. **B) Psychomotor**

    Demonstration of skills is mainly in the psychomotor domain of learning. Cognitive is knowledge; somatic refers to bodily; and affective has to do with values, emotions, and feelings.

53. **D) Concerned, uncomfortable, safety**

    Concerned, uncomfortable, and safety are the three CUS elements taught by TeamSTEPPS to ensure patient safety. Cognitive, uncommunicated, strategies, and scenario are not part of CUS. Cognitive is thinking about what is happening in the patient scenario, and uncommunicated should not happen in teamwork.

54. **A) Cognition**

    A description has to do with cognitive knowledge. The students are not asked to demonstrate so it is not psychomotor, and it does not contain emotions or feelings and therefore it is not affective. Internalization is not a learning domain.

55. **C) Understanding debriefing**

    Much of the learning process in simulation takes place in debriefing. Working with manikins and troubleshooting can be completed by laboratory technicians. Developing scenarios is an important role of the faculty, but debriefing so learning takes place is paramount.

56. **D) An identified leader**

    Not all simulation activities that involve teams need a leader. Everyone on the team must know their role and there does need to be a plan in place for correction and evaluation of the activity.

57. **C) Values**

    Values are one of the core competencies stressed in interprofessional teams. Leadership, delegation, and demonstration are not considered core competencies. The core competencies are role clarification, team functioning, interprofessional communication, patient-centered care, interprofessional conflict management, and collaborative leadership.

58. **C) Internalizing**

    The simulation educator would like to have the learner reflect on the displayed behavior and internalize professional behavior. This is not receiving, valuing, or organizing but a situation where internalization is needed.

59. **A) Provide orientation and training for the people involved**
Standardized patients need orientation and training about how to assist the simulation activity to unfold as planned. It may not be feasible to recruit only trained actors or ensure pay. Following the script is important, but if the activity deviates the standardized patient needs to know what the learning objectives are in order to respond appropriately.

60. **C) Conduct a run-through or field test of the new simulation**
Doing a trial run is important for pacing and effect. Trial runs also ensure that the activity meets the learning goals. Seeking input is important, but understanding the learning goals and ensuring the goals are met are a priority. Having a second faculty look at a scenario is good, but actually doing the scenario may uncover other issues. Students should be included at the time of prebriefing not during the development phase of the scenario. Practice partners may be able to provide cases, but cases can be found in books and also on the web.

61. **B) A curriculum vitae (CV)**
The priority is knowing the person's professional and educational background, which can be determined from a well-written CV. The application, reference, and video are also important, but the CV should be vetted first.

62. **C) "You know this is the wrong way to do this."**
"You know this is the wrong way to do this" sounds accusatory and does not leave room for reflection. The other statements and questions, help me to understand, how do you think, and can you tell me, leave room for reflection and process improvement.

63. **B) Virtual reality**
This is a virtual reality technique. The computer-generated program is not considered high-fidelity. Task-trainer and standardized patient are common modalities used but are not virtual.

64. **D) "Simulation is something that can be done at the last minute if needed for makeup days."**
Simulation is not a last-minute learning activity; it has to be planned and thought out. Simulation learning can be used for hard-to-acquire experiences and for increasing confidence.

65. **D) Simulation<sup>SM</sup> Simulation-Enhanced Interprofessional Education**
Developing simulation activities that involve many disciplines enhances interprofessional education. Using many professionals does not specifically address professional identity. Simulation Design and Outcomes and Objectives are completed because the scenario has been developed.

66. **C) "Recognition and curtailment of unprofessional and unethical behavior during simulation."**
The standard does not include correcting unprofessional behavior as a goal but includes learners reflecting on how they behaved. Debriefing does include critical thinking and learners modifying their behavior based on the experience review.

67. **B) Delegation**

    Delegation is a leadership skill. A shared understanding, balance of work, and mutual trust are team attributes that all team members should demonstrate.

68. **A) Teamwork**

    Teamwork is paramount in interprofessional collaboration. Delegation, prioritization, and demonstration can be a positive part of interprofessional collaboration, but the primary attribute to ensure patient safety is teamwork.

69. **A) Effective evaluation tools that are valid and reliable**

    Evaluation tools need to be valid and reliable in order to promote fair assessment and grading. Videotaping, rubrics, and content that has been covered in class are important, but if the evaluation tool is not adequate then the assessment will be flawed.

70. **B) Self-reporting surveys**

    Self-reporting surveys will help the simulationist gather the perceptions of the students, especially if animosity is maintained. Skills list, direct questions, and OSCEs usually yield quantitative data.

71. **A) "I will have students arrive at 7:00 a.m., and we will see how long the simulation takes."**

    The simulation activity time should be established in the planning phase. Small learning groups are good, as is developing objectives in the planning stage. Prebriefing and debriefing should also be included in the planning.

72. **D) "Debriefing is an effective method for evaluating skill acquisition with task trainers."**

    Debriefing is for reflective learning and process improvement and not skill acquisition. IV arms are low fidelity, and high fidelity can be used in a complex patient scenarios for beginning students. Task trainers can be used for skill practice.

73. **B) Professional career attainment**

    CPD assists simulationists in advancing their career either in academia or in the business sector. It does not directly assist with learners' knowledge, teach simulation educators how to use high fidelity, or promote critical analysis.

74. **C) Reliability**

    Reliability is demonstrated when a tool or instrument works consistently group after group. Validity and content validity are tools that elicit the information that is intended. Creditability is when a tool logically addresses the issue being evaluated. Content does not relate to tool assessment.

75. **A) "The simulation educator moves people toward the future by providing us with what simulation can do for learners."**

    Moving people forward is transformational. Organizing, developing scenarios, and scheduling are managerial-type activities and do not always assist team members to reach their potential.

76. **A) Sharing knowledge**
    Sharing knowledge is a transformational characteristic. Demonstrating, delegating, and prioritization are managerial or top-down leadership styles.

77. **D) Psychological safety**
    Psychological safety is necessary to open conversations and decrease vulnerability. Mutual respect and straightforwardness are important but not the main climate-creating concept, while shared perspectives provides time for the standardized patient or simulation educator to give students their observations.

78. **B) Applying**
    This student learning outcome applies knowledge through demonstration. The student learning outcome expects more than understanding and comprehension because it needs to be incorporated into the behavior. It is not at the level of analysis because it is straightforward and educators do not have to induce or deduce the elements.

79. **C) Has to be renewed every 3 years**
    The certification has to be renewed every 3 years and is not an automatic lifelong certification. It does not get revoked and it does demonstrate a level of expertise, not just proficiency.

80. **B) Organize the simulation laboratory so it is easy for students to learn**
    Organization and scheduling are associated with transactional leadership, whereas futuristic thinking, providing resources, and maintaining the mission are associated with transformational leadership.

81. **D) Expert**
    It is at the expert level that intuition can be used in the practice setting. Proficient means patterns are followed, and if this situation did not occur before there may have not been a pattern. Advanced beginner and competent level practitioners usually follow procedures to produce outcomes.

82. **C) Reasonable accommodations**
    Educators are obligated to follow the instructions on the letter from the Americans With Disabilities Act (ADA) officer. The ADA officer decides if the accommodations are reasonable and the educator enacts the reasonable accommodations as stated. The simulation educator only provides special equipment, additional time, and one-to-one instruction if the accommodation letter states they should do so.

83. **B) Positively impacted by the use of simulation**
    National studies demonstrate that learning is positively impacted by simulation. Simulation does not negatively affect outcomes or obscure learning experiences.

84. **D) Learning which can take place for all under the guidance of experienced simulation educators**
    An experienced simulation educator can create "brave space" where all learners can be respected and accepted. Manikins and SPs are part of the environment but by themselves do not set the culture. The learners or anyone cannot leave social determinants behind; they need to be recognized and reflected on.

85. **A) Feeling like an imposter**
The first step in learning a healthcare profession is feeling like an imposter. Later steps include understanding the role and then gaining confidence. Trial and error should not be part of role development.

86. **D) Acclimating to the primary frame**
The learner is socializing or acclimating to the primary frame or being aware of the surroundings, which include the equipment and the people in the simulation laboratory. Modulation includes reflective practice, while unstructured time in the laboratory is usually included in prebriefing. Role assimilation is usually done by enacting the scenario.

87. **A) Minority students may do just as well in simulation because they will join in**
Simulation educators cannot assume that minority students will react to simulation in the same way as nonminority learners. Minority students may feel marginalized and need additional resources. Minority students may feel they do not belong unless the environment is inclusive.

88. **A) Refer the student to the university's Americans With Disabilities Act (ADA) officer**
The student needs to present the request to the ADA officer, and if the request is granted the student needs to show the letter to the simulation educator. The simulation educator cannot make accommodations without the ADA officer evaluating the request and determining if it is reasonable. Providing a private place and more time needs to be stated by the ADA officer. The request may be reasonable, which is determined by the ADA officer.

89. **D) Provide safe patient care**
The ultimate goal of interprofessional education is safe patient care driven by teamwork. Understanding roles, making environments more congenital, and learning about different perspectives are all part of the ultimate goal.

90. **D) Learning theories**
How students learn by storing and recalling information is a topic of learning theories. Teaching theories have to do with how educators promote knowledge acquisition and worldviews, while philosophies are broad constructs about how and why education fits into human existence.

91. **B) Behaviorism**
This student learning outcome is in the behaviorism realm because it is a demonstration or observable behavior. Constructivism builds behavior from past experiences, idealism is using knowledge to get to a perfect world, and realism uses science as the foundation of education.

92. **D) Mixed simulation**
A mixed simulation has more than one patient care need even if it is hybrid. Task trainer simulation is stand-alone, as is human patients or high-fidelity simulation.

93. **C) Implementation**
This is the implementation stage that is done with the learners. The designing and planning stages are done before the learners arrive, while the debriefing takes place after the activity.

94. **A) Constructivism**

The simulation educator is using constructivism, relating past experiences to new experiences. Scaffolding is building on previous knowledge, while realism is a theory/philosophy that science and empirical data can build knowledge. Behaviorism is knowledge being demonstrated in behavior.

95. **D) Seek out theoretical knowledge**

Adult learners prefer knowledge that is applicable to their goal, not theoretical knowledge. Adult learners are self-directed, motivated, and independent in decision-making due to their past life experiences which they can apply to the new learning situation.

96. **C) Modulation frame**

This is a modulation frame in simulation. Although the learner reflects or remembers past experiences, they are judging this environment with the past experience as a reference. Reflection occurs after the scenario. It is not an expert frame because they are learners, while a primary frame has to do with the environmental equipment itself.

97. **B) "Using simulation for basic science is difficult."**

Simulation can be used effectively for basic sciences. Anything learners learn in the classroom can be demonstrated in a simulation laboratory if innovation is applied. Simulation can be used for pharmacology practice, skills, and crises management. Practicing skills on a part-task trainer is an effective simulation learning process.

98. **D) Active experimentation**

Practicing a skill is the active experimentation stage of Kolb's experiential learning theory. Concrete experience is learning about things that are tangible, abstract conceptualization is taking in learning from different perspectives, and reflective observation is thinking about learning before reacting.

99. **A) Constructivism**

The learning in constructivism is based on reality and the SP is part of the student's learning reality. Behavioralism is displayed in observable performance, scaffolding is building from simple to complex when learning concepts, and realism is using science to justify the learning being facilitated.

100. **C) "Please let me know what you heard me say about the treatment plan."**

The person is requesting the other person to communicate back so that they both understand the same instructions. "Did you get a regular heart rhythm, if so how did it sound?" "Please provide the patient with a shock when I motion with my hand," and "Are you going to tell me what you would like first?" are just one-way communications; they ask a question but do not provide feedback about what was communicated.

101. **D) Promote positive patient outcomes**

The goal of simulation education is to promote positive patient outcomes and improve healthcare. Making up clinical hours, using it for didactic content, and creating innovative therapies are things that can be done with simulation, but they are not the goal.

102. **C) Reflective observation**

The student is demonstrating reflective observation because by recording they can observe the situation. The learner is not using a tangible (concrete) or abstract style because they are not the "doer" or reflecting during the scenario. The student is not actively experimenting because they are not hands-on in this scenario.

103. **D) Predictive**
Validity between responses and expectations is predictive validity; content validity verifies the appropriateness of each item; face validity demonstrates that the tool measures what it is supposed to measure; and construct validity establishes that an action accurately represents the concept being evaluated.

104. **A) Designing**
Developing the scenario and the assessment mechanism are parts of the designing stage. Planning to use the tool and implementing the scenario and tool come after the design. Evaluation and postsimulation take place after the scenario is completed.

105. **A) Displaying professional values related to simulation**
Part of the role of a Certified Healthcare Simulation Educator (CHSE) is to display professional teaching–learning values related to simulation and appropriate to academia and their role as a "role model." Knowing debriefing methods and providing staff professional development can be completed in the role of initial CHSE certification as well. Technical maintenance is under the realm of the simulation technician role.

106. **B) Abstract conceptualization**
The learner is demonstrating abstract conceptualization because they are thinking about a different perspective. Reflection happens, in this theory, before reaction. This is not concrete or tangible, and there is no active experimentation because at the point the student approached the simulation educator there was no hands-on event.

107. **C) "Simulation is spontaneous learning."**
Simulation learning is planned and organized. It is usually less anxiety-provoking than direct patient care and is a safe space for learning that teaches safe patient care.

108. **A) Concrete experience**
Concrete experience is learning that is applied to a situation and is tangible with a cause and effect. It is not abstract, taking in different perspectives, or is reflective because the learner reacted. It is not active experimentation because the action was predicated by the situation and not trial and error.

109. **C) Scaffolding**
Scaffolding is building knowledge through accessing resources and stretching learners to the next level of understanding. Constructivism is building on what is known and does not always include introduction of new resources. Behaviorism is stimulus-response learning that is displayed in changed behavior. Realism is using research as the truth of knowledge.

110. **D) "Encourage students to learn skills using peer tutoring."**
Kneebone's elements include expert tutoring, not peer tutoring. Kneebone's elements include deliberate practice, making simulations as real as possible, and keeping learning student-centered.

111. **A) Frame of reference**
Reflective debriefing techniques assist the standardized patient in better understanding the learners' frame of reference rather than concentrating on social determinants, prior learning, or students' role. Understanding the student's frame of reference can promote feedback that is individualized to the learner.

112. **D) Improving interprofessional collaboration**
Simulation Operations standard addresses interprofessional collaboration. This standard does not address student performance, advancing the simulation program, or designating essential and nonessential team members. Improving interprofessional collaboration is a goal of simulation.

113. **C) Establishing a peer study group**
Establishing a peer group is a good method of studying. Reviewing the website and handbook is a good idea, as well as inquiring about test statistics, but actual studying takes time and can be accomplished more effectively with a group for many candidates.

114. **C) "To get the real feel of the puncture site."**
The haptic trainer provides learners with the touch sensation of a real patient. If the activity was just to visualize, learners could use a computer or nonhaptic part-task trainer. The haptic trainer will help them place the line and learn the technique. 3D is learning by visualization. Many of the simulation techniques can demonstrate the invasive technique and demonstrate anatomically where to place the line, but haptic technique has the feel that is needed.

115. **D) "It is mandated in order to conduct any simulation activity."**
This statement is incorrect. Certification is not mandated to run a simulation scenario. Certification does demonstrate the ability to develop interdisciplinary scenarios, collect data for publication, and demonstrate professional competence.

116. **B) Identify alternatives including renting or borrowing an IV pump from another simulation center or purchasing a refurbished pump**
Identifying alternatives can often meet competing budget and learning needs. Reallocating money from another account within the budget may not be legal if it is earmarked for specific items. Creating a low-fidelity IV pump will not meet the learning objectives of programming and setting up the pump. Asking the educator to change their simulation is the least desirable option. Be creative and collaborative in solving problems.

117. **C) Answer the questions asked by the student**
The standardized patients should answer the questions asked by the learner. The simulation educator should instruct the standardized patient with questions that are likely to be asked. Telling the learner how they feel about the experience is done during the feedback, not during the session. Sharing personal experiences is not appropriate, nor is going off script.

118. **A) Complete a probability impact risk matrix and risk register**
Creating a risk register and probability risk impact matrix will help you track, classify, and score the risks of doing or putting off the purchase or repair of equipment and durable goods. This quantitative method combines probability and impact scores and a visual grid which can help synthesize, prioritize, and rank items for the donor. Conducting an audit and updating the business plan, reviewing and revising the annual report and strategic plan, and starting an issues log may not show the impact that no future resources will have.

119. **C) Increases realism**
Moulage promotes realism. Moulage does not ensure meeting the objectives or student learning outcomes, decrease anxiety, or promote reactive learning.

120. **C) 3 hours 5 minutes**
     (2:00–5:05) Rounds refers to the number of times the OSCE is needed to repeat in order for all students to complete the simulation activity. Begin by identifying how many rooms can run (in this case, there are nine rooms that are up and working, and there are nine graders and nine SPs to fully staff the nine rooms). Then take the total number of students and divide them by the number of available rooms (number of students / number of rooms = number of rounds): 45/9 = 5.

| Time | | | 3:00–3:15 | 3:20–3:35 | 3:40–3:55 | 4:00–4:15 | 4:20–4:35 |
|---|---|---|---|---|---|---|---|
| | **Grader** | **SP** | | | | | |
| Room 1 | Grader 1 | SP 1 | Student 1 | Student 10 | Student 19 | Student 28 | Student 37 |
| Room 2 | Grader 2 | SP 2 | Student 2 | Student 11 | Student 20 | Student 29 | Student 38 |
| Room 3 | Grader 3 | SP 3 | Student 3 | Student 12 | Student 21 | Student 30 | Student 39 |
| Room 4 | Grader 4 | SP 4 | Student 4 | Student 13 | Student 22 | Student 31 | Student 40 |
| Room 5 | Grader 5 | SP 5 | Student 5 | Student 14 | Student 23 | Student 32 | Student 41 |
| Room 6 | Grader 6 | SP 6 | Student 6 | Student 15 | Student 24 | Student 33 | Student 42 |
| Room 7 | Grader 7 | SP 7 | Student 7 | Student 16 | Student 25 | Student 34 | Student 43 |
| Room 8 | Grader 8 | SP 8 | Student 8 | Student 17 | Student 26 | Student 35 | Student 44 |
| Room 9 | Grader 9 | SP 9 | Student 9 | Student 18 | Student 27 | Student 36 | Student 45 |

- Arrive: 2:00 p.m. (1 hour to set up and instruct SPs and graders).
- Start: 3:00–4:35 (nine rooms, five rounds at 15 minutes each and 5 minutes in between).
- Cleanup: 4:35–5:05 (30 minutes to clean up).

121. **D) Repeat what was said out loud**
     In closed-loop communication, the prescription, command, or order is restated out loud so everyone is clear on what needs to be accomplished. Addressing each team member is time-consuming and unnecessary if it is said out loud. Making eye contact is good, as is addressing each team member when needed, but does not close the loop. Documentation is necessary but not the priority in an emergency.

122. **C) Close the gap between theory and practice**
     Closing the theory–practice gap promotes quality patient care, which is the goal of simulation learning. Providing standard evaluations processes, reflection, and innovative teaching are also parts of simulation learning, but patient care quality and safety is the major goal.

123. **A) Implement a timeline and checklist for each simulation**
     Creating and implementing a timeline and checklist for each simulation can help standardize the quality of simulation services that users and learners receive. Checklists have been used successfully to reduce and eliminate errors in the airline industry and in hospitals and operating rooms around the world. Implementing them in a simulation center can also increase quality and reduce error. Reviewing the center's past 18 months of user complaints and assessing the center's scheduling practices can assist the manager/leader in gaining a better understanding of the extent of the issue but do not address or fix the problem. Planning a staff retreat that emphasizes good customer service can help increase morale and refresh the principles of customer service, but it does not address the inherent system issues that a standardized timeline and checklist can.

124. **B) Add descriptions**

Adding descriptions will assist all graders in knowing what to observe so they will know if the students have met the benchmark. Using one evaluator may not be feasible and asking for input from a student or a standardized patient on a summative evaluation makes it very subjective.

125. **D) Develop improvement strategies**

Debriefing is a time to reflect on the simulation event and identify areas of improvement. Some critiquing of the event does occur but does not always lead to stated improvements. Peer interactions may also be addressed and so may be a point that needs consensus building, but they are not the main concept of debriefing.

126. **B) Have the student approach the assessment using what they have learned and discuss later**

Having students use what they have learned builds on previous knowledge. Having the student repeat a pediatric assessment several times to get the procedures correct reflects behaviorism through demonstration of repetition. Developing a scenario that changes the child's status if an assessment is performed wrong and changing the child's status to mimic a healthy child if the assessment is done correctly is a stimulus-response method or behaviorism.

127. **D) Schedule a time in the near future to meet with the STS to discuss the incident**

Schedule a time to resolve the incident with the individual first, at a time when there is adequate time to listen and understand. Eventually, the incident may have to be reported to the director, but always try to resolve the issue with the individual first. Confronting is not an appropriate leadership reaction. The situation cannot be ignored because it affects student learning.

128. **C) Approaching the patient as if we have no information**

Approaching the patient without information is incorrect because it does not build on previous knowledge. "Using the material we learned yesterday and applying it today," "Starting with what we know about this situation and then assessing the patient," and "Relating what is similar in this case to other cases we have worked through" all relate to the constructivist approach as they mention building upon previously learned knowledge.

129. **A) Speak with the scheduler to find out why this action was taken**

Although you might reschedule the events, restoring the initial schedule for the high-priority user and canceling the second group, this should not be the initial action because there may be other pieces of information the scheduler had when taking this action. Take time to find out why the decision was made to cancel the high-priority group before moving forward with other actions. The director might do a resource assessment and, if able, negotiate so that both groups can use the center. The least desirable but sometimes very necessary action would be to remove scheduling privileges until the scheduler undergoes retraining on scheduling policies. As a manager and leader, it is important to conduct an analysis to determine if the issues with scheduling arise from a deficiency in knowledge, tools, system errors, or attitudes, and then address the core issues.

130. **D) Active experimentation (AE)**
     The student is using hands-on skill development by taking the blood pressure. CE—taking the initiative to obtain the blood pressure—is not an example built from reality. AC—taking the initiative to obtain the blood pressure—is not thinking about what to do. RO—taking the initiative to obtain the blood pressure—is not a reflective activity.

131. **D) Perform a gap analysis on the accreditation standards**
     The gap analysis will help identify where the simulation center is now and what items need improvement to meet the required standards. Downloading the accreditation application is highly advised, but just downloading it is not enough. Submitting your application is one of the last steps in a nearly 2-year process of preparing for accreditation.

132. **C) Constructive feedback**
     Constructive feedback may be a missing element in the students' inability to construct a plan. The four components of Vygotsky's scaffolding learning theory are constructive feedback, explanations, reflection, and revision of knowledge. Instructor presence is not warranted to construct a plan. Realism is not part of formulating a plan. Knowledge is present but there is no indication that a revision of knowledge is necessary.

133. **B) Five rounds**
     Rounds refers to the number of times needed to repeat the OSCE for all students to complete the simulation activity. Begin by identifying how many rooms can run (in this case nine—because there are physically nine rooms that are up and working, and nine graders and nine SPs to fully staff the nine rooms). Take the total number of students and divide by the number of available rooms (number of students / number of rooms = number of rounds): 45/9 = 5.

| Time | | | 3:00–3:15 | 3:20–3:35 | 3:40–3:55 | 4:00–4:15 | 4:20–4:35 |
|---|---|---|---|---|---|---|---|
| | **Grader** | **SP** | | | | | |
| Room 1 | Grader 1 | SP 1 | Student 1 | Student 10 | Student 19 | Student 28 | Student 37 |
| Room 2 | Grader 2 | SP 2 | Student 2 | Student 11 | Student 20 | Student 29 | Student 38 |
| Room 3 | Grader 3 | SP 3 | Student 3 | Student 12 | Student 21 | Student 30 | Student 39 |
| Room 4 | Grader 4 | SP 4 | Student 4 | Student 13 | Student 22 | Student 31 | Student 40 |
| Room 5 | Grader 5 | SP 5 | Student 5 | Student 14 | Student 23 | Student 32 | Student 41 |
| Room 6 | Grader 6 | SP 6 | Student 6 | Student 15 | Student 24 | Student 33 | Student 42 |
| Room 7 | Grader 7 | SP 7 | Student 7 | Student 16 | Student 25 | Student 34 | Student 43 |
| Room 8 | Grader 8 | SP 8 | Student 8 | Student 17 | Student 26 | Student 35 | Student 44 |
| Room 9 | Grader 9 | SP 9 | Student 9 | Student 18 | Student 27 | Student 36 | Student 45 |

134. **B) Vicarious experience learning**
     The student is observing the simulation educator's demonstration of chest tube insertion. Mastering experience learning is incorrect because the student is not demonstrating their own history of success and is inactive during this simulation. Verbal persuasion is incorrect; there is no evidence that the healthcare simulation educator is providing verbal encouragement. Physiologic state is not correct because there is no evidence that either the simulation educator or the student expressed success in achieving IV line insertion.

135. **A) Transformational**
Transformational leaders inspire others and have vision; they have a tremendous impact on the decision of the employees to stay in their positions. Transformational leaders focus on vision and empowerment. Democratic leaders consult many people and govern by consensus. Authoritarian leaders are predictive and decisive. Laissez-faire leaders are excellent for highly autonomous and specialized teams. They are characterized by a very loose control with a hands-off approach.

136. **D) Andragogy**
The student is demonstrating andragogy because the student is advancing self by building on past experiences. Pedagogy is a method of learning used to teach passively, mostly to younger students without previous knowledge. Realism refers to the fidelity of the simulation and does not apply in this situation. Behaviorism is not correct because there is no evidence that the student is demonstrating learning through a behavior change.

137. **A) Human resources personnel**
Human resources personnel usually have the responsibility and expertise to advise on personnel issues. Policies and procedures are a good reference, but the human resources department can help managers work through problems and are there to provide guidance during challenging personnel issues. Resource allocation usually refers to supplies and equipment, not personnel. A benefits specialist can help with benefits such as insurance, vacation, pay rates, and so on.

138. **C) Teacher-centered**
Kneebone's simulation principles include student-centered, not teacher-centered simulations. Additional principles include simulations occurring in a safe environment, having tutors available for the student learners, and the simulation mimicking real life.

139. **B) Apply the learning to patient care with positive outcomes**
Apply the learning to patient care with positive outcomes is level 4, the highest level in Kirkpatrick's pyramid. Reacting to the debriefing questions is an example of level 1 or participant reactions. Learning through a premodule requirement is level 2. Demonstrating a change in behavior is level 3.

140. **B) Transference**
Transference is the last step in Doerr and Murray's simulation teaching–learning process, taking the knowledge learned in simulation and applying it to actual patients. Debriefing is the third step, developing learning outcomes is the first step, and creating the situation is the second step.

141. **C) Prioritizing the intervention**
Prioritizing the intervention is an application level objective according to Bloom's taxonomy. Defining the hybrid simulation procedure would be a recall objective. Discussing the clinical decision for starting CPR would be an objective at the understanding level. Evaluating the intervention's effect would be an objective at the evaluating level, higher than application.

142. **C) Inappropriate because the scenario's purpose was for learning**
This action would be considered inappropriate because the scenario's purpose was for learning and this reaction following a formative simulation scenario would not be considered the ideal way to discuss the actions/inactions of the learners. There are appropriate and reflective debriefing methods to have the students understand that they need to improve.

143. **A) The simulation educator can determine what the students know before starting**
Prior to an emotionally stimulating simulation scenario, the simulation educator should determine what the student's experience with death has been and what they know. Students need to know what the expectations are and how to deal with their emotions as they may arise during the scenario and/or the debriefing. It should not be treated as just "real life" and crying may happen, but this scenario should not "shock" or bring up negative emotions by surprise.

144. **A) A microethical situation or dilemma**
A microethical dilemma is an everyday situation that has the potential to cause harm and that requires an individual to make a decision. It should not be addressed during the scenario but at debriefing. It is not difficult or harmless and not the appropriate intervention for a healthcare professional.

145. **C) Learners to have signed a consent agreement to be recorded**
Learners need to be informed about being recorded and have an opportunity to think and decide about being recorded prior to beginning simulation-based experiences. Ethically, there should be full disclosure. Simulation educators should already know how to use the equipment. It is great if technical support can be available, but if not it is the responsibility of the simulation educators. The recording should just record the event, not be enhanced.

146. **C) Every 3 years**
Certified Healthcare Simulation Educator (CHSE) recertification for both the initial and advanced certifications is every 3 years. Recertification is not 5, 4, or 2 years.

147. **D) "It demonstrates that my expertise is ongoing."**
Renewal of certification indicates that the person maintains expertise in the area of certification; this is an internally driven, lifelong learning attribute. Certification may increase job prospects and be an expectation, but these are external motivating factors, as is not wanting to sit for another examination.

148. **A) Formative**
Formative simulation scenarios are held for the purpose of learning to help learners move toward achievement of a goal or objective. Summative evaluation or assessment is at the end or produces a grade. Cumulative means grades are added and usually averaged over time. Additive is when grades build on each other to achieve the 100% or final grade.

149. **D) Has met the minimum standards in the discipline of simulation learning**
Certifications demonstrate minimal competencies. Maximum competencies are ever evolving in a person's professional career and a person can be certified without a course on the subject matter or developing scenarios.

150. **C) Being an expert in the field through practice initiatives**
Some people can achieve a level of expertise without the qualifying university or college degree and this is recognized by certification agencies. Developing a simulation laboratory, promoting simulation, and speaking at conferences are not qualifying criteria by themselves.

# Index